LOVESICKNESS AND GENDER
IN EARLY MODERN ENGLISH LITERATURE

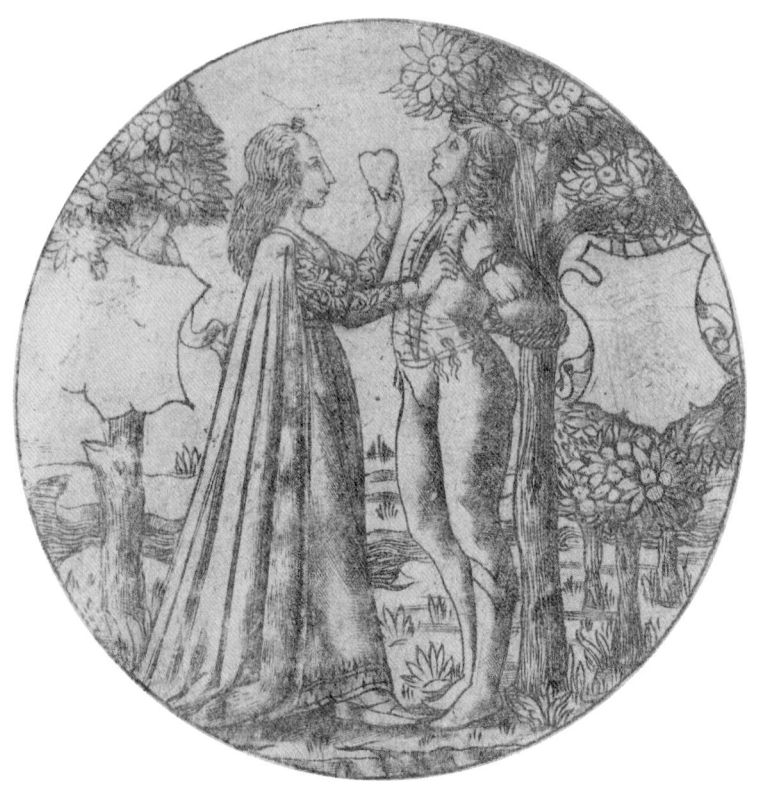

Frontispiece. *The Cruelty of Love*, anonymous fifteenth-century Florentine engraving, (*c*.1465–80.)

Lovesickness and Gender in Early Modern English Literature

LESEL DAWSON

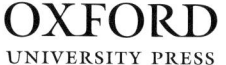

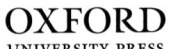

Great Clarendon Street, Oxford OX2 6DP

Oxford University Press is a department of the University of Oxford.
It furthers the University's objective of excellence in research, scholarship,
and education by publishing worldwide in

Oxford New York

Auckland Cape Town Dar es Salaam Hong Kong Karachi
Kuala Lumpur Madrid Melbourne Mexico City Nairobi
New Delhi Shanghai Taipei Toronto

With offices in

Argentina Austria Brazil Chile Czech Republic France Greece
Guatemala Hungary Italy Japan Poland Portugal Singapore
South Korea Switzerland Thailand Turkey Ukraine Vietnam

Oxford is a registered trade mark of Oxford University Press
in the UK and in certain other countries

Published in the United States
by Oxford University Press Inc., New York

British Library Cataloguing in Publication Data

Data available

Library of Congress Cataloging in Publication Data
Dawson, Lesel.
Lovesickness and Gender in Early Modern English Literature / Lesel Dawson.
p.   cm.
Includes bibliographical references and index.
ISBN 978–0–19–926612–8
1. English literature—Early modern, 1500–1700—History and criticism.   2. Lovesickness in literature.
3. Melancholy in literature.   4. Women in literature.   5. Gender identity in literature.   6. Literature
and medicine—England—History—16th century.   7. Literature and
medicine—England—History—17th century.   I. Title.
PR428.M4D38   2008
820.9′353–dc22   2008022056

Typeset by SPI Publisher Services, Pondicherry, India
Printed in Great Britain
on acid-free paper by
Biddles Ltd., King's Lynn, Norfolk

ISBN 978–0–19–926612–8

1 3 5 7 9 10 8 6 4 2

Acknowledgements

This book was a long time in the making and I have many people to thank for their academic advice and support. It started life as a dissertation written at Oxford University, where I benefited from the supervision of Katherine Duncan-Jones and Margarita Stocker, and from the guidance of John Carey, Natsu Hattori, Emrys Jones, and Andrew Wear. My examiners, Roy Porter and Emma Smith, offered excellent advice on how to turn the dissertation into a book. Jacqueline Baker, my editor, was patient and helpful throughout the process, and Mary Worthington, my copy-editor, and the anonymous readers at Oxford University Press read the script with rigorous care. I am grateful to the Leverhulme Foundation for granting me an early career Fellowship and to Bristol University for giving me a semester of research leave during the final stages. An earlier version of Chapter 3 was published in *Early Modern English Studies* 8/1 (2002), and Chapter 6 appeared originally in *Women's Studies* 34/6 (2005). I am grateful to the editors of these journals for permission to reprint this material.

Many friends and colleagues have also made valuable suggestions and given me encouragement during the writing process. Former colleagues at Worcester College, Oxford, David Bradshaw, Roger Dalrymple, Kate Tunstall, and Edward Wilson have been valuable friends and allies. More recently, colleagues at Bristol University have listened to me talk through my ideas, looked at drafts, or have translated passages of Latin, including Jo Carruthers, Stephen Cheeke, George Donaldson, David Hopkins, Stephen James, John Lee, John Lyon, Ad Putter, Tom Sperlinger, and Jane Wright. My thinking about lovesickness has been enriched and refined by my students, particularly those in my 'Gender, Desire, and the Renaissance Stage' course, and by my conversations with (and sometimes awkward questions from) many of my friends, notably: Richard Chamberlain, Marie-Louise Coolahan, David Cunnington, Rachel Gaul, Meraud Grant Ferguson, Tom Freshwater, Dan Hedley, Clark Lawler, Jason Lawrence, Simon Mealor, Jodie Medhurst, Tim Milnes, Steve Loosley, Mel Ord, Kevin Perera, Daren Randell, Dave Reed, Larissa Strauss, Philip Schwyzer, Beth Williamson,

Alex Wilson, and Winkie Wilson. Laurence Publicover did an excellent job on the index, and my family—Elaine, Roger, Jack, Li, Leslie, Dean, and Cleo—supported me throughout my Ph.D. and beyond. Elizabeth Archibald, Charles Brayne, and Anna Brown were incredibly generous with their time, reading many drafts, spotting errors, and acting as my intellectual interlocutors and collaborators. My husband, Mark, shared his interpretations of metaphysical poetry, cooked me lovely meals, and made the days off enjoyable. Finally a special thank you is due to my mother, for her friendship, love, and encouragement. This book is dedicated to her.

Contents

Acknowledgements   v
List of Illustrations   ix

Introduction: Sweet Poison   1

1. 'My Love is as a Fever': Medical Constructions of Desire in
   Early Modern England   12

   The Physiological Construction of Lovesickness: Origins,
      Symptoms, and Cures   13
   Historical Accounts of the Experience of Erotic Melancholy   27
   The Look of Love   33

2. 'A Thirsty Womb': Lovesickness, Green Sickness, Hysteria,
   and Uterine Fury   46

   Green Sickness, the Disease of Virgins: 'A Gamesome
      Bedfellow, Being the Sure Physician'   49
   Hysteria, or the Suffocation of the Mother   60
   Uterine Fury   68
   Shakespeare's Ophelia   72
   A Tale of Two Virgins: Shakespeare and Fletcher's *The Two
      Noble Kinsmen*   79

3. Beyond Ophelia: The Anatomy of Female Melancholy   91

   Historical and Literary Examples of Melancholic Women   94
   Masochism and Revenge in Beaumont and Fletcher's *The
      Maid's Tragedy*   112
   'Divorce Betwixt my Body and my Heart': Starvation in
      Ford's *The Broken Heart*   118

4. Lovesickness and Neoplatonism   127

   Neoplatonic Interpretations of Love and the Female Beloved   131
   Seeing Double: Neoplatonism and Narcissism in John Ford's
      'Tis Pity She's a Whore   140
   'New Sects of Love': William Davenant's *The Temple of Love*
      and *The Platonick Lovers*   150

5. 'Griefs Will Have their Vent': Physical and Psychological
   Remedies for Lovesickness   163
   Physical Cures: Purging the Lover's Body   164
   Psychological Cures   177
6. Menstruation, Misogyny, and the Cure for Love   191

Bibliography   212
Index   237

List of Illustrations

Frontispiece. The Cruelty of Love, anonymous fifteenth-century Florentine engraving, (*c*.1465–80), © the Trustees of the British Museum

1. *Inamorato*, detail from the frontispiece of Robert Burton's *The Anatomy of Melancholy* (1628), © British Library Board, reproduced by permission of the Board of Trustees of the British Library 35

2. Nicholas Hilliard, *Henry Percy, 9th Earl of Northumberland* (*c*.1590–5), reproduced by permission of the Rijksmuseum, Amsterdam 39

3. Nicholas Hilliard, *Unknown Man against a Background of Flames* (*c*.1588), reproduced by kind permission of the Board of Trustees of the Victoria and Albert Museum 40

4. Gerard van Honthorst, *Lucy Harrington, 3rd Countess of Bedford* (*c*.1620), by permission of His Grace the Duke of Bedford and the Trustees of the Bedford Estates 99

5. *Democritus*, detail from the frontispiece of Robert Burton's *The Anatomy of Melancholy* (1628), © British Library Board, reproduced by permission of the Board of Trustees of the British Library 100

6. Attributed to Simon Kick, *Lady Seated at a Table* (*c*.1630), reproduced by permission of the Ashmolean Museum, University of Oxford 101

Introduction
Sweet Poison

In Act IV of John Ford's *The Broken Heart* (1633), Penthea appears on stage looking like a typical lovesick woman: she enters with 'her hair about her ears', speaking in an oblique manner about her sexual desires and her longing for death. Ithocles, her brother, has forced her to marry Bassianus, breaking off her engagement with Orgilus, the man she loves. No longer able to endure her unhappy marriage, she resolves to starve herself. Standing before her former lover, looking like the very picture of frustrated love, she asks Orgilus, 'Like whom do I look, prithee?'[1] Her question, a direct borrowing from John Webster's *The Duchess of Malfi* (acted before 1614), draws attention both to her resemblance to the long line of lovesick women who have appeared on the stage before her, whilst also suggesting her self-conscious performance of her grief.[2] 'To say I love you is always a quotation' not only because expressions of love are to a large extent culturally coded, but also because of the frequency with which they echo literary precursors.[3] The evolving literary configuration of the lovesick woman in early modern England should be read not only as a product of complex intertextual relations in which authors take up, transform, and challenge earlier literary models, but also as a response to developing medical ideas. The discourse of love, which is subjective, private, and instinctive, but also culturally constructed, public, and learned, emphasizes the way in which the expression of

---

[1] Ford, *Broken Heart*, ed. Spencer, IV.ii.114; all quotation are taken from this edition.
[2] Webster's Duchess asks her servant Cariola, 'Who do I look like now?' while imprisoned by her brother Ferdinand (Webster, *Duchess*, IV.ii.30). The stoical self-mastery Penthea demonstrates before going mad owes something to the Duchess, as does her penchant for self-dramatization.
[3] Culler, *Deconstruction*, 120.

reflexive feelings is bound up in wider historical narratives about bodies and interiority. In sixteenth- and seventeenth-century medical texts, intense unfulfilled erotic desire is classified as a species of melancholy, with mental and physiological etiologies and cures. Rather than dismiss lovesickness as a literary trope and decode its symptoms as an artificial display of exaggerated despair, early modern medical authors held erotic obsession to be a real and virulent disease.

The principal focus of this book is on literary depictions of lovesickness in early modern literature. Through a series of close textual readings, I examine figures afflicted with erotic melancholy, providing an historical context for their malady, and discussing how the literary representation of lovesickness relates to wider issues of gender and identity in the early modern period. My aim is to capture something of the complexity and variation in how lovesickness is imagined, exploring the different ways that desire is believed to take root in the body, how gender roles are encoded and contested in courtship, and the psychic pleasures and pains of frustrated passion. Just as today there are a number of ways of explaining and categorizing obsessive love—it has been understood as a form of depression, as a chemical imbalance, as a type of obsessive compulsive disorder, or as a product of our childhood experiences and/or our underlying drives and instincts[4]—so too early modern writers variously describe lovesickness as a burning in the blood and liver, as a humoral imbalance, as an image fixed in the mind, or as the product of seed or sperm. Moreover, during this time medical ideas about love coexist with those derived from Neoplatonism, so that the same physical and mental symptoms could be viewed as either a debasing, animalistic passion or an elevated state of rapture. My study will explore all of these aspects of lovesickness, outlining its medical construction, its divergent moral meanings, its social and seductive functions, and the contradictions that arise when medical ideas about love intersect with those of Neoplatonism. I will also examine the relationship between female lovesickness and uterine disorders (such as

---

[4] For modern approaches to lovesickness see Tallis, *Love Sick*. Tallis observes that, although lovesickness is no longer recognized as a medical condition, 'many of the symptoms of lovesickness can be found distributed through the ICD (the International Classification of Diseases and Related Health Problems) and DSM (Diagnostic and Statistical Manual of Mental Disorders) classification systems . . . being in love produces a symptom profile that would ordinarily suggest significant psychiatric disturbance' (p. 54).

green sickness and hysteria), asking whether it is identical to one or more of these illnesses and if it can resemble the 'heroic melancholy' generally said to be exclusively male. Finally, I will consider how anxieties concerning love's ability to emasculate the male lover emerge indirectly in remedies for erotic melancholy. The blatant misogyny of some of these cures, in which the man is encouraged to hate his mistress or to find her physically disgusting, suggests wider cultural anxieties about the gendered power reversals that accompany courtship, whilst also uncovering the male lover's oscillating emotions towards his mistress. The oxymoronic description of love as bittersweet encapsulates the psychic contradictions of the impassioned lover, who loves and hates, who is tormented by passion but wishes to prolong its delicious agony, who suffers from the disease of love but has no wish to find a cure.

The Renaissance marks a turning point in the gendering of lovesickness. Although there is no shortage of lovesick women in classical and medieval literature, lovesickness was nonetheless generally understood to be a male malady by medical writers. This changed, however, in the Renaissance from which point the lovesick sufferer is increasingly figured as a woman 'whose insanity [is] an extension of her female condition'.[5] As Mary Wack observes, 'Historians of medicine have noted a tendency among medical writers of the Renaissance not merely to consider women subject to morbid love, but to deem them ... the primary victims of the malady, or at least particularly susceptible to it'.[6] This change anticipates, and is related to, a wider transformation in the symbolic gendering of insanity, in which the chief stereotypes of madness, quintessentially masculine in the early modern period, are 'effectively "feminized" ' from the mid-eighteenth century onward.[7] In Elaine Showalter's words, 'the appealing madwoman gradually displaced the repulsive madman, both as the prototype of the confined lunatic and as a cultural icon'.[8] However, a number of modern critics see this new category of women's lovesickness as distinct from that which afflicts men. Indeed, it has become something of a truism to claim that in the

---

[5] Small, *Love's Madness*, p. vii. Wells discusses female lovesickness in relation to the romance tradition in *Secret Wound* (pp. 220–59). Unfortunately, Wells's work came to my attention after my manuscript was completed, so I have been unable to take it into account in my study.

[6] Wack, *Lovesickness*, 175.   [7] Porter, *Social History*, 104.

[8] Showalter, *Female Malady*, 8.

early modern period men and women were thought to experience erotic passion in fundamentally different ways, in which the quality of one's love, its edifying or degrading affect, and its potential for spiritual sublimation are all directly dependant on the lovesick sufferer's gender. Men's and women's passions are not only held to be different in quality, but also to derive from entirely different medical and philosophical traditions. Whereas male lovesickness is classified as a form of melancholy— a malady associated with creativity, interiority, and intellect—the female version is considered a disorder of the womb.[9] This paradigm of gender and illness depends upon a key assumption: that in early modern England 'heroic melancholia' is a specifically masculine affliction, the cerebral and philosophical connotations of which automatically exclude women. Male lovesickness thus comes to be associated with creativity, interiority, and intellect, attributes that allow men's disappointments in love to be placed within a wider cultural context of courtly romance, Neoplatonic philosophy, and Petrarchan poetry. Whereas the masculine intellect is capable of converting sickness and sorrow into an elevating understanding of life, women, it is said, are barred from such privileged forms of expression because they lack the faculty of reason, which interprets and sublimates bodily and emotional disturbances.[10] Far from being the hallmark of a noble mind, a woman's erotic melancholy bespeaks her lack of reason and her subjugation to her body's sexual demands: women's illnesses are constructed as bodily and passionate rather than intellectual and creative.[11]

One of the principal concerns of this book is to challenge this model of gender and illness, exploring alternative models of female lovesickness and melancholy, and suggesting that conditions that we often think of as overwhelmingly debilitating can function, at times, as either sites of pleasure or forms of empowerment. The tendency to collapse hysteria, green sickness, and lovesickness into one disease obscures the specific cultural connotations of each malady, promoting a false, gender-based dichotomy between female and male illness. Although this paradigm is

---

[9] Dixon, for example, regards female lovesickness as having 'a purely physical origin in the uterus' and Peterson claims that 'Desire in female virgins is understood as a pathology, in pointed contrast to the construction of desire in men as relatively chivalric and heroic'. Dixon, *Perilous Chastity*, 109; Peterson, 'Fluid Economies', 42.

[10] Schiesari, *Gendering of Melancholia*; Paster, *Embarrassed*, 25.

[11] Showalter, 'Representing Ophelia', 81; Schiesari, *Gendering of Melancholia*, 14.

not wrong, it creates a clear-cut opposition between women's and men's lovesickness that fails to take into account both the complexity of early modern ideas about the malady and the way the disorder varies in its symptoms and cultural meaning for both sexes. After all, the sexual organs were considered a cause of lovesickness in *both* men and women, and once lovesickness was thought to be a disease of women it was by no means confined to this negative, pathological form. Early modern medical texts readily aggregate different types of lovesickness; as Robert Burton comments in *The Anatomy of Melancholy* (1621–38), '*Proteus* himselfe is not so divers, you may as well make the *Moone* a new coat, as a true character of a melancholy man'.[12] This aggregation of models extends to the physiological construction of female lovesickness, which could *either* be associated with the sexualized behaviour and incoherent speech of uterine disorders *or* with the introspective brooding and philosophical temperament of melancholy. Critics are correct to suggest that the type of sufferer influences the category of malady being experienced, but the type of sufferer is defined, not just by gender, but also by social rank, ethical constitution, time of birth, physical make-up, and age.

In fact, rather than confining individuals to strict gender roles, lovesickness often releases them from conventions of gender and sexual orientation; as Carol Neely writes, 'because it can strike anyone and fasten on anything, it has the effect of making gender roles and erotic object choices fluid and the relation between them unstable'.[13] This aspect of lovesickness has long been understood in relation to Renaissance men, for whom love is regarded as an emasculating force that leads to a reversal of the traditional gender hierarchy.[14] No longer governed by reason, the lovesick man is dominated by both his 'feminine' passions and his newly empowered mistress. Laurentius in the 1599 English translation of his work on melancholy describes how desire wages war on the body and mind, until the lovesick individual's body and rational

---

[12] Burton, *Anatomy*, i.407.   [13] Neely, *Distracted Subjects*, 113.
[14] Jackson suggests that this may be one of the chief reasons why romance (as a genre) and courtship (as a practice) are held to have such a specific appeal for women: both centre upon the transitory phase in which the woman is afforded a position of dominance within the relationship. She argues: 'to be in love is to be powerless, at the mercy of the other, but it also holds out the promise of power, of enslaving the other in the bonds of love' ('Women and Heterosexual Love', 54).

self-control are overcome. Gendered feminine and 'weake', passion is
nevertheless able to tame the male lover:

fearing her selfe too weake to incounter with reason, the principal part of the
minde, [love] posteth in haste to the heart, to surprise and winne the same:
wherof when she is once sure, as of the strongest holde, she afterward assaileth
and setteth upon reason, and all the other principall powers of the minde so
fiercely, as that she subdueth them, and maketh them her vassals and slaves.
Then is all spoyled, the man is quite undone and cast away, the sences are
wandring to and fro, up and downe, reason is confounded, the imagination
corrupted, the talke fond and sencelesse; the sillie loving worme cannot any
more look upon any thing but his idol.[15]

Love captivates and enthrals the male lover, so that even the 'bravest
souldiers and most generous spirits are enervated with it'. Male lovers
are thus 'voluntary servants'; as Burton asks, 'Is he a free man over whom
a woman domineers?'[16]

However, although love can disempower the male lover, threatening
his agency and self-control, it does not inevitably follow that men felt
unequivocal discomfort from such reversals of power, seeking either to
avoid such relationships or re-establish a sense of emotional self-mastery.
Men who are in love may be their mistresses' slaves, but, as Burton
points out, this servitude is 'voluntary' and may even be pleasurable.
Catherine Bates argues that

the traditional courtly scenario of the groveling lover seems an obvious place
from which to explore the other side of masculinity—the side that rejects
mastery and rehearses instead the alternative roles of debility and ruination;
the side that shuns domination and luxuriates rather in sexual ambivalence and
epistemological doubt.[17]

Readings that resuscitate the abject male, restoring him to emotional
self-mastery, fail to take into consideration the masochistic enjoyment
of the eroticized lover, whose agonies are simultaneously experienced

[15] Laurentius, *Preservation of the Sight,* 118.   [16] Burton, *Anatomy*, iii.42, 170.
[17] Bates, 'Abject Male', 9; she criticizes a number of interpretive strategies that attempt
to recuperate the abject male in Petrarchan poetry and restore him to a position of
power; frequently this is achieved by emphasizing the distance between the skilled,
confident poet and his helpless, desolate *persona*. However, as Bates points out, 'this
formulation virtually writes out the psychology of submission' (p. 5). For a discussion of
Petrarchanism and masochism see Marshall, *Shattering*, 13–84.

as extreme pleasure. Love pleases even as it causes pain, a bittersweet quality said to spring from its proximity to death.[18] Early modern Petrarchan poetry, in which the lover's anticipatory longing is also an addictive form of delight, vividly encapsulates love's contradictory, self-destructive aspect as well as the lover's conflicted psyche. Pain within this context is not an impediment to erotic pleasure but an important constituent feature. As Musidorus explains to Pyrocles in Sidney's *Arcadia*, it is the pain that the beloved's beauty causes that makes her sight so wished for. Describing himself as 'a foolish child that, when anything hits him, will strike himself again upon it', Musidorus seeks out his beloved, not despite his pain, but because of it.[19] Within this context, the obstacles that the male lover encounters (such as the beloved's chastity, her indifference, her unavailability, her death) might not be obstacles at all, but the very means through which the individual's delicious agony is prolonged and intensified.

The masochistic aspect of desire, which has as its aim intense emotion and sensation, rather than resolution and consummation, uncovers the narcissistic and solitary aspect of lovesickness, which centres not on the beloved but on the lover. Here, the mistress's inaccessibility is a mere pretext, allowing the lover to romanticize the beloved as an abstract ideal, and to engage in intense, private contemplation. This activity is afforded an educative meaning in Neoplatonic philosophy, instigating the lover's psychic journey, in which sexual longing is sublimated in order to achieve an elevated state of rapture. Within this context, the beloved's real identity is ultimately irrelevant, acting, as Philippa Berry suggests, as 'little more than an instrument in an elaborate game of *masculine* "speculation" and self-determination' for the lover, who is his own preferred object.[20] Lacan, who regards desire as constituted through lack and incapable of satisfaction, regards the state whereby the beloved is inaccessible or indifferent as desire's most authentic expression; here love is either unreciprocated or impossible to achieve, and intimacy is eschewed in favour of a painful but enriching solitude.[21]

The female lover is also depicted as experiencing a delicious pleasure in her psychic disintegration; as Shakespeare's Cleopatra says of her

---

[18] Ficino suggests that Orpheus 'called love *gluchupichron*, that is "bittersweet"' because love is a 'voluntary death' (*Commentary on Plato's Symposium on Love*, II.viii).
[19] Sidney, *New Arcadia*, ed. Skretkowicz, 108.   [20] Berry, *Chastity*, 2.
[21] Lacan, 'Jouissance'. Vice, 'Addicted to Love', 122–3.

own death, love is like 'a lover's pinch, | Which hurts and is desired' (V.ii.290–1). In plays, female characters frequently luxuriate in their afflictions, evoking a form of amorous suffering that is contemplative, elevated, and self-controlled.[22] And in dedications, diaries, and letters from the period, elite women indulge in their lovesickness as well as that 'selfe-pleasing, yet ill easing humour of never glad melancholie' as a means of advertising their contemplative nature and inwardness.[23] Here it is not gender but social rank that is relevant in determining the malady's classification and its ennobling status.[24] Literary representations of lovesick women can thus either confer positive connotations, or, in depicting lovesickness as a negative condition, nonetheless suggest that women have the rational resource to overcome their passions.

For women, lovesickness also provides a vital means to express anger, allowing individuals to criticize those who have mistreated them whilst still appearing as passive victims. Female-voiced complaint poems may be the origin of this particular formulation, in which a woman's self-reproaches combine with condemnation of her lover's false oaths and fickle heart,[25] and the strategy is also employed by Gaspara Stampa and Mary Wroth. As Ann Rosalind Jones argues, these 'poets turn what might appear to be a masochistic dwelling on loss into resistance', so that in their poetry the posture of victim is turned into an attack on the victimizer.[26] Given the social, ethical, and linguistic difficulties encountered by early modern women seeking to establish a voice—which Gary Waller ascribes to 'the structures of power within the language . . . that create [women] as subjects, denying them any owned discourse'— lovesickness can thus be seen to open up a space for women's protest.[27] The lovesick woman's vocabulary of devotion paradoxically facilitates the expression of otherwise impermissible emotions, such as anger and sexual frustration. By turning destructive impulses inward, the lovesick woman acts upon the only sphere she can harm without feelings of guilt or social retribution. Revenge is thus achieved through self-punishment, in which masochism acts as a displaced form of aggression. Like

[22] See Ch. 3.   [23] Tofte, 'Laura', in *Poetry of Robert Tofte*, ed. Nelson, 3.
[24] MacDonald, *Mystical Bedlam*, 152–3, 243.
[25] See Kerrigan, *Motives of Woe*.
[26] Jones, *Currency*, 154. See also Miller, *Changing*, 18–63.
[27] Waller, 'Struggling into Discourse', 246.

Francis Bacon's revenger, who 'keepes his owne Wounds greene, which otherwise would heale and doe well', abject women, such as Beaumont and Fletcher's Aspatia, cultivate their lovesickness, resisting the natural process through which pain fades and wounds heal.[28] Lovesickness within this context recalls Freud's account of melancholy in 'Mourning and Melancholia' (1917), where the sufferer's self-recriminations both disguise and indirectly express accusations of a different sort:

If one listens patiently to the many and various self-accusations of the melancholic, one cannot avoid the impression that often the most violent of them are hardly at all applicable to the patient himself, but that with insignificant modifications they do fit someone else, some person whom the patient loves, has loved, or ought to love ... the self-reproaches are reproaches against a loved object which have been shifted on to the patient's own ego.[29]

The psychological process that Freud describes, in which anger is expressed at a loved object through self-accusation and self-harm, is particularly relevant to the experience of early modern women, whose ability to articulate anger and opposition was restricted by a whole host of cultural expectations. Whereas men in early modern England were encouraged to express their disappointments in love through hostility and aggression—converting desire into disgust, and rejection into self-righteous anger—women were more limited in their expressions of rage. A woman's *self*-harm, on the other hand, 'shades easily into altruism's noble self-sacrifice, so prized socially'.[30] This is reflected in the literature, where ignoble women in early modern literature generally strike out at others, whereas virtuous female characters hurt themselves instead. The cultural and psychological benefits of such behaviour are easy to understand: by harming herself, the lovesick woman expresses her anger in a way that adheres to noble ideals of femininity, and is able to retain, on some level, her love for her betrayer. Masochism, within this context, is 'a psychic strategy that makes the best of a bad business, that insists on wresting identity and self-affirmation from a biased social contract that traumatizes women'.[31] Channelling their anger and

[28] Bacon, 'Of Revenge', in *Essayes*, 17.
[29] Freud, 'Mourning and Melancholia' (1917), in *Complete Psychological Works*, xiv.158.
[30] Massé, *Masochism*, 42.   [31] Ibid.

frustration into their self-destructive behaviour, they simultaneously elevate themselves into 'Love's martyrs'.[32]

My study will explore lovesickness as a recognizable category of illness and the lovesick figure as an important literary type. My primary focus is on Renaissance drama, but I also explore representations of lovesickness in poetry and prose, alongside other primary material (including medical texts, accounts of amorous suffering found in private letters and diaries, Richard Napier's case notes describing the clinical treatment of lovesick patients, and modes of lovesick self-fashioning found in portraiture). Chapter 1 provides an introduction to medical and literary constructions of lovesickness, giving an overview of the malady's aetiologies, symptoms, and cures, its social and intellectual meaning, and its seductive function. The next two chapters explore the lovesick woman as a new medical category and literary archetype; Chapter 2 outlines the complex relationship between lovesickness and female diseases of the reproductive organs, and Chapter 3 examines the correlations between women's lovesickness and intellectual melancholy, and also its links with anger. As well as examining characters who become mad through love (such as Shakespeare's Ophelia) and thereby embody the paradigm of gender and illness for most contemporary critics, I also examine characters who challenge or reinvent this paradigm, for whom melancholy is an instrument of female self-authorship, signifying a woman's refined intellect, or employed as a passive-aggressive means of revenge. Chapter 4 investigates how the pathological conception of love as a physical disease interacted with Neoplatonic models of love as a spiritual and ennobling force; I argue that, as well as advancing different ideas about sexuality within amorous relationships, the discourse of Neoplatonism and erotic melancholy promoted incompatible gender power hierarchies. Chapters 5 and 6 focus on the divergent ways in which playwrights reinvent the medical treatments for lovesickness in order to give them a charged dramatic meaning; here I explore aspects of the sexual double standard and suggest that there is often more to curing the male lover than simply returning him to bodily health.

The discourse of lovesickness emphasizes the way in which the expression of intimate, reflexive feelings is bound up in wider cultural narratives. The physiological constructions of lovesickness not only

---

[32] Ford, *Broken Heart*, IV.iv.153.

furnished writers with a vivid language through which to describe erotic desire, but also influenced early modern ideas about emotion, interiority, sexuality, and gender. As Thomas Lacqueur writes, 'Experience, in short, is reported and remembered so as to be congruent with dominant paradigms.'[33] This is especially true in earlier periods, such as the Renaissance, when illness was conceptualized 'not as a random assault from outside, but as a deeply significant life-event, integral to the sufferer's whole being—spiritual, moral, physical and life-course—past, present and future'.[34] Renaissance literature not only offers a repository of important cultural stereotypes about erotic melancholy, but is also instrumental in forging and challenging these stereotypes. As Sander Gilman observes:

We learn to perceive the world through those cultural artifacts which preserve a society's stereotypes of its environment. We do not see the world, rather we are taught by representations of the world about us to conceive of it in a culturally acceptable manner . . . it is not art which imitates insanity, but the perception of insanity which imitates art.[35]

As well as reflecting the scientific thought of the day, literary depictions influence our understanding of our bodies and ourselves. Early modern representations of lovesickness expose contemporary cultural constructions of love, revealing the relation of sexuality to spirituality, the formation and disruption of gender roles in courtship, and the creation and shattering of the self in love.

---

[33] Laqueur, *Making Sex*, 99. This observation has particular significance in relation to love. As Jackson argues: 'Fantasies do not emerge fully formed into our consciousness. They are actively constructed by us, in narrative form, drawing on the cultural resources to hand' ('Women and Heterosexual Love', 57). See also Rosaldo, who suggests that our feelings are 'structured by our forms of understanding', including the 'stories that we both enact and tell' ('Anthropology of Self', 143).

[34] Porter, *Disease*, 25.   [35] Gilman, *Seeing*, pp. xi–xiii.

1

'My Love is as a Fever': Medical Constructions of Desire in Early Modern England

> Love is the tyrant of the heart; it darkens
> Reason, confounds discretion; deaf to counsel,
> It runs a headlong course to desperate madness.
>
> (John Ford, *The Lover's Melancholy*, III.iii.105–7)

The literature of early modern England abounds with examples of melancholy lovers, who burn with passion, die of breaking hearts, or simply waste away. Deprived of the 'cure' of their beloveds' arms, on-stage lovers become mad or violent; away from the stage, abject poets wallow in delicious torture. The expressions of pain and conflagration that inform the discourse of love in early modern England are of course not unique to the period. Images of burning fires and breaking hearts are found in both classical and medieval literature and, revived in the popular melodramas of the nineteenth century, have since become a staple ingredient of modern romantic fiction. However, whereas contemporary readers interpret such declarations of physical suffering as formulaic metaphors, indicating a state of psychological disquiet, the early modern subject understood the lover's melancholy to be a dangerous physical illness. Lovesickness, in the Renaissance, is considered a species of melancholy, which could inflame the body, take possession of the mind, and overthrow an individual's rational self-control. Like the salamander, with its mythical delight in scorching flames, those suffering from erotic melancholy appear careless of their own well-being, fanning and embracing the fiery passions that consume them.

This chapter is divided into three sections that analyse, in turn, the physiology of lovesickness, historical accounts of individuals experiencing the disease, and the self-fashioning of the melancholy lover. The first section details the physical construction of lovesickness, cataloguing its origins, symptoms, and cures, and suggesting how the four aetiologies of lovesickness offer different ways of conceptualizing desire and its bodily impact. I then turn to a consideration of the ways in which individuals employ the medical discourse to express desire, offering examples of men and women who describe themselves (or are described by others) as lovesick in diaries, letters, and doctors' case notes. The final section examines the dress, posture, and behaviour of the lover, detailing the social and intellectual connotations of lovesick display as well as its seductive function. Lovesickness is an effective tool in courtship, providing an important means of expressing desire and of engineering its fulfilment: by displaying his suffering, the lovesick man was able to exert psychological pressure on the beloved and justify the need for sex. For women too lovesickness provided an important means of expressing desire, and of exerting one's own sexual preferences in the face of resistance.

THE PHYSIOLOGICAL CONSTRUCTION OF LOVESICKNESS: ORIGINS, SYMPTOMS, AND CURES

The Disease of Love

Lovesickness—also known as heroical love, erotic melancholy, and erotomania—was considered a genuine physiological malady in early modern England. Whereas moderate affection was deemed both moral and reasonable, the unfulfilled desires of the lovesick subject engendered a harmful physiological reaction. The power to incite violent emotions and disrupt the equilibrium of mind and body made erotic melancholy more than a psychological condition: it was a destructive sickness, which could result in chronic melancholy, mania, or even death. Letters, doctors' case notes, and personal diaries attest to the fact that a large number of men and women believed themselves to be suffering physically from the effects of excessive erotic passion. The increasing prevalence of such self-diagnosis was no doubt influenced by the growing number of scholarly works devoted to the study of melancholy, of which lovesickness was deemed to be a particular species. Following the translation into English of a treatise by Levinus Lemnius in 1576, Timothie Bright, Thomas Wright, Thomas Walkington, and Robert Burton all published works that included a discussion of erotic melancholy.[1]

The Renaissance construction of lovesickness as a physiological affliction was influenced by the writings of the ancients, almost all of which categorized love as an illness, either defining it as a form of melancholy or associating it with mania and frenzy. Galen treats love as a disease; Greek poetry, from Homer onward, defines eros as a disease (*nosos*) and as madness (*mania*); and stage representations of Phaedra, Medea, and Hercules dramatize the bodily dissolution and mental impairment of erotic passion.[2] As Donald Beecher and Massimo Ciavolella observe, 'Sappho wrote of love in the terms of the symptoms of disease, the early humoral writers explained madness and all emotional disturbances in the brain in terms of the invasion of black bile, Plato spoke of sexual love as a disease of the soul, and Aristotle assigned the origins of eros not to the soul but to a boiling of blood around the heart.'[3] The perceived connection between lovesickness and melancholy was reinforced by Arabic treatises on melancholy, which were eventually absorbed into the medieval medical school of Salerno and disseminated throughout the west. Both Rhazes (al-Rasi) (*c*.850–923 or 924) and the Persian physician Ibn al-Jazzār (Alī ibn al-'Abbās al-Majūsī), known in the Latin West as Haly Abbas (fl. 950), treat lovesickness, lycanthropy, and melancholy as one disease. And love is treated as a physiological disorder in Constantine the African's *Viaticum*, an adaptation of the popular medical handbook of Abu Jafar Ahmed Ibn Ibrāhīm ibn Alī

---

[1] Lemnius, *Touchstone*; Bright, *Treatise*; Laurentius, *Preservation of the Sight*; W[right], *Minde*; W[alkington], *Optick Glasse*; Burton, *Anatomy*; Ferrand, *Erotomania*. For a modern translation of *ΕΡΩΤΟΜΑΝΙΑ* see Ferrand, *Treatise*, trans. and ed. Beecher and Ciavolella. For a recent survey of the medical and philosophical traditions that underpin the early modern construction of lovesickness see Beecher and Ciavolella, 'Ferrand'. For melancholy see Klibansky, Panofsky, and Saxl, *Saturn*. For medieval studies of lovesickness see Wack, *Lovesickness*, and Solomon, *Literature of Misogyny*. For early modern constructions of lovesickness see Beecher and Ciavolella, 'Ferrand'; Beecher, 'The Lover's Body'; Babb, 'The Lover's Malady in Medical Theory', in *Elizabethan Malady*, 126–42; and MacDonald, *Mystical Bedlam*.

[2] Cyrino, *Pandora's Jar*, 2; Pigeaud, *Maladie*, 375–439.

[3] Beecher and Ciavolella, 'Ferrand', 42.

Khālid, often called Ibn Eddjezzar (d. *c*.1004), *Zād al-musāfir wa-qut al-hadir* (*Provisions for the Traveller and the Nourishment of the Settled*).[4] Early modern writers tended to consolidate these different historical traditions, regarding the entire literature from a nearly two-thousand-year span as offering 'a single set of definitions, symptoms and cures'.[5] Lovesickness was also open to occult explanations (such as astrology, sorcery, spells, charms, and witchcraft) in the early modern period, a time in which the discourses of medicine and magic grew closer together.[6] Although early modern medical writers are often hostile to non-natural explanations of lovesickness, the period nonetheless saw 'the infiltration of occult causes, some of them the legacy of folk medicine, others the result of an intensified interest among theologians in demonology and witchcraft'.[7] Demonologists drew upon medical explanations of lovesickness as a means of highlighting the waywardness of the imagination and its susceptibility to manipulation by the devil and witchcraft, and ordinary men and women used charms and spells in an attempt to manipulate the desires of others.[8]

Early modern explanations of the causes, effects, and cures of lovesickness are predicated upon the existence of an inescapable interrelationship between the mind and the body. The physical and emotional selves, tied together in 'a true love knot', were held to be inseparably unified: a bodily imbalance could result in a negative emotion and a mental condition could cause physical harm.[9] As F. N. Coëffeteau explains in *A Table of Humane Passions* (1621), 'there riseth no passion in the soule, which leaveth not some visible trace of her agitation, upon the body of man'.[10] Like other illnesses, love is represented as an infectious malady; it is caught through the eyes and triggers an immediate physical

---

[4] Klibansky, Panofsky, Saxl, *Saturn*, 83. See also Beecher and Ciavolella, 'Ferrand', 62–70.

[5] Beecher and Ciavolella, 'Ferrand', 39.

[6] For a discussion of the relationship between lovesickness and the occult see Beecher and Ciavolella, *Eros and Anteros*, and Beecher and Ciavolella, 'Ferrand', 83–97. Wack argues that 'the emergence of visual species in causal analyses of *amor hereos* in the late thirteenth and fourteenth centuries placed lovesickness in a fertile nexus of debates on imagination and magic in natural philosophy and theology'. See 'From Mental Faculties to Magical Philters', 14.

[7] Beecher and Ciavolella, 'Ferrand', 83.

[8] MacFarlane discusses several trials in which men and women are accused of using love magic. See *Witchcraft*, 77, 288, 292, 303.

[9] Bright, *Treatise*, 35.   [10] Coëffeteau, *Table*, 17.

reaction: the spirits grow distracted, the liver malfunctions, the blood becomes muddy, and the body deteriorates. James Hart suggests that excessive passion had the power to 'emaciat, dry up and exhaust all the radicall moisture of the body', casting the lover into an 'irrecoverable consumption'.[11] Similarly, in John Alday's 1581 translation of Pierre Boaistuau's *Theatrum Mundi*, love is represented as a smouldering flame, desiccating the sufferer's body and damaging the internal organs, so that the lover's secret passion is plainly visible to the eye of the anatomist:

> I have seene a Natomie made of some of those that have dyed of this malady, that had their bowels shrunke, their poore heart all burned, their Liver and Lightes all vaded and consumed, their Braines endomaged, and I thinke that their poore soule was burned by the vehement and excessive heat that they did endure, when that the rage of love had overcome them.[12]

The lover's claim to burn in passion could thus be explained in somatic terms: as desire grew, so the body rose in temperature, causing combustion of the humours, and producing melancholy. It is thus fitting, according to Burton, that 'a moderne writer of amorous Emblems, expresse Loves fury by a pot hanging over the fire, and *Cupid* blowing the coales'—such images not only express metaphorically how the lover feels, but also encapsulate the bodily effects of erotic desire: 'As the heat consumes the water . . . so doth Love dry up his radicall moisture.'[13]

While the physiological effects of intemperate desire were believed to pervade the whole body, the heart was thought to be particularly susceptible to the influence of emotion. According to Coëffeteau, the heart either 'dilates it selfe, or shrinkes up', according to the emotion felt; in joy 'the heart melts with gladnesse; in grief 'it shrinks up and freezeth'.[14] Many of the standard clichés concerning languishing or broken-hearted lovers were thus held to have a biological foundation. In a letter of November 1600, written by a minor courtier, Philip Gaudy, to his brother in the country, the correspondent reports news of 'the tragycall death of Mrs Ratcliffe', a maid of honor to Queen Elizabeth, who

---

[11] Hart, *Klinike,* 348.   [12] Boaistuau, *Theatrum Mundi,* 192.
[13] Burton, *Anatomy,* iii.159.   [14] Coëffeteau, *Table,* 13, 17.

ever synce the deathe of Sr Alexander her brother hathe pined in such straunge manner, as voluntarily she hathe gone about to starve her selfe and by the two dayes together hath receyved no sustinaunce, which meeting with extreame griefe hathe made an end of her mayden modest dayes at Richmond uppon Saterdaye last, her Mae^tie being [present?] who commaunded her body to be opened and founde it all well and sounde, saving certaine stringes striped all over her harte. All the maydes ever synce have gone in blacke.[15]

Despite the fact that Mrs Ratcliffe 'voluntarily...hathe gone about to starve her selfe', Queen Elizabeth orders her autopsy, which reveals the physiological effects of her 'extreame greife'; the outer layers of her heart are found to be ruptured—she has died, it seems, of a broken heart. Literary texts also suggest that extreme or violent emotions can break or crack the heart. Calantha and Florio are depicted as dying from broken hearts in Ford's *The Broken Heart* and *'Tis Pity She's a Whore* (1633) respectively, as are Lear and Gloucester in Shakespeare's *King Lear* (1610). And in *Antony and Cleopatra* (1606), Enobarbus dies on stage, with the command:

> Throw my heart
> Against the flint and hardness of my fault,
> Which, being dried with grief, will break to powder,
> And finish all foul thoughts.
>
> (IV.x.14–17)

Grief and guilt desiccate Enobarbus' heart, which shatters when he calls to mind his betrayal of Antony.[16]

Many of the symptoms of erotic melancholy described in early modern texts correspond to clichés about lovesick behaviour that are still employed today: those suffering from lovesickness are said to be afflicted by insomnia, loss of appetite, exhaustion, depression, mental fixations, and speechlessness.[17] Lovers are pale and emaciated; they have hollow, sunken eyes, and are subject to intense, fluctuating emotions: sometimes

---

[15] Bodleian Library, Egerton MS 2804, fo. 127, cited in Gawdy, *Letters*, 103. For the relation of this anecdote to John Ford's *'Tis Pity She's a Whore* see Neill, 'What Strange Riddle's This?', 156; and 'New Light', 249–50.

[16] At times, even joyful news could impact the body in dangerous ways; Shakespeare's Pericles, for example, seeks to mitigate his joy upon learning that Marina is his lost daughter, 'Lest this great sea of joys rushing upon me | O'erbear the shores of my mortality | And drown me with their sweetness!'; *Pericles* (1607), Scene xxi.179–82.

[17] Gilman, *Disease*, 1–6.

they are 'gaye, cheerful and plesant', at other times they are 'drowned in teares, making the ayre to sounde with their cryes', and at other times still they become 'cold, frozen and in a traunce, their faces pale and chaunged'.[18] Captivated by the image of the beloved, lovers avoid the company of others, 'loving solitarines, the better to feed & follow [their] foolish imaginations'.[19] Even when they are in company, they are distracted and have difficulty conversing about anything other than their beloved. Enclosed in their private obsession, they are 'carelesse of their persons', of their dress, and of the outside world; in fact, only activities related to their passion are of interest, such as writing love poetry or 'singing amorous songs and ditties'.[20] If the melancholy persists and there is little chance of their love being fulfilled, lovesick individuals may become mad, tearing their clothes, ranting in sexually explicit language, or becoming violent or suicidal.

Lovers are blind to the imperfections of their beloved, transforming any physical flaw into a distinguishing asset. Burton writes, 'If she be flat-nosed, she is lovely; if hooke-nosed, kingly; if dwarfish and little, pretty; if tall, proper and manly, like our brave Brittish *Bunduica*; if crooked, wise; if monstrous, comely'.[21] Sometimes the lover's judgement is so impaired that he will dote on anything associated with the beloved. Unlike the typical lover who might treasure a lock of hair or a glove, melancholic lovers fetishize more unusual tokens. One man kept a case where he gathered and preserved his mistress's spittle, and another wished himself to be 'a saddle for her to sit on'. Such idealization goes hand in hand with the lover's fantasies of submission and self-abasement, in which 'it would not grieve him to be hanged, if hee might bee strangled in her garters'. Often the thoughts of melancholy lovers turn to suicide; Burton writes: ''Tis the common humour of them all . . . to wish for death.'[22]

The cure of lovesickness could be effected by pharmaceutical, surgical, dietary, or psychological means: the patient's bodily humours, diet, emotional life, and the movement of the planets were all seen

---

[18] Boaistuau, *Theatrum Mundi*, 194.

[19] Ferrand, *Erotomania*, 125; Laurentius, *Preservation of the Sight*, 118. For a modern translation of Ferrand's *Erotomania* see Ferrand, *Treatise*, ed. Beecher and Ciavolella.

[20] Burton, *Anatomy*, iii.160, 190.

[21] Burton's source for this is Lucretius, *De rerum natura*, iv.1157–69.

[22] Burton, *Anatomy*, iii.58, 167, 174, 179.

as interrelated, giving clues to the source of the problem and possible means of its cure. Often a number of different methods were used in conjunction with one another, so that phlebotomy (bloodletting), clysters, vomits, change of diet, and an examination of the individual's astrological chart could be combined with practical and psychological advice when treating a patient.[23] Bloodletting is a principal cure for lovesickness; it released the lover's excess blood and the corrupt melancholy, and thus restored the balance of the four corporeal substances.[24] Sex could similarly have a purging effect, releasing excess seed and returning the individual to physical health; as Burton writes, "Tis the speciall cure, to let them bleed *vena Hymenea*, for love is a pluresie'.[25] Lovesick individuals were encouraged to keep busy, to engage in strenuous exercise, and to confess their passion to a trusted adviser or friend.[26] Music was held to have beneficial effects, inducing harmony in the mind and rousing sagging spirits, and travel was thought to expel the harmful vapours that intensified the disease and to provide a distraction for the lover's troubled imagination.[27] Some cures for lovesick men centred upon inducing an aversion to the beloved, either through vilifying the body of the desired mistress, or by denigrating love itself as infantile or effeminizing.[28] And finally, writers sometimes suggest 'Divelish and forbidden means' of curing those afflicted with erotic melancholy.
• Laurentius suggests that individuals 'drinke of the blood of him or her which is the object of the mischiefe' to extinguish the passion.[29]

Four Medico-Philosophical Traditions of the Origin of Lovesickness

Donald Beecher argues convincingly that the plurality of explanations used to describe the physiological course of erotic love is attributable not to a lack of scientific rigour on the part of early modern authors, but rather to a multiplicity of medico-philosophical systems. Each is 'potentially a complete pathological sequence with its own set of physiological causes leading to a crisis that independently accounts for the emergence

---

[23] Beecher and Ciavolella, 'Ferrand', 82; Babb, *Elizabethan Malady*, 138–40.
[24] Burton, *Anatomy*, iii.206.   [25] Ibid. 243.   [26] Bright, *Treatise*, 123.
[27] Burton, *Anatomy*, ii.114. See also Bright, *Treatise*, 248.
[28] Burton, *Anatomy*, iii.220; See Ch. 6.
[29] Laurentius, *Preservation of the Sight*, 124. See also Hart, *Klinike*, 347.

of a common disease with its common symptoms'.[30] Lovesickness can thus be explained via four separate and often mutually exclusive systems which coexist in medical and literary texts. Each of these traditions represents a separate way of conceptualizing love, providing a different physiological account of what desire is and how it takes root in the body. This multiplicity of explanations contributes to the rich vocabulary inherited by early modern writers for imagining erotic passion.

The primary tradition underlying the early modern understanding of lovesickness draws upon the humoral view of human health in the Hippocratic and Galenic schools, which provided a general model for European conceptions of disease and illness from classical times to the seventeenth century. According to the humoral model, health is determined by the admixture or commingling of the four humours—blood, phlegm, black bile, and yellow bile—which in turn affect a person's disposition, well-being, morality, and temperament. Illness is the result of a disruption of the isonomic state, which occurs when there is either a disproportionate quantity of one of these physical substances, or when the dominant humour is scorched.[31] In this system, lovesickness either causes, or is the result of, a humoral imbalance: intense sexual desire and passion may scorch the humours, producing melancholy in the body, or alternatively this physiological combustion may begin in the body, producing a corporeal state predisposed to lovesickness. In addition, anything which affects the humours can influence erotic appetite, rendering one more or less prone to lovesickness. Diet, sleeping habits, climate, and exercise can heat or cool the body, allowing for the accumulation or release of malignant humours.

Lovesickness in this system is often characterized as having two phases: a hot, moist sanguine stage, in which the lover abounds in blood and is overwhelmed by fiery passion, and a cold, dry melancholy stage, during which the lover feels fear and sorrow. These phases, however, are not always clearly distinguished, but may blur together or fluctuate.[32] There are several reasons why the lover, who is initially hot and moist, eventually becomes melancholic. Fear and sorrow (cold and dry passions) engender natural melancholy, while turbulent, fiery emotions can produce melancholy by scorching the humours. The lover's mental

[30] Beecher, 'The Lover's Body', 4.
[31] For a summary of the humoral system see Wear, *Knowledge*, 37–40.
[32] Babb, *Elizabethan Malady*, 143.

fixation on the beloved also consumes heat and moisture, making his or her brain dry and cold. As the emotional state of the lover swings erratically between love and hate, fear and hope, so too does the body alternately burn and freeze. Early modern playwrights frequently depict lovers as burning in passion for the beloved; characters complain that desire is a fire, 'Burning mine entrails with a strong desire'; they love 'With liver burning hot', or feel 'a continuall burning in all my bowels, and a bursting almost in every vaine'; they have 'scalding veins,' 'hot itching veins', and 'lust-burnt veins'.[33] Petrarchan poetry, on the other hand, characteristically focuses on the lover's contradictory, fluctuating states; in Sonnet 26, for example, Wyatt writes, 'I fere and hope I burne and freise like yse', and in *Astrophil and Stella* Philip Sidney parodies this convention, writing of 'living deaths, deare wounds, faire stormes and freesing fires'.[34]

The humoral system is the principal tradition used to explain and detail the effects of lovesickness in early modern England, but within this framework other medical ideas are integrated. A second aetiology suggests that lovesickness is primarily a mental malady, which stems from the lover's mental fixation which takes root when he or she gazes upon a beautiful form. This tradition emphasizes the powerful visual effect of beauty, which triggers the lover's mental fixation and takes hold of the imagination to the exclusion of anything else.[35] This system is described by Gerard of Berry in his thirteenth-century commentary on the *Viaticum* from the *Zād al-musāfir* of Ibn Eddjezzar, translated by Constantine the African late in the eleventh century; it draws on both Aristotle's concept of phantasms and Avicenna's account of mental faculties, in which 'images of the mind are extracted from matter and passed from ventricle to ventricle of the brain and from faculty to faculty of the soul'.[36] According to this theory, the brain is divided into

---

[33] Chapman, *Blind Beggar* (1598) I.232; Shakespeare, *Merry Wives*, II.i.112; Lyly, *Endimion*, in *Complete Works*, iii., V.iii.98–9; [anon], *Lust's Dominion*, V.ii; Dekker, *Honest Whore* II, V.33; Webster, *Appius and Virginia*, in *Works*, ii. V.iii.111. All quotations taken from Babb, 'Physiological Conception', 1026–32.

[34] Wyatt, Sonnet 26, l. 2, in *Collected Poems*; Sidney, Sonnet 6, *Astrophil and Stella* (1582), in *Poems*, 4.

[35] Tallis argues that the tradition of lovesickness derived from Avicenna and Aristotle is comparable to modern day obsessive-compulsive disorders (*Love Sick*, 54–5).

[36] Beecher, 'The Lover's Body', 6; Wack, *Lovesickness*, 56–7. See also Burton, *Anatomy*, i.152.

three sections, or ventricles, of which each takes charge of two specific mental functions: the first ventricle, at the front of the head, contains the common sense (which receives from the eyes the forms of sensory objects) and the fantasy (which preserves these forms once they are no longer present); the second ventricle, in the middle of the head, contains the imagination (which converts the forms provided by the fantasy into *phantasms*, or mental pictures) and the estimative faculty (which judges instinctively whether objects should be pursued or avoided); and the third ventricle, in the back of the head, contains the faculties of memory (which retains the forms) and bodily motion.[37] The imagination (or *phantasy*) thus provides the link between the external world and its internalized forms, translating sensory input into a pictorial mental language. This reconfiguration is possible due to the presence of a refined vapour called spirit, or *pneuma*, which transforms messages from the external senses into *phantasms* perceptible to the soul.

According to this aetiology, the sight of the beloved is so pleasing to the lover that his or her estimative faculty malfunctions and 'overestimates' the object of desire, who is judged to be more desirable and worthy than s/he actually is. The imaginative faculty thus becomes fixated on the mental image of the beloved (or *phantasm*), which dominates the mind of the lover. As Arnald of Villanova explains:

Because of the violent desire, he retains the form imprinted upon his mind by the fantasy, and because of memory, he is constantly reminded of the object. From these two actions a third follows: from the violent desire and from the constant recollection arises compulsive cogitation. The lover dwells on how and through which methods he will be able to obtain this object for his own pleasure so that he may come to the enjoyment of this destructive delight that he has formulated in his psyche.[38]

• The phantasmic image of the beloved is thus detached from the real presence of the amorous object and exists autonomously in the melancholic's mind, displacing all other sensory impressions. As Ioan P. Coulianu observes, 'When Eros is at work, the phantasm of the loved object leads its own existence, all the more disquieting because it exerts a kind of vampirism on the subject's other phantasms and

---

[37] Wack, *Lovesickness*, 56–7; Beecher and Ciavolella, 'Ferrand', 78–9.
[38] Arnald of Villanova, *De amore heroico*, trans. Beecher and Ciavolella, 46–7; quoted by Beecher and Ciavolella, 'Ferrand', 79.

thoughts.'[39] Here sexual intercourse is recommended as much to dispel the lover's mental fixation as to supply a physical release. The lover dotes obsessively, not on the true physical form of the beloved, but on the *phantasm*: the perceived, spiritual image that is impressed upon his or her mind. Falling in love is ultimately a solitary process—the lover is not only besotted by an external object, but also by an inner vision.

The apprehension of the beloved thus has the power to corrupt imagination, pervert reason, provoke appetites, and dominate memory. At times, the lover is so overwhelmed by this inner vision as to be unable to see the real physical features of the beloved, a phenomenon that gives new significance to the idea that love is blind. Burton describes one 'young gallant, that loved a wench with one eye' whose parents sent him travelling for many years to cure him of his lovesick affliction. After many years he returned and met his former beloved, and asked her how she had lost her eye. Her response plays on the trope of love as a form of blindness: '*no said she, I have lost none, but you have found yours*'.[40] Sometimes the image of the beloved is etched so strongly upon the lover's mind that he sees his love constantly before him; Burton describes 'one, that through vehemency of his love passion, still thought hee saw his mistris present with him, she talked with him...still embracing him'.[41] Like Tantalus, the lover is teased by an ever-present yet elusive image of the beloved. He will run after it, 'kissing this his idoll in the ayre, daintily intertaining and welcomming it as though it were present', or else he will attempt to flatter and seduce his own shadow.[42] Although this effect is most common amongst those who are lovesick, any excessive contemplation of a person or object could conjure its presence or image. It is to this notion that Gertrude refers when Hamlet claims to see his father's ghost: Hamlet's excessive mourning for his father gives credence to his mother's claim that the ghost is 'the very coinage of your brain' (III.iv.128–30).

There are a number of lovesick subjects in early modern drama whose passion provokes imaginary visions of the beloved object. Characters such as Memnon in Fletcher's *The Mad Lover* see their mistresses perpetually before them, so deeply ingrained is the beloved's image. The

---

[39] Coulianu, *Eros*, 30–1.   [40] Burton, *Anatomy*, iii.213.
[41] Ibid. iii. 156. See also Vaughan, *Directions*, 233.
[42] Laurentius, *Preservation of the Sight*, 120–1.

longed-for image eclipses the outer world, so that even in its absence, the imaginary presence of the loved one is keenly felt. Often this is the occasion of some comically ineffectual wooing. In Fletcher and Middleton's *The Nice Valour* (*c*.1615), for example, the Passionate Lord bows chivalrously to the empty air. The 1st Gentleman notes:

> … his love fit's upon him;
> I know it, by that set smile, and those congies.
> How courteous hee's to nothing? …
>
> .   .   .   .
> See how it kisses the fore-finger still.[43]

The motif of the lover's mental fixation also accounts for characters whose love-struck minds obscure their vision, causing faults in recognition. Although the 'bed trick' is often regarded as an unrealistic plot device, medical texts suggest that lovers are easily tricked into mistaking a stranger for their lover: enraptured by an inner vision, the sufferer displaces all other sensory impressions, projecting the beloved's image onto others. Lovers see what they want to see, or more precisely, they see the object of desire, revealing the extent to which the fulfilment of erotic desire is achieved as much in the head as in the bed. In Sidney's *The Arcadia*, for example, Basilius' belief that he is having sex with 'Cleophila', rather than Gynecia, his wife, transforms his own sense of the amorous encounter; 'O who would have thought there could have been such difference betwixt women?' he comically asks himself.[44] And in Shakespeare and Fletcher's *The Two Noble Kinsmen* (1634), the Jailer's Daughter is persuaded that the rough country wooer who comes to court her is actually Palamon, her beloved. The Doctor explains to the Jailer:

That intemperate surfeit of her eye hath distempered the other senses. They may return and settle again to execute their preordained faculties, but they are now in a most extravagant vagary. This you must do: confine her to a place where the light may rather seem to steal in than be permitted; take upon you, young sir her friend, the name of Palamon; say you come to eat with her, and to commune of love. This will catch her attention, for this her mind beats

---

[43] [Fletcher and Middleton], *Nice Valour,* in Beaumont and Fletcher, *Dramatic Works,* vol. vii, I.i.184–90.
[44] Sidney, *Old Arcadia,* ed. Robertson, 275.

upon—other objects that are inserted 'tween her mind and eye become the pranks and friskins of her madness.   (III.iv.128–30)

The mind of the Jailer's Daughter is so dominated by the image of her beloved that it has corrupted her judgement; 'Her mind beats upon' the image of Palamon, obscuring the sight of real objects and people in the world. Her mental impairment illustrates how she is ultimately captivated by a product of her imagination; even if the Jailer's Daughter were being courted by Palamon rather than the simple country wooer who comes in his place, Palamon would still be overlaid with her idealistic vision of him.

The third aetiology of lovesickness focuses directly on the lover's need for sexual satisfaction; this aetiology posits seed, or sperm (*sperma*), as the corporeal origin of erotic melancholy, which was held to be produced by both men and women in Galenic gynaecology. According to this theory, the desire for sex is the product of the seed itself, which 'tickles the seminal vessels by means of the airy vapors and spirits of which it is composed', provoking libidinous appetites and causing an instinctive craving for coitus.[45] As Burton writes, 'ita ut nisi extruso semine gestiens voluptas non cessat, nec assidua veneris recordatio' [until the ejaculation of semen is achieved the pleasure does not cease, nor the constant awareness of lust].[46] This is the case for both sexes; as William Vaughan writes, in women accumulated seed triggers 'secret flames and unbrideled affections which dispose their mindes to waiwardnes and extravagant imaginations'.[47] The eroticized lover thus craves sex as a physiological cure for his or her psychosomatic affliction, as it expels excess seed and distracts him or her from the object of desire. Here, the identity of the sexual partner is less vital than the achievement of sexual release. If, however, the seed is not released it will turn malignant, poisoning the body and deranging reason 'by sending up divers noysome vapours to the Braine'.[48] Because sperm is simply blood that has been refined and whitened from heat, this third aetiology can be easily integrated within the primary humoral model, which suggests that the lover produces an excess of blood while in the

---

[45] Fregosos, *L'anteros*, 140, quoted in Beecher and Ciavolella, 'Ferrand', 125. See MacLean, *Notion*, 35–7.
[46] Burton, *Anatomy*, iii.57 (trans. vi. 41).   [47] Vaughan, *Directions*, 113.
[48] Ferrand, *Erotomania*, 261; Hart, *Klinike*, 325.

sanguine state of erotic melancholy: 'when blood abounds in a body, seed also abounds', and this in turn increases the amorous disposition of the lover, creating the instinctive craving for coitus.[49]

• The final theory explaining the physical origin of lovesickness is found in Marsilio Ficino's *Commentary on Plato's Symposium on Love* in Speech Seven, where he contrasts noble, spiritual love with pathological forms of desire.[50] Like the second aetiology of lovesickness, Ficino's model focuses on the powerful effect of viewing a beautiful form. But whereas the aetiology derived from Avicenna's account of mental faculties focuses on the lover's incessant contemplation of an internal mental image, Ficino focuses on the act of gazing, which infects the lover and depletes his or her blood. According to Ficino, lovesickness is the result of a condition that he terms *fascination*, in which love enters through the eyes, infecting the body and initiating the pathological sequence of erotic melancholy. In this sequence, the lover's hungry gaze acts as a magnet, drawing a thin vapour of blood out of the eyes of the beloved and towards the image in the mind.[51] These vapours are received into the eyes of the lover, where they travel through the body into the liver, turning into alien blood. Alday's translation of Boaistuau's *Theatrum Mundi* provides a summary of Ficino's theory:

• When we cast our sight upon that which we desire, sodainly certaine spirits that are engendered of the most perfectest parte of bloud, proceedeth from the heart of the partie which we doe love, and promptly ascendeth even up to the eyes, and afterward converteth into vapours invisible, and entreth into our eyes, which are bent to receive them ... and so from the eyes it penetrateth to the heart.[52]

The lover is thus infected by a foreign blood that can attack the liver, heart, and blood. S/he is enervated by the loss of blood, which is similarly drawn to the beautiful image in the mind, desiccating the body and leaving a melancholy residue.

Poetry and drama contain numerous examples of individuals transfixed by the lover's gaze, and Petrarchan poetry and pictorial traditions

---

[49] Babb, 'Physiological Conception', 1021.

[50] Ficino, *Commentary on Plato's Symposium on Love*, VII.iv–v. See Ch. 4 for a discussion of Neoplatonic philosophy.

[51] As Ficino writes, 'a ray which is sent out by the eyes draws with it a spiritual vapour, and that vapour draws with it blood' (*Commentary on Plato's Symposium on Love*, VII.iv).

[52] Boaistuau, *Theatrum Mundi*, 192. See also Burton, *Anatomy*, iii.88.

going back to the Middle Ages are rich in images of the lover being shot with arrows from the beloved's eyes. Wyatt's Sonnet 47 describes how 'The lyvely sperkes that issue from those Iyes | Against the which ne vaileth no defence | Have prest myn hert', linking the arrows fired from the beloved's eyes to those of Cupid.[53] And in cases where the love is mutual, the lovers' interlocked gaze can allow for the physical exchange of blood. Donne creates a graphic image of this gaze in 'The Ecstasy': 'our eye-beams twisted, and did thread | Our eyes, upon one double string'.[54] And in William Davenant's play, *The Platonick Lovers* (1636), the doctor Buonateste uses a very similar image when he explains how 'the Opticks' give insight into the origin of abstract affection. Buonateste explains how

> Amorists oppos'd in levell to
> Each others sight, unite and thridd their beames,
> Untill they make a mutuall string, on which
> Their spirits dance into each others braine,
> And so beginne short Journeys to the heart.[55]

Here, the lovers' interlocked gaze allows for a form of spiritual intermingling: desire unites the lovers, setting off a chain reaction which involves their eyes, minds, and hearts.

HISTORICAL ACCOUNTS OF THE EXPERIENCE OF EROTIC MELANCHOLY

Evidence from the early modern period suggests that lovesickness was more than just a literary construction. Portraiture, doctors' case records, letters, and diaries all attest to the fact that men and women viewed themselves, or were represented, as suffering from melancholy as a result of love. Indeed, the association of melancholy with intelligence, alienation, depression, and ecstatic rapture made such posturing both fashionable and culturally resonant. Such visual and verbal texts testify to the interaction of societal codes and personal experience: whilst being

---

[53] Wyatt, Sonnet 47, 1–3.
[54] Donne, 'The Ecstasy', in *Donne*, ed. Patrides, 7–8. All references to Donne are taken from this edition.
[55] Davenant, *Platonick Lovers*, sig. D3ᵛ.

constructed socially and medically, lovesickness was also an emotion individuals genuinely felt.

The sense of psychological disquiet described in accounts of lovesickness offers insight into the passionate attachments and anxieties that accompanied courtship, anxieties often aggravated by patriarchal assumptions about female modesty, and social restrictions regarding marriage. As social historians have emphasized, courtship was a particularly stressful time in the lives of young men and women in early modern England. Matrimony was an expensive undertaking, and marriageable women outnumbered eligible men, producing a difficult marriage market. Because marriage had serious social and financial consequences, courtship was a period of intense private and public negotiation; it was of crucial importance not only to the couple concerned, but also to the family and wider community. Subject both to psychological pressure and to the approval of their neighbours and kin, young men and women frequently found 'their marriage plans facilitated, inhibited or entirely prevented by their families, by their neighbours and by wider corporate structures like the parish or township'.[56] In the fraught context of courtship, the discourse of lovesickness provided an important means of expressing what was sometimes an intractable conflict between physical desire and familial duty.

The medical dangers of lovesickness are clearly substantiated in historical accounts, many of which recount the death of those afflicted. Aubrey believed that Viscount Falkland deliberately allowed himself to be killed in battle because his mistress had died, and Napier records that Robert Malins 'died poisoning himself for that he could not marry a maid that . . . he loved extremely, as some suppose'.[57] Burton thought the problem very common: 'Goe to *Bedlam* for examples. It is so well knowne in every village, how many have either died for love or voluntary made away themselves, that I need not much labor to prove it . . . Death is the common *Catastrophe* to such persons.'[58]

Lucy Hutchinson's biography of her husband shows how the experience of love is frequently articulated through the discourse of melancholy. It is a category to which Hutchinson seems drawn: she describes

---

[56] O'Hara, *Courtship*, 165. See Stone, *Family*, 127–36.

[57] Aubrey, *Brief Lives*, 215–16; Napier, Bodleian Library, Ashmole MS 182, fo. 77 (Malins).

[58] Burton, *Anatomy*, iii.199.

herself as exhibiting a 'melancholly negligence both of her selfe and others' (linking this disposition to her scholarly absorption in books and writing), and uses melancholy to express both her husband's innate nobility and his eventual political marginalization.[59] She also describes her husband's love for her in the language of erotic melancholy, especially in the early stages of their courtship before they are married. In one such instance, she describes how he is beset by the physical symptoms of lovesickness, after misunderstanding a conversation over dinner that leads him to believe that she is married:

Mr. Hutchinson immediately turn'd pale as ashes, and felt a fainting to seize his spiritts, in that extraordinary manner that finding himselfe ready to sink att table . . . it was not necessary for him to feigne sicknesse, for the distemper of his mind had infected his body with a cold sweate and such a dispersion of spiritt that all the courage he could at present recollect was little enough to keepe him allive.[60]

Colonel Hutchinson's grief instigates a violent physical reaction, clenching the heart and agitating the vital spirits, so that 'the whole body feeles it selfe mooved, not onely inwardly, but also outwardly'.[61] He retires to his room where he 'recollect[s] his wisedome and his reason' in order to quell his passion, but his 'sick heart could not be chid nor adviz'd into health'. Overwhelmed by the strength of his passion, he begins to wonder if there is not something supernatural about its source. Recalling the stories of tragic love he has heard, he begins 'to believe there was some magick in the place which enchanted men out of their right sences'.[62] Hutchinson associates love and supernatural agency, echoing a popular notion, common in early modern England, that falling in love was similar to a state of bewitchment.[63] Hutchinson's illness is recorded retrospectively by his wife and should not, therefore, be read in the same way as a first-person narrative: his experiences are shaped by Lucy with specific purposes and interests in mind. Regardless of this, however, the fact that Lucy constructs her husband's love as an illness shows the extent to which the common experience of love was mediated by the language of erotic melancholy, providing a vocabulary

---

[59] Hutchinson, *Memoirs*, 31.   [60] Ibid. 30.
[61] Coëffeteau, *Table*, 16–17.   [62] Hutchinson, *Memoirs*, 30.
[63] Burton, *Anatomy*, iii.89. For the relationship between lovesickness and magic see Beecher and Ciavolella, *Eros and Anteros*.

for expressing private passion, and at times influencing and shaping what the lover actually felt. Throughout the *Memoirs* his 'illness' is figured as the dramatic prelude to his union with Lucy, emphasizing the happiness and 'health' of their eventual marriage.

Historical evidence also exists elsewhere to suggest that love was commonly experienced and regarded as a medical affliction. The manuscript case notes of Richard Napier, a doctor who treated several patients suffering from unrequited love, reveal the emotional and physical anguish lovesick individuals experience.[64] Almost 40 per cent of the men and women who describe their anxieties and dilemmas to Napier complain about the frustrations of courtship and married life, and a number of them experience the physical sensations and disturbed mental state that can be characterized as symptoms of erotic melancholy.[65] Lovesick patients often complain of digestive problems: they are 'loose bodied' (diarrhoeic) and cannot eat; they frequently have nightmares or are troubled with insomnia; and sometimes they lose the will to live. Thomas May of Rishden, for example, treated by Napier in May 1629, threatened suicide: Napier records that Thomas had 'grief taken for a wench he lovd. he sayth if he may not have her he will hang him selfe. 10 dys ill, semes mopish, loose bodyed, cannot sleep well.'[66] Napier's diagnostic response is to prescribe his patient a purge.

Jane Travell of Gothurst visited Napier five times between November 1615 and May 1617 for her unhappiness in love. Piecing together Napier's case notes, we see some of the social pressures that must have aggravated normal courtship practices. Upon her first visit Jane, then 24, does not mention the cause of her malady. Napier writes that she is 'full of melancholie' and 'fancies', and so very 'Troubled in mind [she] can take no rest nor joy of any thing'.[67] Two years later, in her second visit, Jane complains of insomnia as well as an aversion to music: she 'cd not like Song. [and could] no longer endure hir troubles'. However, although Jane remains silent about the cause of her distemper, a seemingly inexplicable nocturnal vision suggests that the cause of her illness may originate either in erotic longings or her unmarried state. Napier's notes elliptically record that 'in a night a thing sayd unto her y^t he would

[64] For an excellent overview of Napier's practice see MacDonald, *Mystical Bedlam*.
[65] Ibid. 88.
[66] Napier, Bodleian Library, Ashmole MS 406, fo. 21^v (May) (punctuation added).
[67] Napier, Bodleian Library, Ashmole MS 196, fo. 140^r (Travell).

be her husb'.[68] Thirteen days later Jane complains of being 'mightily tempted [and] ready to goe out of her wits', and is sent away with the prescription for a clyster.[69] A month later still, Napier reports that she is 'much troubled with wind in hir bowels and guts', complaining that 'no body can tell the sorrow y^t she indureth. hir fansyes much troubled. Sometymes will sing 3 hours. otherwise as heavy and as sad as can [be]'. She 'should have maryd on[e] and they were at words as if she would not sute him. and then bydding him to marry else wher fell into this passion. She knoweth y^t she shall never have him.'[70]

The mysterious cause of Jane's refusal to marry her lover is clarified only upon the occasion of her final visit. One month later, she returns and edges towards a confession. Jane, Napier writes, 'was in love. full of fond and strong concits and sayth y^t noone but god can cure it'. Her despair is combined with a sense of alienation, both from herself and from her lover; Jane 'hath a concit y^t tis hir lover dissembleth, but it is not soe. she sayth that she is a spirit and not her selfe'. Disoriented and confused, Jane reveals the identity of her former lover to be 'hir mothers serv', in which 'serv' could mean household attendant or lover. Napier's final notes are provocative: Jane 'made as if she [her mother? Jane?] could not have him and yet it semeth she [Jane?] did'.[71] Whether we interpret Jane's beloved as her mother's servant or lover, either way she would have been placed in a frustrating position of powerlessness, trapped in a relationship that crossed class or familial boundaries. She could not require the man to behave in a certain way without exposing her sexual and social indiscretion, and so is forced to hide her feelings which re-emerge as an illness.

Given the pressure placed upon individuals to marry in a socially and economically advantageous manner, lovesickness could function as a form of complaint against parents and guardians who treat their dependants as passive objects of exchange. As well as exerting psychological pressure on the beloved, a sufficiently virulent attack of lovesickness might prompt one's parents and friends to tolerate a suitor previously deemed unacceptable. Lovesickness can thus articulate the sufferer's own emotional and sexual preferences in the face of opposition, providing a

---

[68] Napier, Bodleian Library, Ashmole MS 198, fo. 87^r (Travell).
[69] Ibid., fo. 140^r (Travell).   [70] Ibid., fo. 116^v (Travell).
[71] Ibid., fo. 146^r (Travell).

physiological imperative for the sufferer to be united with the beloved; the malady was even used 'in a number of legal cases that granted daughters the right to marry without their father's consent'.[72] The potentially fatal consequences of lovesickness make it imperative (in at least the doctor's eyes) for the lover to be united with his beloved, lest he or she die or go mad, so that the display of lovesickness becomes an indirect means of engineering its fulfilment.[73] An example of this is found in Napier's treatment of a man named Fettyplace. Fettyplace, who is besotted with his mother's servant, is prevented from marrying her due to their class difference. Originally, he is forced to visit Napier by his mother and he seems very much against any treatment that Napier might offer. In their first meeting on 16 May 1620 Napier records: 'Mr. Fettyplace came to me not of his own accord but by the appoytment of his lady mother a young gentleman | [he] lovd on[e] y^t his mother despised | He is by fits in his head mopish and will not speake a word . . . a quartr of a year ill 2 y by fits'. The next day Fettyplace complies with Napier by sending a urine sample, but still seems hostile to therapy: he 'would talke little, no good could be done, mopish and will speak litle, by fits very unruly, wil be outragius sometyms'.[74]

A month later Fettyplace's lovesickness turns violent. In a moment of rage, he beats his servant senseless. It is unclear whether the servant is an amorous rival, or simply a random victim of Fettyplace's mental estrangement and bottled-up anger; what is clear, however, is that the act of violence is bound up with his lovesickness. Napier's case notes record: 'not a week since furious, & struke his ~~master~~ svrt & made him black & blue, & then told him y^t now he will fight no more, & sayd y^t he will have his wench ann & wisheth y^t he had.' Fettyplace's emotional declaration precipitates a change in the doctor–patient relationship. Fettyplace is recorded as suddenly going to visit Napier of his own free will, and on one occasion Napier writes that 'Mr. Fettyplace came to me & borrowed an english book in folio with sundry aphorismes made for prince henrye his use Aug 1, 1620'.[75] The change in Fettyplace's

---

[72] Dixon, *Perilous Chastity*, 219.
[73] It is in this way that the well-known classical story of Antiochus' lovesickness for his stepmother is resolved. See Bright, *Treatise*, 121.
[74] Napier, Bodleian Library, Ashmole MS 414, fo. 38^r (Fettyplace) (punctuation added).
[75] Ibid., fo. 130^v (Fettyplace).

demeanour coincides strikingly with evidence of Napier's support for him; a week later, Napier records his judgement on the case, presumably an opinion he would have conveyed to Fettyplace's parents: he 'shall prv a good husb . . . [he should] marry ~~the~~ poore myd his mothers mayd though but poor or to continue still foolish & idle headed . . . purge him well with vomits or purges or clystirs or all . . . & then let him mary wher his mynd is set'.[76] Melancholy provides Fettyplace with a means of protest, as well as an imperative for being united with his love. By making sexual desire a real matter of life or death, lovesickness proves an effective form of emotional blackmail.

THE LOOK OF LOVE

In William Shakespeare's *Love's Labour's Lost* (*c*.1594–5), the kings of Navarre, Biron, Longueville, and Dumaine each in turn read sonnets they have composed for their mistresses. The men have previously sworn that for three years they will avoid women, devoting themselves instead to their studies, but have broken their vows in order to pursue the Princess of France and her ladies, Rosaline, Maria, and Catherine. For each of the four men, falling in love causes them to act in precisely the same manner: they become melancholy, send the women gifts, and go to the woods to write love poetry. To be 'infected' with the disease of love makes one appear oddly 'affected', as Boyet puns, not only in the sense that love is powerful in its impact, but also because it can make one's behaviour seem oddly artificial and contrived (II.i.230, 232). Biron finds it ironic that having been 'love's whip' he is nonetheless transformed into a conventional lover (III.i.169). He knows that cupid is 'Regent of love rhymes, lord of folded arms' but this does not prevent him from conforming to this role: 'I do love', he complains, 'and it hath taught me to rhyme and to be melancholy' (III.i.176; IV.iii.11–12). Love is not only culturally codified, but also oddly anonymous, so that in moments of intense inwardness one's own words can seem horribly clichéd. As Terry Eagleton writes, 'in its very moment of absolute, original value, the self stumbles across nothing but

---

[76] Ibid., fo. 187ʳ (Fettyplace).

other people's lines, finds itself handed a meticulously detailed script to which it must slavishly conform'.[77]

Early modern constructions of lovesickness depict the malady as physically internal (located in the subject's very blood, mind, genitals, and liver) and psychically enclosed. 'Inamorato' on the frontispiece of the 1628 edition of Burton's *Anatomy of Melancholy* (Fig. 1), for example, draws himself inward with his crossed arms, hides his face under a floppy hat, and directs his gaze, not at the world around him, but at an invisible world within. Nevertheless, while the clothing and bearing of the lovesick individual suggest that the symptoms of erotic melancholy were privately felt, the fact that this inwardness is expressed through recognizable conventions of posture, dress, and behaviour indicates the way in which lovesickness was a role performed as well as an emotion experienced. To be taken seriously as a lover one must look and dress the part. As Rosalind playfully advises Orlando in *As You Like It* (1599–1600), to be a lover requires

A lean cheek, which you have not; a blue eye and sunken, which you have not; an unquestionable spirit, which you have not; a beard neglected which you have not . . . Then your hose should be ungartered, your bonnet unbanded, your sleeve unbuttoned, your shoe untied, and everything about you demonstrating a careless desolation.   (III.ii.361–9)

While desire may be instinctive, its expression is bound up in culturally determined forms. Beyond being simply a disposition, erotic melancholy is a pose which proclaims to the world one's status as a lover.

Burton's *Inamorato* (Fig. 1) is a typical example of the lover's persona with his contemplative and dishevelled demeanour.[78] He wears a large, floppy hat, and around him are the '*symptomes of his vanity*': his books, poetry, and a lute. A similar image appears in Samuel Rowlands's *The Melancholie Knight* (1615), in which a lovesick man slumps in an identical posture, 'his head hung downe', his face 'masked with his hat pull'd down', his arms crossed, 'And in his hat a cole-blacke feather stucke'.[79] The large feather and the ribbons—possibly favours given to him by

---

[77] Eagleton, *Shakespeare*, 18–19.

[78] Gilman suggests that Burton's frontispiece 'serves as a seventeenth century summary of visual icons of mental illness' (*Seeing*, 17).

[79] R[owlands], 'To Respective Readers', *Knight*, pp. v, vi; Laurentius, *Preservation of the Sight*, 90.

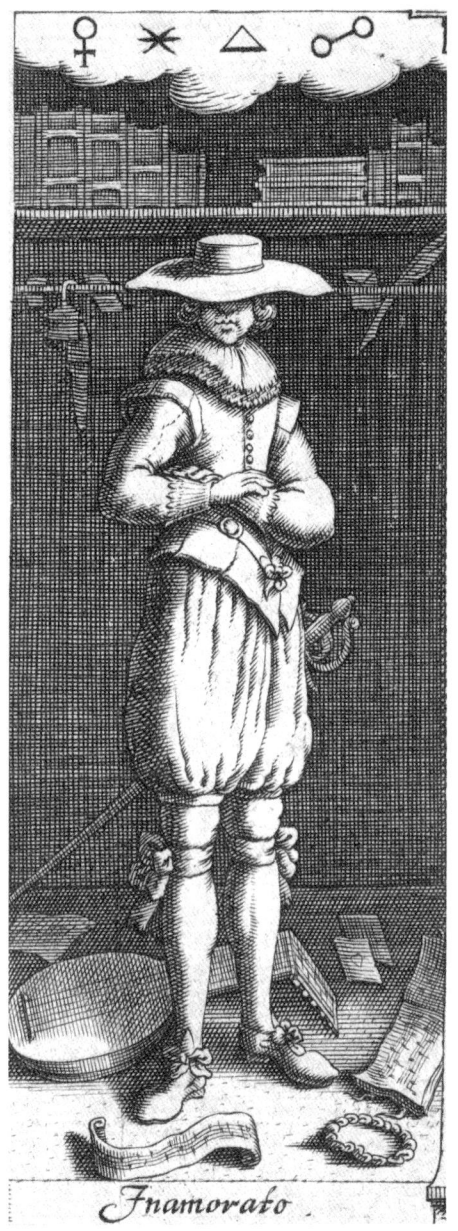

Fig. 1. *Inamorato*, detail from the frontispiece of Robert Burton's *The Anatomy of Melancholy* (1628).

his mistress—suggest a carefully constructed aura of neglect. Women also expressed their amorous discontent in socially codified ways. Like their male counterparts, women crossed their arms and appeared dishevelled and distracted when in love, frequently appearing with their hair undone.[80]

In Elizabethan and Jacobean literature, willows signify unrequited love and those who are jilted wear the willow garland.[81] In Shakespeare's *Othello* (1603–4), for example, on the evening of her death Desdemona sings a 'song of willow', which is said to be 'an old thing' that she had learned from Barbary, her mother's maid; Barbary 'was in love, and he she loved proved mad | And did forsake her', and 'she died singing' this song (IV.iii.26–9). Similarly, in 'The Seeds of Love', a seventeenth-century song attributed to Mrs Fleetwood Habergham of Lancashire, Mrs Fleetwood Habergham describes her love as a red rose that harbours a 'sharp thorn'. The speaker describes how she 'oftentimes plucked at the red rose bush | Till it pierced me to the heart' and she 'gained the willow tree'.[82] Male characters could also use willows to denote their lovelorn status. In Lyly's *Sappho and Phao* (1584), for example, Phao, bewitched by the beauty of Sappho, is instructed to wear 'willow in thy hat and bays in thy heart', and in Sidney's *The Countess of Pembroke's Arcadia*, the disguised Pyrocles writes his love lament in a sandy bank with a 'willow stick'.[83]

Because the melancholic lover conformed to a recognized model of dress and behaviour s/he was easy to spot; as Ferrand suggests in *Erotomania*, 'the Lover still beleeves his desires are so closely carried, as that the quickest apprehension cannot discover them: whereas indeed they lye open, and exposed to every eye'.[84] In the drama, conventions of lovesick dress and behaviour act as a convenient shorthand for characterization, enabling lovers to display their passion without saying a word. In Shakespeare's *Hamlet* (1600–1), for example, Ophelia describes Hamlet as the very picture of diseased love when he appears visibly distraught after she has returned his letters: he is described by

[80] Female lovesickness is discussed in more detail in Chs. 2 and 3.

[81] Willows were thought to be medicinal in early modern medicine (rightly, as they are the source of aspirin), and Psalm 137 associates the plant with grief.

[82] Sedley (ed.), *Seeds of Love*, 138–9. I am grateful to Peter and Jane Freshwater for this reference.

[83] Lyly, *Sappho and Phao*, II.iv.24–5; Sidney, *Old Arcadia*, ed. Robertson, 118. See also Shakespeare, *Twelfth Night*, I.v.253, 257–8.

[84] Ferrand, *Erotomania*, 104.

Ophelia as entering her closet sighing and trembling 'with his doublet all unbraced, | No hat upon his head, his stockings fouled, | Ungartered, and down-gyvèd to his ankle' (II.i.78–80). However, although Hamlet's appearance gives some justification to Polonius's claim that Hamlet is in 'the very ecstasy of love' (II.i.103), it is important to note that the audience does not actually see Hamlet 'unbrac'd', 'ungart'red', and 'pale as his shirt', but only hears this from Ophelia. It is therefore possible that this picture of Hamlet is one that Ophelia imagines (and wishes for), indicating not Hamlet's amorous malady, but Ophelia's own.

For individuals whose love is deemed unacceptable, erotic melancholy may be a means of articulating desire in an oblique fashion. Such assumptions govern criticism today, so that Antonio's melancholy in Shakespeare's *The Merchant of Venice* is often read as the sign of his frustrated love for Bassanio.[85] The same strategy can be used when one's beloved is of a different social rank. In Lyly's *Sappho and Phao*, when the lowly Phao falls in love with Sappho, the queen, he is advised by Sibylla to express his passion visually; Sibylla tells him to 'Look pale and learn to be lean, that whoso seeth thee may say the gentleman is in love'.[86]

As the Burton frontispiece shows, examples of lovesick and melancholic self-fashioning are not confined to the realm of literature. The vogue for melancholic affectation in portraits is identified by Roy Strong in a series of paintings whose subjects are depicted as either melancholy or lovesick.[87] Paintings such as that of Sir Robert Sidney (*c*.1585), the younger brother of Sir Philip Sidney, reveal the popularity of the melancholy pose. Robert Sidney bears all of the typical attributes of the melancholic individual. Attired in black, with his arms folded, he stands in a solitary field that is distanced from the cityscape behind him. His body is slumped over—in a mixture of grief, fatigue, and meditation—and his drooping head wears an expression that is at once downcast and contemplative. His pose recalls not only that of the 'Inamorato',

---

[85] See e.g. Auden, *Dyer's Hand*, 229. For an early modern example of lovesickness resulting from same-sex desire see Diethelm, *Dissertations*, 65; for early modern ideas about homosexuality see Smith, *Homosexual Desire*; Bray, *Homosexuality*; Bredbeck, *Sodomy and Interpretation*; and Goldberg, *Sodometries*.

[86] Lyly, *Sappho and Phao*, II.iv.112–13.

[87] My discussion of representations of lovesickness in portraits relies on Strong, *Monarchy*.

but also that of the allegorical figure of melancholy in Albrecht
Dürer's engraving *Melancholia I* (1514); as in Dürer's engraving the
subject's gaze is directed not at us or at the world around him, but at
an invisible world within. Preoccupied with internal visions, the melancholy pose suggests a disengagement with the petty material realm, rendering the subject elevated and removed. Nonetheless, Sidney's averted
gaze, while emphasizing his own subjective and private realm, simultaneously transforms him into an object to be gazed at and admired.

Portraits by Nicholas Hilliard and Isaac Oliver also present their
subjects with melancholic trappings; the miniature of the young man
by Hilliard which is believed to be the ninth Earl of Northumberland (Fig. 2), and Oliver's Lord Herbert of Cherbury (*c*.1610–14)
depict their sitters in melancholic poses, rapt in deep contemplation.[88] There are also several portraits of melancholic lovers. One
miniature by Hilliard depicts a man clasping his lady's hand let down
from heaven. And the portrait sometimes called 'Christopher Marlowe'
(1585), held at Corpus Christi College, Cambridge, includes the motto
Quod me nutruit me destruit (that which nourishes me destroys me).
But the most famous of all the love-portraits is that of the poet John
Donne (1595):

A Latin inscription on the portrait implores his lady, to whom he owes a
saint-like devotion, to lighten the shadows which envelop his love-sick misery:
Illumina tenebras nostras domina. Donne has all the usual trappings: a large
hat with a floppy brim, arms folded across his chest, black dress, his collar
negligently left undone.[89]

A few portraits of lovesick individuals stress their fiery passion rather
than their melancholy. A miniature by Isaac Oliver, *Man with a Background of Flames* (*c*.1610), and another by Nicholas Hilliard, *Unknown
Man* (1590), both depict the lover amid a burst of fire, providing a
compelling visual image to Adams's claim that the lover 'lives like a
Salamander in the flames of lust, and quencheth his heat with fire'.[90]
In the Hilliard portrait (Fig. 3), the cause of the man's grief is made
explicit: around the sitter's neck, and in his grasp, is a miniature of his
mistress.[91]

---

[88] Ibid. 299.   [89] Strong, *Monarchy*, 301.
[90] Adams, *Diseases of the Soule*, 46.   [91] Ashelford, *Dress*, 103.

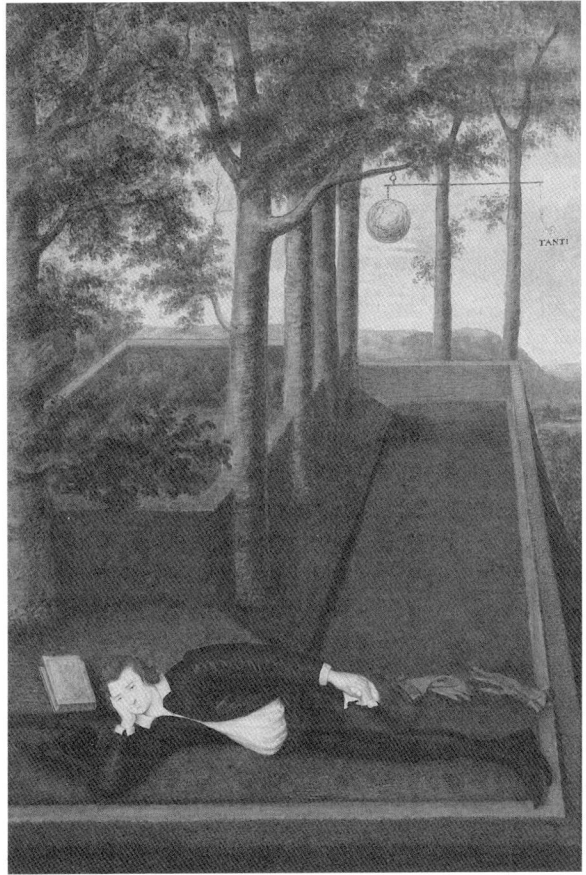

Fig. 2. Nicholas Hilliard, *Henry Percy, 9th Earl of Northumberland* (*c*.1590–5).

Part of the appeal of lovesick self-fashioning in early modern England was that, like melancholy, it was an affliction associated with an introspective, philosophical disposition and was held to afflict the social and intellectual elite. Lovesickness was termed '*Heroicall* because commonly Gallants, Noblemen and the most generous spirits are possessed with it'; typical lovesick sufferers are 'young and lusty, in the flowre of their yeares, nobly descended, high fed, such as live idly and at

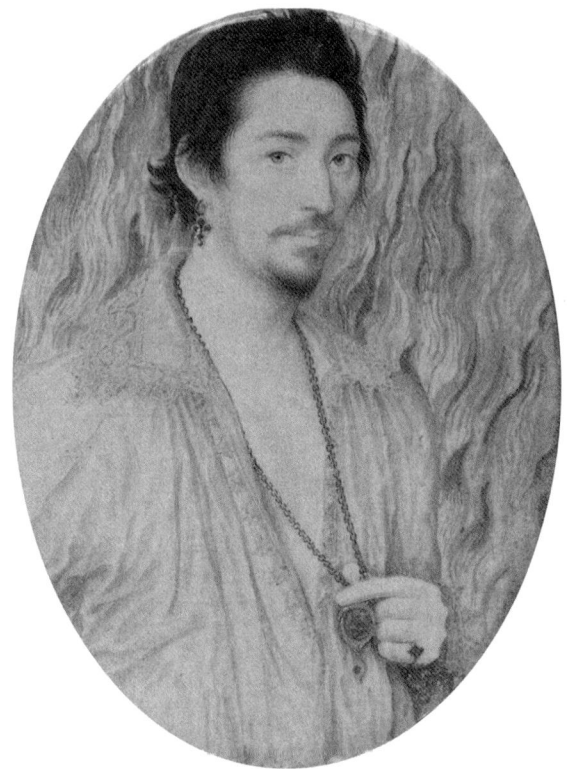

Fig. 3. Nicholas Hilliard, *Unknown Man Against A Background of Flames* (*c*.1588).

ease'.[92] Richard Napier's case notes reveal that his melancholy patients were from a significantly higher class than most of his other patients; more than 40 per cent of them were peers, knights and ladies, or masters and mistresses. The term 'melancholy' was reserved for the social elite, whereas those lower down the social ladder evincing similar behaviour would be classified as 'mopish' or as 'troubled in mind', rather than 'melancholic'.[93] Thus, although lower-class individuals might feel

[92] Burton, *Anatomy*, iii.39, 56.   [93] MacDonald, *Mystical Bedlam*, 151–2.

alienated and depressed, to claim to be melancholic was seen as socially pretentious. In Lyly's *Midas* (1592), for example, when Motto, a barber, complains of feeling 'as melancholy as a cat', he is reproached for his impudence. 'Is melancholy a word for a barber's mouth?' Licio asks him: 'Thou shouldst say heavy, dull and doltish. Melancholy is the crest of courtiers' arms, and now every base companion, being in his mubble-fubbles, says he is melancholy.'[94]

Lovesick self-fashioning was also a key means of communicating one's affection to one's mistress. By simply donning a floppy hat and wandering about sighing and ungartered, a man could proclaim his lovelorn status. As Ashelford observes in her study of Elizabethan dress, 'the expression of an abstract idea through a visual image was an essential part of Elizabethan life, for the love of allegory was all-pervasive and an accepted part of everyday life'.[95] A man could wear his mistress's colours as a means of signalling his affection, or wear particular shades that had symbolic meaning.[96] Thomas Whythorne, for example, in his autobiography of 1576, describes how he wore russet to suggest to his beloved that he lived in hope.[97] To aid in devising designs on garments or other items, 'drawers' could be consulted whose job it was to produce patterns on materials for individuals to embroider.[98]

Melancholy could thus function as the visual idiom through which one could express passion, providing an indirect means of articulating desire. Such unspoken forms of communication were particularly useful if the union with the beloved was in any way obstructed due to class, marriage, or family ties. In fact, the extent to which melancholy was associated with erotic desire could cause real confusion. Lucy Hutchinson describes how a young woman mistook Colonel Hutchinson's melancholy for love:

---

[94] Lyly, *Midas*, V.ii.102, 103–8; quoted in MacDonald, *Mystical Bedlam*, 151.

[95] Ashelford, *Dress*, 90.   [96] Ibid. 98.

[97] Whythorne, *Autobiography*, 40.

[98] For example, in the anonymous *Faire Maide of the Exchange* (1607) Phillis seeks the aid of a drawer, with whom she is in love, for a handkerchief. Choosing a design that conveys her emotions, she hopes that the drawer will guess the love that she feels for him (sig. [D4^r]). See also the coverlet known as *The Shepherd Buss* (*c*.1590), which depicts a lovelorn shepherd, surrounded by a rebus indicating how 'False *cupid* with misfortunes *wheel* hath wounded *hand* & *heart*' (in Ashelford, *Dress*, 93–4).

At that time there was in the Towne a young maid, beautifull, and esteemed
to be very rich, but of base parentage and penurious education, though else
ingenuous enough . . . his greate heart could never stoope to thinke of marrying
into so meane a stock; yet by reason of some likenesse apprehended betweene
them and the melancholly he had with some discontents at home, she was
willing to flatter her selfe, and others to perswade her, that it was love for her,
which, when she discover'd her mistake, was a greate griefe to her.[99]

Melancholy, read as the repressed expression of desire, is as convincing
as an amorous declaration. In the formal and restricted domain of
male–female friendships, melancholy comes to be understood as a silent
expression of love.

  The display of erotic melancholy, which could act as a powerful
form of communication, also had certain rhetorical and psychological
advantages in courtship, offering the wooer an effective means of seduction. By adopting a melancholic persona, lovers exert psychological
pressure on the beloved while simultaneously displacing responsibility
for their behaviour, either by blaming their illness ('I am sick; I can't
help myself'), or their beloved ('you made me this way'). As Beecher
and Ciavolella suggest, there is a fine line 'between the despairing lover
as passive victim and as *animateur* of a last desperate ploy to possess
the lady'.[100] As the gendered terms in the quotation imply, this is
generally a male activity, in which the suitor takes control of his malady,
exaggerating or feigning his symptoms in order to woo his mistress by
eliciting sympathy from her. This stratagem derives from Ovid, who
recommends to the lover in the *Ars amatoria* 'swear that you are dying
of frantic love', and it appears in the Renaissance as a staple rhetorical device in seduction.[101] Letter-writing manuals advise the lover to
describe his passion as an illness, representing desire as a fire that must
blaze forth 'into words and actions' or burn the lover to death.[102] In
Lyly's *Sappho and Phao* (1584), Sibylla advises Phao in the 'rules for poor
lovers' set forth in Ovid's *Ars amatoria*, telling Phao to 'Flatter—I mean
lie', make promises, praise lavishly, write letters, dress well, dance, and
play music.[103] Similarly, in Ford's *Love's Sacrifice* (c.1632), Fernando

---

[99] Hutchinson, *Memoirs*, 26.   [100] Beecher and Ciavolella, 'Ferrand', 162.
[101] Ovid, *Ars amatoria*, I.374, quoted by Oestreich-Hart, 'Prove a Lover', 246.
[102] F[lesher], *Cupids Messenger*, 167.   [103] Lyly, *Sappho and Phao*, II.iv.67, 118.

uses his erotic melancholy as a seductive strategy, complaining that he cannot find any 'Physic strong to cure a tortured mind' and citing his emaciation as physical proof of his intense desire: 'That passion, and the vows I owe to you, | Have changed me to a lean anatomy', he tells her.[104] Significantly, by insisting that the beloved holds life and death sway over him, the male lover is able to displace psychological responsibility for his affliction. As Shore's Wife complains in Drayton's poem, 'Shores Wife to King Edward the Fourth' (1597), men exaggerate both their physical malady and their mistress's perfection in order to 'lay the fault on beauty, and on us', a trick derived from 'Romes wanton Ovid'.[105]

Lovesickness, as well as being a corporeal illness, was also interpreted within a moral framework in early modern England: no longer governed by reason, lovesick individuals were enslaved by their passionate impulses. As Lawrence Babb observes, 'Because of the physical tortures which love inflicts, the mental aberrations which it causes, and the spiritual calamities which rise from it, the physicians and moralists of the Renaissance find it a matter for grave concern'; lovers act under an 'irresistible compulsion', which drives 'the most reasonable and most virtuous person into sin and calamity'.[106] Lust, often explicitly associated with lovesickness, is also depicted in terms of its animalistic effects and could equally tyrannize reason and enslave the individual. Nevertheless, lovesickness and lust should be treated as distinct passions, for although desire is an important constituent of lovesickness, sexual desire devoid of love is invested with a very different cultural meaning. Lust is associated neither with melancholy nor with introspective brooding, and individuals afflicted with lust are driven by the desire to dominate and subjugate another, rather than being prone to subjection, as is the case with lovesick individuals. Lust is thus associated with aggressive ambition in early modern literary texts, evident in the political valency often ascribed to rape in early modern literature, in which the lust of the governor is linked to the despotism of his government.[107] In Shakespeare's *Titus*

---

[104] Ford, *Love's Sacrifice*, II.iii.62, II.i.130–1.
[105] Drayton, 'Shores Wife to King Edward the Fourth', in Kerrigan (ed.), *Motives of Woe*, 102–3.
[106] Babb, 'Physiological Conception', 1024–5; 1034.
[107] See Levin, 'Lust Being Lord', 255–78.

Andronicus (1592), for example, Saturninus' initial seizing of Lavinia
to be his wife prefigures her later rape, and emphasizes the arbitrary
and barbaric nature of Saturninus' rule, and in Shakespeare's *The Rape
of Lucrece* Tarquin's indulgence in his passion goes hand in hand with
his abuse of political power.[108] And where lustful men are generally
depicted as tyrannous, lustful women are depicted as ambitious, as in
Beaumont and Fletcher's *The Maid's Tragedy* in which Evadne's sexual
desire for the King springs from his political position rather than his
person; as she tells her lover, 'I love with my ambition, | Not with my
eyes'.[109]

   As we have seen, lovesickness was represented in ways that seem contradictory in the early modern period. Lovesickness can be considered
a morally destructive and dangerous affliction, corrupting judgement,
polluting the body, and, at times, leading to the sufferer's death. In men
it is seen as dangerously emasculating. Given these pejorative associations, lovesickness would seem to be a wholly negative affliction with
destructive effects upon one's ethical being, gender identity, and body.
However, like melancholy, lovesickness was associated with a sensitive
disposition, and was thought to afflict the social and intellectual elite in
particular. Lovesickness could also have a positive ethical meaning due
to its association with Neoplatonism, which constructed amatory desire
as ideal, chaste, and spiritual, rather than disorderly and pathological.
That lovesickness could alternatively be depicted as either a shameful
illness or an ennobling fervour renders its ethical meaning paradoxical
at best. Furthermore, the humanist tradition—more concerned with
recovering ideas than challenging them—does not reconcile these conflicting notions but stresses that love can be either a debilitating illness

---

[108] Shakespeare, 'The Argument', in *Rape of Lucrece*, 238; Platt, 'Republic', 59–79;
Kuhl, 'Shakespeare's *Rape*', 352–60. Early modern poets could thus employ depictions
of lust as a way of critiquing despotic government, as in Wyatt's *A Paraphrase of the
Penitential Psalms* (*c*.1536), in which King David's desire for Barsabe prompts him to
exercise his royal power over Uriah to fatal effect, making him forget 'the wisdome
and fore-cast | (Wych wo to Remes when that thes kynges doth lakk)' (ll. 17–18). As
Greenblatt glosses, 'David's abuse of his political power—the monopoly of legitimate
force that enables him to send Uriah to his death—is the result of the sensual usurpation
of reason's power within him' (*Renaissance Self-Fashioning*, 126).
[109] Beaumont and Fletcher, *Maid's Tragedy*, ed. Craik, III.i.174–5; all references to
The Maid's Tragedy are from this edition. See also Brome, *Queen and Concubine*, 12.

or a state of ecstatic rapture (or even, at times, both).[110] The sense of lovesickness's complexity and variation is further increased when we turn our attention away from the dominant model of lovesickness (which by and large takes the male subject for granted), to female lovesickness, which, as well as embodying some of the same tensions within male melancholy, has its own unique set of problems, due to its relationship to other female disorders, such as green sickness, uterine fury, and the suffocation of the mother.

[110] Burton, *Anatomy*, iii.12.

2

'A Thirsty Womb': Lovesickness, Green Sickness, Hysteria, and Uterine Fury[1]

One of the aspects of women's lovesickness which has caused the most confusion is its relation to three other female maladies: hysteria (known in the early modern period as 'the suffocation of the mother', or just 'the mother'), green sickness, and uterine fury. Most critics tend to assume that lovesickness is a version of one or several of these illnesses, rather than a separate malady with its own physiological construction and cultural meaning. Laurinda Dixon, for example, sees female lovesickness as the exact equivalent of hysteria, defining it as 'an illness with a purely physical origin in the uterus'; alternatively, Ronald McFarland regards green sickness as the 'complementary feminine ailment' to men's erotic melancholy.[2] Ophelia is the focus of many of these discussions, in which her symptoms are read as a 'document in madness', typifying female erotic disorders and setting a model for stage representations that follow (IV.v.178).[3] Carol Neely maintains that Ophelia's 'restlessness, agitation, shifts of direction, "winks and nods and gestures" suggest the spasms of the mother', and Kaara L. Peterson calls her 'a textbook medical subject of hysterical illness'.[4] Such studies foster the idea that

[1] Marston, *Sophonisba* (1604–6), V.i.8.
[2] Dixon, *Perilous Chastity*, 109; McFarland, 'Rhetoric of Medicine', 252.
[3] Neely describes Ophelia in this manner in her essay 'Documents in Madness'. Showalter has shown how in later periods Ophelia is interpreted as suffering from hysteria, and many modern critics argue that this is indeed the malady she suffers from ('Representing Ophelia', 84–7). Along with Neely and Peterson, Rousseau and Camden both suggest that Ophelia is suffering from hysteria. See Rousseau, 'A Strange Pathology', 108; Camden, 'On Ophelia's Madness', 254–5.
[4] Shakespeare, *Hamlet*, IV.v.11; Neely, *Distracted Subjects*, 52; Peterson, 'Fluid Economies', 46.

'Desire in female virgins is understood as a pathology, in pointed contrast to the construction of desire in men as relatively chivalric and heroic'.[5] However, contrary to critical opinion, lovesickness, hysteria, green sickness, and uterine fury are understood as separate maladies in the early modern period, with their own unique set of symptoms, stereotypical sufferers, and cultural associations.

The failure to differentiate between the symptoms of discrete diseases in early modern texts, compounded by the tendency to regard Shakespeare's Ophelia as the embodiment of a single authoritative pattern of female illness, has obstructed a more elaborate critical investigation of the varied patterns of female sickness in late Tudor and early Stuart literature. This chapter disentangles maladies that are often conflated, whilst clarifying the points at which they overlap in order to establish a more accurate and detailed understanding of female sickness.[6] As literary texts make clear, despite the similarities in symptoms and cures, each disease holds a distinct place in the early modern imagination: green sickness emphasizes the dangers of virginity, intersecting with the *carpe diem* tradition; hysteria resembles the wild behaviour of those thought to be possessed; and uterine fury is similar to the modern concept of nymphomania. There is, however, an important caveat to lovesickness being established as a separate malady. When a woman's lovesickness develops into full-scale madness (as in the case of Shakespeare's Ophelia), her illness is frequently seen to be related to her menstrual cycle and is thus represented as being similar to uterine disorders. Those critics who argue that Ophelia's madness resembles uterine disorders are correct, but I dispute the idea that this is the pattern for *all* female lovesickness. For lovesickness, like melancholy, is a disease that can be manifested *either* as a destructive, bodily illness, *or* as an ennobling, intellectual affliction. The reasons for this are similar to those given in the Aristotelian 'Problem 30' (second century BCE), which explains how the same physiological substance

---

[5] Peterson, 'Fluid Economies', 42.

[6] My research is supported by a number of recent studies that have aimed to recapture the historically specific ways that maladies are constructed and envisaged. I have benefited enormously from a number of works; these include: Wack, *Lovesickness*; Gilman *et al.* (eds.), *Hysteria Beyond Freud*; King, 'Green Sickness' and *Disease of Virgins*; Ferrand, *Treatise*, trans. and ed. Beecher and Ciavolella; Neely, *Distracted Subjects*.

(melancholy) can have a diverse range of bodily affects according to both the quantity of the substance in the body and the unique physiological make-up of the sufferer. While a little melancholy (like a little wine) can improve the mind and senses, making a person witty and observant, too much will stupefy the sufferer.[7] The same is true of lovesickness, which can either enhance or overwhelm one's rational faculties.

The discourses surrounding green sickness, hysteria, and uterine fury suggest that women are dependent upon sex to maintain their physical and emotional health: women who refuse sex, or who have sex withheld from them, are depicted in literary accounts as either dying, or being driven mad by their sexual needs. While some critics valorize these maladies, suggesting that they provide women with an indirect means to express sexual desire,[8] uterine disorders also offer a rationale with which to coerce women into taking up roles as wives and mothers, indirectly implying that young women who are not married are in danger of becoming sick: whereas men can survive without women, women without men risk being driven to madness by their uncontrollable bodies.[9] When lovesickness is represented as a uterine affliction, it too is represented as pathological, irrational, and destructive. My study aims to give a sense of both forms of female lovesickness: in this chapter I focus on instances in which a woman's lovesickness resembles uterine disorders, and in Chapter 3 I focus on examples of lovesickness which are aligned with intellectual melancholy. I begin this chapter by outlining the medical constructions and literary representations of green sickness, hysteria, and uterine fury, before turning to a more detailed examination of Shakespeare's *Hamlet* (1600–1) and Shakespeare and Fletcher's *The Two Noble Kinsmen* (1613), two texts that associate lovesickness with uterine disorders and thus support the dominant critical model of gender and illness.[10]

---

[7] Aristotle, *Problem XXX, i*. There is considerable doubt as to whether the *Problems* is by Aristotle.

[8] Simon, *Mind and Madness*, 242.

[9] See King, who argues that the discourse surrounding green sickness supports 'ideas of women's innate weakness and proper roles' ('Green Sickness', 386). See also Maaskant-Kleibrink, 'Nymphomania', 286.

[10] For alternative models of female lovesickness see Ch. 3.

GREEN SICKNESS, THE DISEASE OF VIRGINS:
'A GAMESOME BEDFELLOW, BEING THE
SURE PHYSICIAN'[11]

Green sickness, also known as the white fever, the disease of virgins, and from the seventeenth century onwards chlorosis, was thought to be an exclusively female malady, which was caused by suppressed menses and seed (also called sperm, or *sperma*).[12] According to early modern theories, when the menstrual flow was obstructed an excess of blood and seed would collect within the body and eventually putrefy. Illness would ensue, either as a direct result of this blockage in the body, or from the noxious vapours emitted from the blood and seed; according to the anonymous *A Rational Account of the Natural Weaknesses of Women* (1716), 'when the Courses do not flow at all in Maids, and the Obstruction is of long standing, it is then called the Green-sickness'.[13] Women afflicted with this disorder are held to exhibit a variety of symptoms: they are pale or badly coloured, have puffy faces and bodies, and suffer from headaches, nausea, impaired respiration, heart palpitations, and a racing pulse. They also have strange appetites, either craving odd and unusual food (a symptom known as *pica*) or having no appetite whatsoever:

the Person becomes pale and dull, unwilling to stir about, and is afflicted with Loss of Appetite, loathing of Food, desire after things not fit to be eaten, bad Digestion, Pain in the stomach, which in some Patients is so violent by Fits, as hardly to be borne, Shortness of Breath, often swelling about the Ankles, sometimes vomiting, and universal Disorder.[14]

The absence of menstruation, however, remained the illness's defining symptom, as is evident in the casebooks of Richard Napier: women

---

[11] Fletcher [and Massinger], *Elder Brother*, in Beaumont and Fletcher, *Dramatic Works*, vol. ix, I.i.50–1.

[12] Although Johannes Lange claimed in 1554 that his description of the disease was derived from Hippocrates, there is no exact equivalent for the malady he describes in any classical texts, so that he appears to be the disease's inventor rather than its reviver. For a discussion of Lange, the origin of green sickness, and its representation in medical texts, literature, and art from the mid-sixteenth to the early twentieth centuries see King, 'Green Sickness', 372–87, and *Disease of Virgins*, 43–66.

[13] [Anon.], *Rational Account*, 4.   [14] Ibid. 3, 4.

who were labelled as 'green sick' but who subsequently menstruated were rediagnosed as having an 'obstruction of the spleen'.[15] Although a variety of remedies could be suggested (including phlebotomy, physical activity, a change of diet and various medicines), sexual intercourse was thought to be the most effective cure as it would open up the veins of the womb, releasing the trapped menses and seed. Young women who were believed to be green sick were thus advised to get married as soon as possible. As Helen King writes in her study of green sickness, 'the cure for the disease of virgins was to cease to be a virgin'.[16]

Contemporary theorists have sometimes tried to discover the 'real' malady behind green sickness. Clearly it has some affinity to what we now call premenstrual tension, and in later periods it is increasingly associated with anaemia and eating disorders. However, given the fact that the chief symptom of green sickness is the absence of menstruation, the condition that it most clearly resembles is pregnancy. In fact, it seems likely that, in certain circumstances, women disguised unwanted pregnancies as green sickness, an illness which simultaneously provided a justification for a speedy marriage.[17] Once married, the hidden pregnancy could then be 'discovered', retrospectively confirming the doctor's original diagnosis of green sickness; within this context, pregnancy would appear as the *cure* of the woman's puffiness, nausea, exhaustion, and disorderly appetites, rather than their *cause*. Alternatively, women who were pregnant, but who claimed to be green sick, could ask doctors for the means with which to provoke menstruation, seeking remedies which would in effect cause an abortion.

Of the three uterine disorders under discussion, green sickness is the malady most relevant to lovesickness. Like lovesickness, green sickness is associated with a young woman's emerging sexual appetites, emphasizing a woman's readiness for marriage and providing a rationale for her contrary, unsettled emotions. The discourse surrounding green sickness also provides an alternative, negative way in which to imagine a woman's virginity, countering Petrarchan and Neoplatonic traditions which grant virginity an elevated ethical and spiritual

---

[15] King, *Disease of Virgins,* 9; Sawyer, 'Patients, Healers, and Disease', 491 n. 41, quoted by King, 'Green Sickness', 374.

[16] King, *Disease of Virgins,* 80.

[17] For a literary example of this see Ford's *'Tis Pity,* in which Anabella's pregnancy is thought to be a case of green sickness, necessitating a speedy marriage (III.iv.8).

meaning.[18] As such, green sickness reinforces the misogynistic view that women are fundamentally incomplete without men, suggesting that a woman's virginity, rather than being the sign and source of her rational self-mastery, is an unnatural state prone to illness. Green sickness thus provides a physiological imperative for women to marry, suggesting that a woman must renounce her dangerous virginity for the health and fecundity of marriage.

Green sickness bears a certain affinity to lovesickness, and is increasingly associated with erotic melancholy in the early modern period. Called 'love fever' by the women of Brabant, it is linked explicitly to a lack of sexual activity, aggravated by strong sexual desire, and cured via coitus.[19] Moreover, green sickness and lovesickness share an aetiology (trapped seed), and green sickness is occasionally given an amatory origin.[20] Burton, for example, suggests that the physiological consequences of erotic melancholy can trigger an attack of green sickness: 'the Liver doth not performe his part, nor turnes the aliment into bloud as it ought', indirectly causing green sickness in women.[21] In addition, lovesickness, like green sickness, is sometimes represented as the inevitable consequence of puberty. Ferrand observes that 'young Girles, when they now begin to be ready for Marriage, are apt to fall into a kinde of Melancholy, or Madnesse', and Burton similarly links a young woman's sexual urges with her physical growth, suggesting that at 'fourteene yeares old, then they doe offer themselves, and some plainely rage ... many amongst us after they come into the teenes, doe not live without husbands, but linger'.[22] Such features allowed for a significant amount of overlap between the two maladies, upholding King's claim that 'for some girls, green sickness could be seen as a form of love sickness in which there is no specific love object'.[23]

Green sickness and lovesickness also have some key symptoms in common. Although the 'greenness' of the green-sick sufferer's

---

[18] Elizabeth famously used her virginity as a means of legitimating her sovereignty. See Marcus, 'Shakespeare's Comic Heroines'. For a discussion of Neoplatonic constructions of virginity and erotic desire see Ch. 4.

[19] King, *Disease of Virgins*, 36–42, 47.

[20] Trapped seed, which could cause green sickness, was also held to incite sexual desire; see Ch. 1.

[21] Burton, *Anatomy*, iii.139.

[22] Ferrand, *Erotomania*, 96; Burton, *Anatomy*, iii.54.

[23] King, *Disease of Virgins*, 40.

complexion could be interpreted in several different ways (from suggesting that the sufferer was actually green in colour, to her being 'ill-complexioned'), it was frequently taken to mean that the sufferer was pale, a typical symptom of lovesickness.[24] Lange certainly seems to understand it this way, suggesting that green sickness is called love fever 'since every lover is pale, and this colour is appropriate for a lover'.[25] In addition, the green sick sufferer's feverish pulse resembles the lover's pulse (which quickens at the sight or mention of the beloved), and her aversion to food corresponds to the lover's inability to eat. Finally, when green-sick women take their own lives, they are reputed either to hang or drown themselves, methods frequently associated with erotic melancholy.[26]

There are, however, important differences between green sickness and lovesickness. Although some writers suggest that green sickness can be triggered by excessive amorous desire (or any other extreme emotion), neither the existence of an erotic object nor sexual desire is necessary to engender the affliction. Instead green sickness occurs solely as the result of a bodily dysfunction. The beloved's function in the cure is likewise entirely physical: intercourse is necessary, not so much as a fulfilment of erotic desire, but because it will unblock the veins of the womb and allow the trapped blood and seed to be released. The specific identity of the lover is thus irrelevant: as long as he possesses a penis he can restore the sickly girl's body to its healthy state. Lovesickness, on the other hand, is wholly engendered by the erotic object, who inflames the body and possesses the mind. Sex is necessary, not only to purge the sufferer's body of excessive seed and malignant melancholy, but also to satisfy and dislodge his or her mental fixation.

Another important difference between green sickness and lovesickness is that, whereas lovesickness has its origin in both the body and the mind, green sickness is primarily a physiological disorder.[27] External factors which can aggravate the condition—such as excessive desire, a lack of exercise, or types of food—are always subordinate to the internal causes of the malady, namely the stopped menses and corrupted

---

[24] Vaughan, *Directions*, 113. King, *Disease of Virgins*, 36.
[25] Lange, *Medicinalium epistolarum miscellanea*, trans. and quoted by King, *Disease of Virgins*, 47.
[26] See e.g. Platter and Culpeper, *Histories*, 43.
[27] For the origins of lovesickness see Ch. 1.

seed which putrefy within. While it is impossible for an individual to become lovesick without the mental impression of an erotic object, the emotional and psychological disturbance associated with green sickness is a symptom, not a cause. Whereas lovesickness springs from frustrated desire, green sickness develops with the onset of sexual maturity. Where lovesickness warns of the dangers of amorous obsession, green sickness emphasizes the hazards of a particularly precarious time in life: puberty.

In literature, green sickness varies in its representation: it can be employed to depict virginity as sickly and unnatural, or it can be prettified as an alluring sign of both sexual ripeness and chastity. Regardless of its representation, however, the discourse surrounding green sickness suggests that women are dependent upon sex to maintain their physical and emotional health. Like the *carpe diem* tradition, which advises women 'gather ye Rose-buds while ye may', the discourse surrounding green sickness suggests that a woman's virginity is there to be lost; left too long, it can turn into a debilitating illness, damaging a woman's health as well as her looks.[28] While the majority of literary allusions to green sickness refer to the physical malady itself, there are a number of metaphoric references to green sickness within early modern discourse. On a number of occasions, green sickness is invoked in dedicatory verse as a means of disparaging bad poetry for its immaturity, or to criticize the reading public's desire to consume the 'trash' such poets produce.[29] In addition, early modern writers frequently focus on the *pica* of the green sick woman, describing her strange longings for substances such as ash, charcoal, or clay, or employing the malady metaphorically to describe any other inclination deemed to be abnormal.[30]

[28] Herrick, 'To the Virgins to Make Much of Time', in *Poetical Works*, 1.

[29] Good poets are represented as artistically virile, capable of satisfying the reader's intellectual appetite with wholesome poetry and implanting in them good verse. Bad poets, on the other hand, are depicted as artistically impotent: the poetic process is obstructed and the readers are left unsatisfied. A poet's wit can thus be described as green sick, or poets themselves can be likened to green-sick girls. See Collop, 'The Poet', in *Poesis Rediviva*, 1; Du Bartas, 'Indignis', in *Du Bartas*, 5; Elys, 'To his honest cousin, *E.E.* on his *Dia Poemata*', in *Dia Poemata*, sigs. [A6^v–A7^r]; Bell, 'To the Memory of Mr. William Cartwright', in Cartwright, *Comedies, Tragi-Comedies*, sig. [cii]; and [Cleveland], 'To P. Rupert', in *London-Diurnall*, [49].

[30] For the green sick woman's *pica* see Davenant, *Wits*, 17; and Scot, 'An Irish Banquet', in *Philomythie*, sig. M3^r. For its use as a metaphor for inclinations deemed to be abnormal see Cartwright, 'The Siedge', in *Comedies, Tragi-Comedies*, 155–6. Cleveland uses green sickness to deride a woman's taste for virtue and other intellectual pursuits ('The Antiplatonick', in *Poems with Additions*, 71).

The connotations attached to green sickness also facilitate its use as a metaphor for describing a variety of unripe and unready things, from young wines and spiritual sickness,[31] to descriptions of spring.[32] Because of this, men who are either effeminate or exceptionally chaste are also described as green sick. In Shakespeare's *Henry IV, Part 2* (1597–8), for example, Falstaff criticizes Prince John as having 'a kind of male green-sickness', implying that he is reserved and cold-natured compared with Hal, his brother; while in Fletcher and Massinger's *The Elder Brother* (*c*.1625), Andrew describes his master Charles as being 'tender, | And of a young girles constitution . . . Ready to get the greene sicknese'.[33] Similarly, in John Ford's *The Lover's Melancholy* (1629), after failing in her attempts at seduction, Kala mocks the disguised Eroclea, exclaiming, 'What a green-sickness-livered boy is this! | My maidenhead will shortly grow so stale | That 'twill be mouldy'.[34]

At times, metaphoric uses of green sickness suggest a fairly sophisticated understanding of the origin and symptoms of the disease. One of the most striking examples is found in Matthew Stevenson's poem 'A Visit', in which a chimney is compared to a green sick woman. Here, the speaker of the poem visits his neighbour's house to 'see what Hospitallity he kept' and finds

> his Chimnie like a Maiden
> In the green sicknesse, with her colour fading,
> Blushlesse, and bleath, only herein they sever:
> This a numme Palsie hath, and that a Feaver:
> Neighbour said I, your Chymnies to be let.[35]

Noting the fading colour of the fire, the speaker likens it to a 'blushlessse, and bleath' woman afflicted with green sickness, and cleverly aligns the cause of the fire's extinction to the origin of the disease: like the blocked-up body of the green sick woman which needs to be opened, the speaker suggests that the chimney needs to be 'let' so that it can burn freely.

---

[31] B[enlowes], *Theophilia*, 59. See also Du Bartas, 'Auto-Machia', in *Du Bartas*.
[32] Ford and Decker, *Sun's-Darling*, 11. See also 33.
[33] Shakespeare, *2 Henry IV* (1600), IV.ii.89–90; Fletcher [and Massinger], *Elder Brother*, in Beaumont and Fletcher, *Dramatic Works*, vol. ix, IV.ii.20–2.
[34] Ford, *Lover's Melancholy*, III.ii.17–9.
[35] Matthew Stevenson, 'A Visit', in *Occasions Off-Spring* (1654), 80–1.

The symptoms of green sickness reinforce wider cultural stereotypes about young, virginal women, who are frequently portrayed in early modern texts as having disorderly appetites, not only regarding food, but also in terms of their erotic impulses. Young women are subject to strong sexual urges, but are standoffish and peevish; their virginity makes them ill, but they stubbornly refuse to part from it. Thomas Campion's 'Faine would I wed', for example, focuses on the conflicted emotions of a young woman who would like to marry, but finds her own desires transitory:

> Faine would I wed a faire yong man that day and night could please mee,
> When my mind or body grieved, that had the powre to ease mee.
> Maids are full of longing thoughts that breed a bloudlesse sickenesse,
> And that, oft I heare men say, is onely cur'd by quicknesse.
> Oft have I beene woo'd and prai'd, but never could be moved:
> Many for a day or so I have most dearely loved,
> But this foolish mind of mine straight loaths the thing resolved;
> If to love be sinne in mee, that sinne is soone absolved.
> Sure, I thinke I shall at last flye to some holy Order;
> When I once am setled there, then can I flye no farther.
> Yet I would not dye a maid, because I had a mother:
> As I was by one brought forth, I would bring forth another.[36]

Although the young woman has loved a number of men for 'a day or so' and 'would not die a maid', her sexual appetite alternates between longing and loathing, so that her passion ends each time she reaches the point of consummation ('I have most dearly loved, | But this foolish mind of mine straight loathes the thing resolved'). Although green sickness is not explicitly referred to, the young woman's observation that 'Maids are full of longing thoughts that breed a bloodless sickness' suggests that she suffers from the disease of virgins (and is therefore bloodless because she does not menstruate). The woman must renounce her virginity if she is to achieve what is made to sound like her biological destiny ('As I was by one brought forth, I would bring forth another') and cure herself of an illness, which 'is only cured by quickness'—a phrase that suggests both sexual activity and the process of being made 'quick' or pregnant.

---

[36] Campion, [Faine would I wed] (1617), in *Works*, 1–12.

Green sickness furnished writers with a negative way in which to view virginity, allowing predominately male writers to denigrate overly chaste maidens as sickly or 'stale'.[37] Within this context, virginity is depicted not as a quality that elevates a woman, but one that makes her unnatural or diseased. In a number of instances, women who refuse to marry or to have sex are vilified as being green sick. In *Romeo and Juliet* (1597), for example, when Juliet rejects Paris's offer of marriage, her father cries, 'Out, you green-sickness carrion! Out you baggage | You tallow-face' (III.v.156–7); and in Shakespeare's *Pericles* (1609), Pander exclaims, 'Now, the pox upon her green-sickness for me!' when Marina refuses to become a prostitute (Scene xviii, l. 22). Similarly, in Henry Glapthorne's *The Ladies Priviledge* (1640) green sickness is thought to be a fit punishment for women who are excessively chaste. Frangipan, whose friend Doria will only be released from prison if a virgin claims him as her own, hopes that if the women refuse, they will be 'forc'd to keepe their maiden-heads | Till they be musty and not marchantable'; 'May the green-sicknesse raigne in their bloods,' he exclaims, 'and may they be debar'd of oate-meale, and clay-wall, and fall Ratsbauc'.[38] Like women, maidenheads are clearly imagined to have a brief shelf-life.

The discourse surrounding green sickness warns of the dangerous consequences of too rigid an adherence to chastity, fostering the notion that women need sex in order to remain in physical and psychological health.[39] In Shirley's *Changes: or Love in a Maze* (1632), for example, Master Goldsworth believes that the melancholy of Sir John Wood-homore's niece arises because she 'languish[es] for a husband', and thus warns him to 'Take heed o'th' greene disease'; and in Robert Green's *Mamillia* (1583), one young woman 'beeing at the age of twentie yeeres, would ... fall into the greene sicknes for want of a husband'.[40] Because of this, green sickness could be used as a means of compelling a woman to marry.[41] This is the case in Fletcher and Massinger's *The Elder Brother* (1637), although initially the play takes a critical stance towards green sickness, suggesting that young women's disorders may in fact arise from

---

[37] See, for instance, Aston Cokain's 'A Satyre', in *Small Poems*, 39.
[38] Glapthorne, *Ladies Priviledge*, sig. F1^r.
[39] See also Pecke, *Parnassi Puerperium*, 45; and Glapthorne, *Hollander*, sig. A4^v.
[40] Greene, *Mamillia*, ii. 36.   [41] Cokayn, *Trappolin*, 481.

their boredom and domestic confinement. The play opens with Lewis giving a lengthy speech to his daughter, Angellina, warning her about the pernicious effects of the indolent lifestyle common amongst young 'Virgins of wealthy families'.[42] Their lives, he suggests, are an endless cycle of sleeping and eating, 'Without variety or action', in which even the most mundane tasks, such as dressing, are performed by 'others hands' (I.i.22; 27). In the same way that Burton stresses that a lifestyle of leisure allows for the accumulation of noxious humours that could lead to illness, Fletcher identifies the lifestyle of upper-class women as the origin of their maladies:

> From this idlenesse
> Disease both in body and in minde
> Grow strong upon you; where a stirring nature
> With wholsome exercise guards both from danger:
> I'de have thee rise with the Sunne, walke, daunce, or hunt,
> Visite the groves and springs, and learne the vertues
> Of Plants and Simples: Doe this moderately,
> And thou shalt not with eating chalke, or coales,
> Leather and oatmeale, and such other trash,
> Fall into the greene sicknesse.
>
> (I.i.28–37)

Lewis prescribes both physical and mental activity to preserve his daughter's health: she should get up at dawn and exercise her mind with the study of 'Plants and Simples', activities which not only break up the dull monotony of life without activity, but also expel any noxious humours. Lewis's diagnosis, linking the sociological conditions of young, rich women to their distempers, seems remarkably astute, and is striking for its sympathetic and non-judgemental tone.[43]

However, Angellina's maidservant Sylvia has other ideas of how to safeguard her mistress' health, boasting that 'I could | Prescribe a remedy for my Ladies health, | And her delight too, farre transcending those | Your Lordship but now mention'd' (I.i.38–41). Her 'treatment' is:

---

[42] Fletcher [and Massinger], *Elder Brother*, in Beaumont and Fletcher, *Dramatic Works*, vol. ix, I.i.19; all quotations are taken from this edition.

[43] Compare with Scot, 'An Irish Banquet', in *Philomythie*, sig. M3[r]; and Manuche, *Loyal Lovers*, 10.

> A noble Husband; In that word,
> A noble Husband, all content of Woman
> Is wholly comprehended; He will rowse her,
> As you say, with the Sunne; and so pipe to her,
> As she will daunce, ne'er doubt it, and hunt with her,
> Upon occasion, untill both be weary;
> And then the knowledge of your Plants and Simples,
> As I take it, were superfluous; A loving,
> And but adde to it a gamesome Bedfellow,
> Being the sure Physician.

> (I.i.42–51)

Sylvia assumes that a husband will satisfy all of Angellina's mental and physical needs, rousing her every morning with amorous advances, which will render any intellectual activity 'superfluous'. Sylvia's remedy thus leaves the problem of the boredom and inactivity of upper-class women's lives unresolved, suggesting instead that women are solely driven by their sexual urges. She instructs Lewis, 'Shew no mercy | To a Maidenhead of fourteene, but off with't', warning him:

> fathers that deny
> Their Daughters lawfull pleasures, when ripe for them,
> In some kindes edge their appetites to tast of
> The fruit that is forbidden.

> (I.i.56–7; 58–61)

Lewis approves of Sylvia's suggestion. Marriage was, in fact, his intention for Angellina all along; his complaint about the indolent and monotonous life of upper-class women was merely an excuse to prompt her to a 'noble husband'. Even as Lewis seems to recognize (what feminists will later argue) that uterine disorders are 'caused by women's oppressive social roles rather than by their bodies or psyches', he nonetheless turns away from his insight, urging his daughter to become a wife and mother to avoid becoming ill.[44]

Lewis's derogatory reference to green sickness as a debilitating illness associated with inexperienced young women is the standard way in which the illness is viewed in the early modern period. There are,

---

[44] Showalter, 'Hysteria, Feminism, and Gender', 287.

however, some exceptions. Edward Herbert of Cherbury and Thomas Carew write poems that prettify the malady, depicting it as an erotic innocence that guarantees the woman's sexual purity.[45] Their poems portray green sickness as a state of sexual ripeness, which enhances the woman's ethical status as well as her physical allure.[46] Conventions about the Petrarchan mistress are given an oddly physiological basis, as the woman's stereotypical pale skin and chilly chastity result from her somatic disorder. Herbert writes two poems, both entitled 'The Green-Sickness Beauty'. In the first of these, 'From thy pale look, while angry Love doth seem', Herbert compares his mistress to a statue, insisting that a rosy glow conveying sexual satisfaction would mar her pale perfection ('As then in vain | One should flesh-colouring to Statues add'), and simultaneously throw her sexual scruples into question, as one 'gilding Silver Coin, | Gave but occasion to suspect it more'. Green sickness thus becomes 'an emblem of your mind', offering physical proof of the woman's mental and physical chastity.[47] Far from portraying the green-sick woman as sexually predatory or dysfunctional, green sickness marks the moment of a woman's sexual maturity, charging it with a tantalizing, unthreatening eroticism.

Herbert's second poem, also entitled 'The Green-Sickness Beauty', opens with a description of the beloved's pale face, dim eyes, wandering mind, and short breath, afflictions that only serve to make her unful-filled sexual promise all the more alluring; it is 'as a budding Rose, when first 'tis blown, | Smells sweeter far, then when it is more spread'.[48] Translating sexual sickness into erotic ripeness, Herbert praises her 'green and flourishing estate', in which her 'Virgin leaves' are allowed to grow. Nevertheless, despite this praise, Herbert suggests that she must eventually renounce her sickness for health:

---

[45] See Carew, 'On Mistres N. to the Greene Sicknesse' and 'To Mris Katherine Nevill on her Greene Sickness', in *Poems*, 113, 129.

[46] Dubrow reads Herbert and Carew's poems on green sickness as being part of the 'ugly beauty' tradition (*Echoes of Desire*, 170–97).

[47] Herbert, 'The Green-Sickness Beauty' [From thy pale look, while angry Love doth seem], in *Occasional Verses* (1665), 69; all references to Herbert are taken from this edition. My readings of these poems are indebted to McFarland's 'Rhetoric of Medicine', 250–8.

[48] Herbert, 'The Green-Sickness Beauty' ('Though the pale white within your cheeks compos'd'), 67.

> So, if you want that blood which must succeed,
> And give at last a tincture to your skin,
> It is, because neither in outward deed,
> Nor inward thought, you yet admit that sin
> For which your Cheeks a guilty blush should need.

(p. 68)

Herbert gently puns about his mistress's 'want of blood', conflating her pale cheeks with her virginal state. The sin she will not admit is clearly sexual intercourse, and the poet generously implies that he will do what he can to restore her 'health': his emphasis on her 'want of blood' not only refers to the lack of menstruation associated with green sickness, but also suggests that she 'wants'—that she requires and secretly desires—the blood which she will receive from his orgasm. Just as sexual intercourse will send a guilty blush to the maiden's cheeks and incite the menstrual flow to resume, so will it provide her with the refined blood in the form of sperm. The poet thus depicts a mistress who is at once sexually needy and ready, but who is simultaneously chaste and unthreatening. Moreover, the young woman's malady justifies the poet's attempt at seduction as it is 'for her own good': Herbert ends his poem with an injunction to 'be gather'd rather than to fall', offering his mistress what Ronald E. McFarland has termed a 'therapeutic seduction'.[49] If green sickness reveals the peak of a woman's sexual development, it also warns how quickly this ripeness will transform into rottenness if the sick virgin will not submit herself to her lover's cure.

HYSTERIA, OR THE SUFFOCATION OF THE MOTHER

Hysteria, also known as the suffocation of the mother, or just 'the mother', was thought to be primarily a woman's malady in which 'the mother' signifies the womb.[50] There were a number of different possible explanations as to what triggered hysteria, which corresponded to different medical traditions available to early modern writers. These

---

[49] Herbert, 'The Green-Sickness Beauty', 68; McFarland, 'Rhetoric of Medicine', 258. See also Brathwait, 'An Age for Apes', in *Honest Ghost*, 150.
[50] Jorden, *Briefe Discourse*, fo. 5^r.

include: movement in the womb, pressing upon or obstructing other organs; vapours arising from the womb which disturbed the body and mind; or organs acting in sympathy with the womb.[51] Helen King, who traces the shifts in, and dissemination of, medico-philosophical constructions of hysteria in ancient and medieval medicine, writes:

In the Hippocratic texts a dry, hot, and light womb rises in search of moisture; Soranus believes that the anchoring membranes prevent any movement, while for Aretaeus, although the womb moves it is pulled back by its membranes, thus affecting the higher part of the body only through sympathy. In Galen the problem is a womb filled with retained seeds or menses, rotting to produce coldness. In Arabic medicine a Hippocratic mobile womb becomes a mobile womb with Galenic contents, and vapors as well as sympathy explain its effects on the higher parts. In the Latin West the focus on Soranus had been combined with acceptance of womb movement.[52]

The malady could also be triggered by the failure to discharge menstrual blood or seed, a factor that led some physicians to see green sickness and hysteria as closely related.[53] Robert Pierce, for example, writes that green sickness 'is many times joyn'd [with] the *Hysterick Passion*, or *Fits of the Mother*', noting how the 16-year-old Mrs Elizabeth Eyles, who was afflicted with green sickness, developed 'Mother-fits withal'.[54] In addition, external factors (such as a lack of exercise or diet) and emotional disturbances, or the 'perturbations of the minde' (such as extreme jealousy, love, or anger), could also incite a physiological imbalance that could trigger hysteria.[55] Although it is impossible to know the extent to which this textual preoccupation regarding hysteria reflects a wider tendency amongst doctors to diagnose their female patients as hysteric, Katherine Williams's study of seventeenth-century case records and unpublished manuscripts demonstrates that hysteria was not simply a theoretical condition, but a widely recognized category of illness.[56]

Women afflicted with hysteria are said to suffer from impaired respiration, loss of speech, incoherence, delusions, and a lack of sensation

---

[51] For changes in the medical construction of hysteria see Boss, 'Transformation', 221–34.

[52] King, 'Once Upon a Text', 55. For a fuller discussion of the history of hysteria see Veith, *Hysteria: The History*; and Micale, *Approaching Hysteria*.

[53] Jorden, *Briefe Discourse*, fos. 17ᵛ [19ᵛ], 20ʳ; Hart, *Klinike*, 328.

[54] Pierce, *Bath Memoirs* (1697), 189 [188].

[55] Jorden, *Briefe Discourse*, 22ᵛ.   [56] Williams, 'Case Records', 383–401.

in the limbs; Edward Jorden in *A Briefe Discourse of a Disease called the Suffocation of the* Mother (1603) locates the inability to speak as the reason why the malady is referred to as the suffocation of the mother, as 'most commonly it takes them with choaking in the throat', and suggests that this is caused by the womb pressing against the diaphragm and stomach.[57] Frequently, individuals suffering from hysteria are described as moving in a violent and uncontrolled manner, causing injury to anyone who comes to their aid; for example, one 'Essex Gentlewoman of good note' suffered from 'such violent convulsions, as five or six strong men could scarce hold her down'.[58] In this respect, hysterical women are strikingly different from those afflicted with green sickness: whereas green sick sufferers are weak and submissive, hysterical women are typically violent and aggressive, exhibiting dramatic symptoms that call for physical restraint. In its most extreme form, hysterical women fall into unconscious swoons, in which they 'fetch no breath, but ly like dead people'.[59] Because of this, doctors devised methods to determine whether the individual was actually dead (such as holding a feather or glass in front of a woman's mouth to determine if she still breathed), and advised that a period of time be observed before the hysterical individual be buried.

Cures for hysteria include applying scented oils to women's sexual organs to release the pent-up seed and menses, and using scents to coax the womb back into its accustomed place, a remedy founded on the belief that the womb was sensitive to different odours.[60] In this therapy, sweet smells were held between the woman's legs and foul smells held at her nose as a means of enticing the womb back to its proper position.[61] As in the case of green sickness, sexual intercourse was also recommended as a cure, as it was thought both to moisten the womb and to open up its veins (enabling the corrupted seed and menses to be released). Jorden suggests that sexual intercourse is a fundamental ingredient in a woman's physical health, not because it fulfils her desires, but rather because it expels the malignant humours which gather around the womb:

---

[57] Jorden, *Briefe Discourse*, fo. 5^r; Sadler, *Private Looking-Glasse*, 61.
[58] Jorden, *Briefe Discourse,* fo. 17^r.
[59] Platter, Cole, and Culpeper, *Golden Practice* (1662), 126.   [60] Ibid. 127.
[61] Ibid. Jorden, *Briefe Discourse*, fo. 16^v [23^v]; Beier, *Sufferers and Healers*, 126.

the want of the benefit of marriage in such as have beene accustomed or are apt thereunto, breeds a congestion of humours about that part, which increasing or corruption in the place, causeth this disease. And therefore we do observe that maidens and widdowes are most subiect thereunto.[62]

Bennett Simon argues that hysterical fits could function as an indirect means for women to express erotic desire and acquire a husband, and there are some examples from literature that corroborate this view.[63] However, as in green sickness, the discourse surrounding hysteria also functioned as a means of coercing women into their social roles as wives and mothers, suggesting that young women who remained unmarried were in danger of becoming sick; Felix Platter, for one, offers an example of how a woman's refusal to marry led to her having an hysterical attack.[64]

Hysteria bears some similarity to erotic melancholy, with which it shares an aetiology (retained seed) and a cure (sexual intercourse). Like both lovers and green-sick girls, women afflicted by the suffocation of the mother could be described as 'wan and pale', and like green sickness, hysteria could be induced by psychological distress, including the pain of unfulfilled desire.[65] Nonetheless, hysteria was not as closely linked to lovesickness as green sickness, and was more frequently seen as a purely physical ailment, rather than one with an emotional origin. Indeed, Katherine Williams demonstrates how hysteria was rarely linked to frustrated love, and was instead persistently associated with 'organic pathology' (including fevers, painful white menses, tumours, and symptoms that suggest arthritis), so that 'many cases of hysteria were probably the misdiagnosis of organic diseases'.[66] In addition, when hysteria is associated with an emotion in early modern literary texts, it is more frequently anger than amorous longing. The violent and dramatic symptoms of hysteria, which overwhelm the sufferer, bear little resemblance either to the wistful introspection of the melancholic in

---

[62] Jorden, *Briefe Discourse,* fo. 22ᵛ.

[63] Simon, *Mind and Madness,* 242. See also Rousseau, 'A Strange Pathology', 134.

[64] Platter and Culpeper, *Histories,* 107.

[65] Although Jorden describes one instance in which a woman 'upon love fell into this disease', he also mentions a number of other cases of hysteria that were caused by jealousy, anger, and fear. Jorden, *Briefe Discourse,* 16ʳ; See also Guillemeau, *Child-Birth,* 235.

[66] Williams, 'Case Records', 401. Hysteria has also been linked with epilepsy. See Addyman, 'The Character of Hysteria', 28.

love, or the lyrical sexuality of a woman gone mad. Instead the hysteric's swoons, unnatural strength, and wild movement resemble the wild behaviour of the demonically possessed. It is perhaps the importance of hysteria in latter periods, and the tendency to conflate green sickness and hysteria, which has led critics to see hysteria as associated with lovesickness.

Hysteria had an affiliation with witchcraft in early modern society, and ultimately 'played a major role . . . in the demystification of witchcraft'.[67] In his ironically titled *Discoverie of Witchcraft* (1584), Reginand Scot argues that women who believe they have supernatural powers are actually suffering from melancholy or hysteria, and in the trial of Elizabeth Jackson in 1602, Edward Jorden posited hysteria as an alternate explanation for possession, suggesting the correlation between these two phenomena.[68] During the trial, Elizabeth Jackson, an old woman, was charged with having bewitched Mary Glover, a 14-year-old girl who had fallen into fits. Glover was reported to be periodically blind, speechless, and numb: 'her neck and throat did swell extremely . . . depriving her of speeche'; her left 'hand, arme and whole side, were deprived of feeling and moving'; and 'her belly was swelled and shewed in it, and in the brest, certaine movings'.[69] The dispute centred on whether Glover was suffering from demonic possession or a physical affliction. Edward Jorden, who was sent to study Jackson's case, argued that Glover was experiencing the suffocation of the mother, and suggested that her affliction should not be imputed to the Devil, but rather was the consequence of illness.

Critics such as Veith have hailed this trial as a landmark of scientific progress in which superstitious ideas about witchcraft met the sceptical gaze of scientific reason. However, it is important not to exaggerate Elizabeth Jackson's trial as a scientific watershed. First, despite Jorden's testimony, Jackson was found guilty: Glover was judged to be possessed. Secondly, despite Jorden's emphasis upon psychological counsel and verbal therapy, his suggestions for curing Glover are fundamentally orthodox: Jorden advises, 'In the fit let the bodies bee kept upright, straight laced, and the belly & throat held downe with ones

---

[67] Rousseau, 'A Strange Pathology', 97.
[68] MacDonald, 'Introduction', in *Witchcraft*, ed. MacDonald, pp. xxvi–xxxi; Porter, 'Body and the Mind', 232.
[69] Bradwell, *Mary Glover*, 4–5.

hand ... apply evil smels to their nostrils, and sweet smels beneath tie their legs hard with a garter for revulsion sake'.[70] Thirdly, Veith's reading fails to take into account the political motivation behind Jorden's book. As Michael MacDonald demonstrates, the book, commissioned by the Bishop of London, Richard Bancroft, functioned as a 'work of religious propaganda' in order to provide 'scientific arguments for disputing the validity of cases of possession, witchcraft and dispossession that both Catholics and Puritans were exploiting to win public approval and make converts'.[71] Roy Porter has pointed out that Veith's desire to regard Jorden as a hero of the medical profession reflects her larger historical narrative that regards medical history as 'a progression from superstition to science, ignorance to expertise, prejudice to psychoanalysis'.[72]

Although Veith is right to recognize the similarity between symptoms of hysteria and the signs of possession, her belief that many of the witches and their victims described in the *Malleus Maleficarum* (1494) 'were simply hysterics' is also reductive, ignoring the complex social, theological, and intellectual issues which informed the early modern construction of witchcraft.[73] Nor is it true to say that in the early modern period 'hysteria ... was viewed as a sign of possession by the devil'.[74] The point of Jorden's pamphlet is that Glover was *not* seen by others as suffering from hysteria; instead, the suffocation of the mother is introduced as an alternative means of explaining Glover's odd and violent behaviour, and therefore founded on the assumption that the two conditions are discrete and mutually exclusive. Jorden is thus not reclaiming hysteria as a medical disorder, but rather reinterpreting possession as hysteria; his pamphlet (following Scot's *Discoverie of Witchcraft*) uses medical explanations to discredit behaviour held to have a supernatural origin, marking another instance of the disease's entry into the discourse of witchcraft, rather than pinpointing the moment of its transformation into an organic pathology.

Although there are fewer references to hysteria in early modern literature than there are allusions to green sickness, those instances in which the disease is mentioned suggest that early modern writers were familiar

---

[70] Edward Jorden, *Briefe Discourse*, fos. 16ᵛ [23ᵛ].
[71] MacDonald, 'Introduction', in *Witchcraft*, pp. viii–ix.
[72] Porter, 'Body and the Mind', 232.
[73] Veith, *Hysteria: The History*, 61.   [74] Micale, *Approaching Hysteria*, 20.

with its causes and symptoms.[75] In *Poly-Olbion* (1612–22), for example, Michael Drayton employs hysteria metaphorically, comparing a raging river to a fit of the mother:

> As when we haplie see a sicklie woman fall
> Into a fit of that which wee the Mother call,
> When from the grieved wombe shee feeles the paine arise,
> Breakes into grievous sighes, with intermixed cries,
> Bereaved of her sense; and strugling still with those
> That gainst her rising paine their utmost strength oppose,
> Starts, tosses, tumbles, strikes, turnes, touses, spurnes and spraules,
> Casting with furious lims her holders to the walles;
> But that the horrid pangs torments the grieved so,
> One well might muse from whence this suddaine strength should grow.[76]

Unlike the pale, passive green-sick sufferer, the hysterical woman is violent and physically powerful, more in need of physical restraint than sexual fulfilment. Rather than enhancing her attractiveness, the symptoms of hysteria render the woman frightening and out of control.[77]

Hysteria is frequently represented as the physiological consequence of an excessive passion, in which the violent emotions that disturb the body incite a hysterical attack.[78] Indeed, the most famous example of hysteria in early modern literature represents it in this way. In Shakespeare's *King Lear*, Lear articulates his loss of emotional control by appropriating the symptoms and discourse of hysteria; 'O, how this mother swells up toward my heart!' he cries, '*Histerica passio* down, thou climbing sorrow; | Thy element's below'.[79] Perhaps the earliest instance of a man being described as hysteric, Lear's articulation of his hysterical pains demands a momentary appropriation of the female body, offering

---

[75] See e.g. B[astard], 'Epigram 35', in *Chrestoleros*, 73–4. For the use of the mother in puns see W[roth], *Idle Houre*, 20; Webster, *The Duchess of Malfi*, II.i.108–9, and his *The Devil's Law-Case*, in *Complete Works*, III.iii.258–9. The womb's sensitivity to strong scents is invoked humorously by Mayne (*Citye Match*, 39).

[76] Drayton, *Poly-Olbion*, 102.

[77] Because of the violent symptoms associated with hysteria, the malady could be used as an excuse for any odd or otherwise inexplicable behaviour. See e.g. Part 2 of Dekker's *The Honest Whore* (1630), in which Candido comically attempts to excuse his new wife's violent outburst by telling the assembled company that it is a result of 'the disease called the mother' (p. 133).

[78] See e.g. [Mabbe], *Spanish Bawd*, 88.

[79] Shakespeare, *King Lear* (1623), II.ii.231–3.

physiological proof of the intensity of his feelings.[80] As Janet Adelman argues, 'Suffocated by emotions that he thinks of as female, Lear gives them the name of the woman's part as though he himself bore that diseased and wandering organ within.'[81] As in the case of Lear, it is anger and frustration, rather than love, which most frequently is seen to trigger a hysterical attack. In Part 1 of Thomas Dekker's *The Honest Whore* (1604), for example, Bellafront asks her servant to cut the laces of her dress, asserting that she is 'so vext' that she 'shall ha the mother presently'.[82] And in Thomas Nashe's *The Unfortunate Traveller* (1594) the Countess's hysterical fit is brought on by her anger when she discovers that her prisoner, Jack Wilton, has escaped. Nashe describes her fury with comic exaggeration; she

fared like a franticke Bacchinall, she stampt, she star'd, shee beate her head against the walls, scratcht her face, bit her fingers, and strewd all the chamber with her haire . . . After her furie had reasonably spent it selfe, her breast began to swell with the mother, caused by her former fretting and chafing.[83]

The Countess's enraged behaviour both resembles the symptoms of someone experiencing the suffocation of the mother while simultaneously engendering her physical breakdown; she both causes and 'deserves' her hysterical fit.

Women are sometimes depicted as feigning the suffocation of the mother in order to manipulate others, a representation which corresponds with more recent stereotypes of the hysterical sufferer as histrionic and calculating. In Nicholas Breton's *Grimellos Fortunes* (1604), for example, Grimello tells how a farmer's wife, who has turned her husband's prized giant eel into a pie, simulates a hysterical fit in order

---

[80] Lear's attack suggests a shift in the construction of the malady from an exclusively female illness to one which includes men. Boss argues that while early constructions of the suffocation of the mother were attributed to the womb, after 1600 hysterical afflictions were also linked to hypochondria (the affliction in which the spleen was thought to give off vapours), and to melancholy. Such an interpretation seems affirmed by Harsnett who notes that Richard Maynie 'had a spice of the *Hysterica passio*, as seems from his youth, he himself terms it the Moother', believing it to be a disorder that arose from 'wind in the bottome of the belly'. Nevertheless, hysteria remained a predominantly female affliction. For Maynie's hysteria see Muir, 'Harsnett', 14. For changes in the physiological construction of hysteria see Boss, 'Transformation', 221–34. For Lear as an early example of a male hysteric, see Brain, 'Concept of Hysteria', 321.

[81] Adelman, *Suffocating Mothers*, 114. See also Addyman, 'The Character of Hysteria'.

[82] Dekker, *Honest Whore* I, l. 37.

[83] Nashe, *Unfortunate Traveller*, sig. [N4^r].

to avoid his anger: 'ready to burst with laughing, and yet keeping it in with a fayned sigh', she 'sits downe in a chaire, and hangs the head, as though she had had the mother'.[84] And in Thomas Dekker's *North-ward Hoe* (1607) Kate feigns a fit of the mother in order to get rid of her husband, Greeneshields. She tells Fetherstone, her lover, that such tactics are common amongst experienced wives, who 'can be sick when they have no stomack to lie with their husbands'.[85]

At times hysteria is represented as the only socially tolerated means for a woman to express her passion, corroborating Bennett Simon's claim that hysteria provided 'a socially acceptable means of expressing suppressed desire and protest against social oppression'.[86] In Thomas Tomkis's *Albumazar* (1615), Flavia suggests that women are forced to disguise their passions as physical afflictions:

Alas, our Sex is most wretched, nurst up from infancie in continuall slavery. No sooner able to pray for our selves, but they brayle and hudde us so with sowre awe of Parents, that wee dare not offer to bate at our owne desires. And whereas it becomes men to vent their amorous passions at their pleasure; wee poore soules must take up our affections in the ashes of a burnt heart, not daring to sigh without excuse of the spleene, or fit of the mother.[87]

According to Flavia, there is no difference in the passions that men and women feel, only in the extent to which they are allowed to express their feelings publicly. It is not that women's passions are bodily rather than intellectual, but that women are constrained to represent their emotions as physical afflictions.

UTERINE FURY

Lack of attention to green sickness and hysteria represents a threat to the woman; if the conditions that engender these illnesses are allowed to continue and worsen, they can lead to a condition called uterine fury, also known as *furor uterinus* or 'a fury in the womb'. Ferrand suggests

---

[84] Breton, 'Grimellos Fortunes' (1604), repr. in *Two Pamphlets*, 56–7.
[85] Dekker and Webster, *North-ward Hoe*, sig. E^v.
[86] Simon, *Mind and Madness*, 250.   [87] Tomkis, *Albumazar*, sigs. D3^v–D4.

that the disorder arises either from a problem of temperature in the womb, or from vapours which emanate from corrupted seed:

qui est Desipiscentia Furiosa, proveniens ab extremo Ardore Matricis, sive Intemperaturâ calidâ, cerebro, reliquisq*ue* corporis partibus per spinam dorsi communicatâ, vel per acres Humores emissos à semine corrupto, circa Matricem putrescente.

it is a raging or madness that comes from an excessive burning desire in the womb, or from a hot intemperature communicated to the brain and to the rest of the body through the channels in the spine, or from the biting vapors arising from the corrupted seed lying stagnant around the uterus.[88]

Similar to nymphomania (the condition it eventually becomes) and sexual overexcitation, individuals suffering from this malady lose their minds entirely, and are easily spotted because of their outrageous words and behaviour.[89] Driven mad by their voracious wombs and overwhelming libidinous appetites, 'Mulieres garriunt indesinenter, & nihil aliud vel loquuntur, vel audire cupiunt, quàm Res Venereas' ['such women chatter incessantly and speak about, or like to hear about, sexual matters'].[90] Ambroise Paré links the illness to a choleric disposition and describes how the malady causes women to 'speak all things that are to bee concealed'.[91] Galen believed that the disease was particularly rife among young widows, whose lack of sexual activity brought on the disease. In a similar vein, Felix Platter describes how a newly married woman became sick with 'a grevous fury in the womb' after her husband

[88] Ferrand, *Erotomania*, 95; Ferrand, *Treatise*, trans. Beecher and Ciavolella, 263. Ferrard adds this section to the 1623 edition of *Erotomania*, suggesting that the condition belongs under the general heading of erotic melancholy. However, although 'Ferrard was attempting to extend the range of this thesis by subsuming as many related conditions as possible . . . such diseases [uterine fury and satyriasis] have little to do with passions of the soul provoked by powerful erotic desires fixed upon an object of beauty'. See Ferrand, *Treatise*, 431 n. 1.

[89] For the transformation of the condition in the eighteenth-century see Rousseau, 'Erotic Sensibility', 95–119. See also Groneman, who argues that nymphomania 'embodies the fantasies and fears, the anxieties and dangers connected to female sexuality': *Nymphomania: A History*, 8.

[90] Ferrand, *Erotomania*, 95; Ferrand *Treatise*, trans. Beecher and Ciavolella, 263.

[91] Paré, *Workes of the Famous Chirugion*, 632–3. Quoted by Veith, *Hysteria: The History*, 114.

fell ill. The man eventually died without the couple consummating the relationship, rendering the woman:

a widow and a maid, for he was sick as soon as married; she presently after his death fell into such a fit of madness and lust, that she would not only by words and actions desire to couple with such as came to her to see her, but when they denied her, she would call for the English Mastives to be brought to her to do it with a loud voice. Her Parents hearing those horrid expressions, were very sad, and wondered how from being so chast and godly, she should turn such, and detestable, and she died mad in the same condition.[92]

In *Erotomania*, Ferrand argues that uterine fury is a species of love melancholy, and descriptions of women grown mad from love closely resemble those of uterine fury; as Burton writes, 'Love and *Bacchus* are so violent Gods, so furiously rage in our minds, that they make us forget all honesty, shame and common civility'.[93] Platter records how 'a noble Virgin, that should have been married to a noble Man, that was hindered and kept from her by his friends, she fell mad, and spake and did many beastly and rude words and things, and so died.[94] And Daniel Oxenbridge, who practiced medicine between 1620 and 1640, described one Goodwife Jackson, aged 39, who 'ran up and down the Streets, bare footed, Cloaths torn, Hair loose, was ready to lye down and pull up her Cloaths to every one, pretended Love to one Mr Holland her Master'.[95]

If literary references are anything to go by, uterine fury was the least well known of the uterine disorders. Nonetheless, the behaviour of those suffering from the disease bears a striking similarity to women whose lovesickness has developed into full-scale madness. And in literature, women are occasionally driven mad by their needy wombs, so that sexual desire is depicted as a product of the womb itself.[96] In Brome's *The Antipodes* (1640), for example, Martha becomes mad when Perigrine, her husband, fails to consummate their marriage due to the fact that he is also mad (Perigrine has read too many travel books and is obsessed with going abroad). Like the woman described by Felix Platter who

[92] Platter and Culpeper, *Histories*, 47–8.   [93] Burton, *Anatomy*, iii.197.

[94] Platter and Culpeper, *Histories*, 47.

[95] Oxenbridge, *General Observations*, quoted by Hunter and Macalpine, *Three Hundred Years of Psychiatry*, 123.

[96] See e.g. Marston's *Sophonisba*, in which Ericho, the witch, represents her desire for Syphax as the product of her 'thirsty womb' (V.i.8).

suffers from 'a grevous fury in the womb', Martha is therefore both a wife and virgin. Joyless describes his daughter-in-law:

> she's full of passion, which she utters
> By the effects, as diversely, as several
> Objects reflect upon her wand'ring fancy:
> Sometimes in extreme weepings, and anon
> In vehement laughter; now in sullen silence,
> And presently in loudest exclamations.[97]

Martha is totally overcome by her bodily needs, which are represented as originating in her womb; she talks incessantly about having a child, and even asks her friend Barbara about the possibility of lesbian sex. Barbara sees Martha's madness as a product of sexual frustration:

> To keepe a maidenhead three yeares after marriage
> Under wed-lock and key! Insufferable! Monstrous!
> It turnes into a wolf within the flesh,
> Not to be fed with chickens and tame pigeons.
>
> (I.i.103–6)

Brome describes Martha's womb as an animal with a life of its own, capable of engendering voracious sexual appetites which need to be fed with something more than 'chickens' and 'pigeons'.[98] Given this description, it is perhaps unsurprising that Perigrine is terrified to consummate his marriage. As if responding to the characterization of women's bodies as hungry animals, he asks if he can 'hire…Another man to couple with this bride | To cleare the dangerous passage of a maidenhead' (IV.i.464–5). Sexual intercourse, he worries, might be fatal: 'She may be of that serpentine generation' he observes anxiously, 'That stings oft-times to death' (IV.i.467–8). In the end, Perigrine is cured by Dr Hughball, who satisfies Perigrine's obsession with travel 'by degrees' by making him believe that he has visited all of the places he imagines (V.ii.278). Brome thus offers, as Mathew Steggle suggests, 'a theory of drama almost as therapy as opposed to a site of infection'; Perigrine's mental

---

[97] Brome, *Antipodes*, I.i.160–5.
[98] Martha's behaviour in some ways fits into earlier models of nymphomania, in which the woman becomes 'a half-conscious, animal-like being'. See Maaskant-Kleibrink, 'Nymphomania', 286.

fixation is satisfied through the very theatrical illusion that is the play.[99] However, while Perigrine requires an imaginative engagement with his fantasies and needs, the same cannot be said for Martha, who requires not psychological satisfaction but the physical act of sex to restore her to health. The difference in the couples' illnesses thus conforms to the common critical paradigm of gender and illness, which sees men's distempers as mental and women's as physical: while Perigrine goes mad from an intellectual fascination with foreign places, Martha's sickness arises from her virginity and sexual frustration.

SHAKESPEARE'S OPHELIA

Ophelia's madness occupies a pre-eminent position in modern criticism, and is frequently regarded as the embodiment of a single authoritative pattern of female lovesickness in the Renaissance. In such readings, Hamlet is seen as the archetypal male melancholic and Ophelia is seen to be the paradigm of female disorders: whereas men's illnesses are constructed as cerebral, philosophical, and creative, female illnesses are seen as passionate, sexual, and destructive. Not simply melancholic, her unchecked sorrow has developed into full-scale insanity.[100] Such madness engenders a loss of reason, allowing passion, once unchecked, to become dominant, and intensifying sexual desires. Ophelia's disordered mind is reflected in her unkempt dress, and her sensuality is suggested by her loose hair, an offence against decorum.[101] In fact, each aspect of Ophelia's madness can be unpacked to uncover the social and literary clichés attached to the figure of the abandoned, lovesick woman: the flowers and herbs she enumerates associate her suffering with traditions of mourning; the bawdy songs emphasize her heightened sexuality; and the willow makes her lovesickness explicit. Rejected by Hamlet and in mourning for her father, her madness is eroticized and 'interpreted as something specifically feminine', and eventually she is drawn to the water where she drowns.[102]

---

[99] Steggle, *Brome*, 115. For a discussion of this type of cure in relation to lovesickness see Ch. 5.

[100] As Burton writes, 'For if this passion continue . . . *it makes the blood hot, thicke and blacke; and if the inflammation get into the braine, with continuall meditation and waking, it so dries it up, that madnesse followes*'. Burton, *Anatomy*, iii.198.

[101] Charney and Charney, 'Language of Madwomen', 453.   [102] Ibid. 451.

Ophelia's madness confirms that sometimes female lovesickness is represented as a disorder of the womb: her lovesickness is depicted as a sexual affliction, related to her virginal state, and associated with both her sexual 'ripeness' and the fecundity of nature. However, unlike in *The Two Noble Kinsmen*, in which the Jailer's Daughter's malady is explicitly linked to her menstrual cycle, in *Hamlet* the association between Ophelia's madness and womb disorders is implied by aspects of the play's language and imagery. As Kaara L. Peterson points out, the play 'utilizes agricultural and horticultural images to refer to the female body and its processes', imagining the female body as well as the corrupt world as 'an unweeded garden | That grows to seed' (I.ii.135–6).[103] Green sickness, in which even virginity can be the source of sickness, perfectly suits this fallen world, in which one need not be adulterous, but merely sexual, to be corrupt, as Janet Adelman observes: 'For in the world seen under the aegis of the unweeded garden, the very corporality of flesh marks its contamination.'[104]

Ophelia is likened to, and dramatized with, flowers throughout the play: she gives flowers and herbs away while mad, drowns in flower-filled water, and is covered with flowers in her grave. This association is first evident when Laertes offers his sister words of advice before leaving to go to university. Using floral imagery to suggest that she is on the threshold between youth and adulthood, innocence and sexuality, he warns Ophelia she must be wary of both Hamlet's advances and her own emerging desires:

> . . . keep within the rear of your affection,
> Out of the shot and danger of desire.
> The chariest maid is prodigal enough
> If she unmask her beauty to the moon.
> Virtue itself scapes not calumnious strokes.
> The canker galls the infants of the spring
> Too oft before their buttons be disclosed,
> And in the morn and liquid dew of youth
> Contagious blastments are most imminent.
> Be wary then; best safety lies in fear;
> Youth to itself rebels, though none else near.
>
> (I.iii.34–44)

---

[103] Peterson, 'Fluid Economies', 43. [104] Adelman, *Suffocating Mothers*, 17.

The image of Ophelia as a bud about to open suggests that she is on the point of sexual maturation, a moment in which youthful fecundity is simultaneously in danger of corruption both by external sources ('Contagious blastments'), and from within (as in the image of the canker within the closed bud). As Peterson points out, 'It is the production of blood and seed within the female body upon menarche that means woman's irretrievable fall into pathology', explaining why 'it is possible for young female buds to be galled before "their buttons be disclos'd" '.[105] Women, it seems, are in danger not only from men, but also from their own physiological make-up, so that 'Youth to itself rebels, though none else near'. Laertes' warnings to his sister are echoed, disturbingly, by Hamlet, who, in his first on-stage encounter with Ophelia, denies he ever loved her ('I did love you once . . . You should not have believed me . . . I loved you not') and questions her chastity (III.i.117–21). Asking Ophelia if she is honest, Hamlet suggests that 'the power of beauty will sooner transform honesty from what it is to a bawd than the force of honesty can translate beauty into his likeness'; he warns her, 'be thou as chaste as ice, as pure as snow, thou shalt not escape calumny' (III.i.113–15, 137–8).

Ophelia's madness seems, at least superficially, to confirm the play's anxieties about female sexuality, in which the virginity of the nunnery can paradoxically lead to behaviour more appropriate to the brothel (also called a nunnery in early modern England). Madness heightens Ophelia's erotic impulses, and liberates her from the 'chariness' and modesty expected of her, so that she speaks and acts in a manner typical of one suffering from uterine fury.[106] She sings a song that recounts a young woman's loss of her virginity and distributes flowers, behaviour that suggests either her sexual readiness (that she is ready to be plucked) or her defloration; like the green-sick girl, whose lack of menstruation can either indicate her virginity or hidden pregnancy, Ophelia's mad behaviour is similarly open to conflicting interpretations.[107] The image of Ophelia carrying (and wearing) flowers also associates her with the

---

[105] Peterson, 'Fluid Economies', 43, 45.
[106] Platter and Culpeper, *Histories*, 47.
[107] As in Richard Lovelace's Poem 'Love Made in the First Age: To Chloris' which harks back to a time when 'Lads, indifferently did crop | A Flower, and a Maidenhead' (in *Poems*, 146). For the debate on whether Ophelia's behaviour suggests her sexual frustration or her pregnancy see Neely, ' "Documents in Madness" ', 81.

nymph Chloris, who (like her later persona Flora) is called the 'Queene of the flowers, and Mistreis of the Spring', whilst also being associated with both virginity and (as her name suggests) the colour green. According to Ovid, Chloris was raped by the west wind, Zephyrus, after which she was transformed into Flora and given sovereignty over all the world's flowers.[108] The story of Chloris thus offers an allegory, not only of the seasons, but also of the virginal pubescent girl's entry into sexuality and fecundity; while Chloris embodies the moment at which a woman is on the threshold of sexual maturity, Flora stands as a symbol of fertility and growth. Chloris can thus be read as an apt figure for the pubescent virgin's chlorosis or green sickness and is of particular significance to Ophelia, who is called a 'green girl' and a 'rose of May' and is similarly on the cusp of sexual maturity (I.iii.101, IV.v.158).

Unlike Hamlet's melancholy, which is cerebral, bookish, and philosophical, Ophelia's madness is thus corporeal, emotional, and sexual, a difference that corresponds both to the gendering of reason as masculine and passion as female in Renaissance thinking, and to representations of early modern men as intellectually melancholic and women as madly lovesick by historians and literary critics. Both distempers are also valorized in ways that are gender-specific: where Hamlet's melancholy evinces his philosophical temperament, Ophelia's lovesickness demonstrates her sensitivity. Laertes sees the death of Ophelia's 'wits' as the sign of her emotional delicacy, indicating the depth of her affection for Polonius; he asks, 'O heavens, is't possible a young maid's wits | Should be as mortal as an old man's life?' (IV.v.160–1). As in the tale of the fairy-tale princess, whose sensitivity to the tiny pea under the mattress proves her noble rank, Laertes sees Ophelia's madness as the hallmark, not of a noble mind, but of a fine-tuned sensibility:

> Nature is fine in love, and where 'tis fine
> It sends some precious instance of itself
> After the thing it loves.
>
> (IV.v.162–4)

[108] Lyons discusses Ophelia in relation to the iconography of Flora, suggesting that she calls to mind both the nymph from Ovid and an alternative tradition in which she is a wealthy courtesan ('Iconography', 63–5). As E. K. glosses 'Flora' in *Shepheardes Calender*, she is 'the Goddesse of flowers, but indeed (as saith Tacitus) a famous harlot, which with the abuse of her body having gotten great riches, made the people of Rome her heyre' (in Spenser, *Shorter Poems*, 63).

The positive meaning that Laertes ascribes to Ophelia's madness is complemented by the aesthetic manner of her representation. It is not surprising that later writers and painters have portrayed Ophelia in a poetic and erotic manner, for she is presented in this way in the play; where Hamlet's introspective melancholy allows for an intimate, sympathetic engagement by the audience, Ophelia's madness is presented as a bawdy and bodily spectacle, an erotic performance watched and commented upon by others. Gertrude, Laertes, Claudius, and Horatio watch her mad behaviour with interest and aesthetic appreciation, reflecting on the strange attractiveness of her insanity. Claudius calls her 'Pretty Ophelia' (IV.v.55), and Laertes declares that 'Thought and afflictions, passion, hell itself | She turns to favour and to prettiness' (IV.v.186–7). So able is Ophelia to metamorphose passions and afflictions into 'prettiness' that, as Enobarbus says of Cleopatra, 'vilest things | Become themselves in her'.[109] However, in many respects Ophelia's appeal is due to, rather than in spite of, her madness: it is not that Ophelia transforms vile things into prettiness, but rather it is the vile things themselves that make her so attractive. From her lyrical, sexually explicit songs and loose hair to Gertrude's sensuous rendering of her death, Ophelia's madness is presented as unabashedly erotic, allowing her to fulfil opposing cultural stereotypes of the innocent virgin and experienced whore. Her intense sexual desire is matched by helpless vulnerability, and her vivid sexual language is justified and made unthreatening by the very madness which prompts it.

Gertrude's description of Ophelia's death draws together many of the tropes that recur in Ophelia's madness. Her death by drowning links her madness to womb disorders (victims of these disorders were frequently said either to drown themselves or to plunge themselves into rivers in order to cool their overheated wombs).[110] And the willow tree that Ophelia sits beneath associates her madness with lovesickness and wider conventions of forsaken women. Gertrude describes Ophelia's death in sensuous and lyrical language:

> There is a willow grows aslant a brook
> That shows his hoar leaves in the glassy stream.
> Therewith fantastic garlands did she make
> Of crow-flowers, nettles, daisies, and long purples,

[109] Shakespeare, *Antony and Cleopatra* (1606), II.ii.244–5.
[110] Wack, *Lovesickness*, 50.

> That liberal shepherds give a grosser name,
> But our cold maids do dead men's fingers call them.
> There on the pendent boughs her crownet weeds
> Clamb'ring to hang, an envious sliver broke,
> When down the weedy trophies and herself
> Fell in the weeping brook.
>
> (IV.vii.138–47)

The flowers and herbs she had proffered earlier become the 'fantastic garlands' that she weaves to crown her own watery grave. Appropriately, Gertrude mentions the orchids, or 'long purples', which 'our cold maids' call 'dead men's fingers' and 'liberal shepherds' give a 'grosser name', hinting that both grief and erotic desire are sources of Ophelia's madness. Kaara L. Peterson argues that the flowers encircling Ophelia can also be read as having a symbolic meaning. 'Flowers' was the common term for menstrual blood and seed in early modern England, as the menses go 'before Conception as flowers do before fruit'.[111] Women troubled by disorders of the womb are thus 'suffocated by the suppression of the flowers'.[112] Read within this context, the image of Ophelia sinking among her 'weedy trophies' suggests an internal landscape, in which her virginal body is awash with 'flowers' (trapped menstrual blood and seed). As Peterson argues, 'if flowers are identified with menstruum and "to penetrate the hymen is to deflower", then Ophelia's being surrounded by flowers as she drowns in the brook suggests her literally drowning in "flowers" of blood and seed, not "deflowered" but pathologically "enflowered", to coin a term'.[113]

Ophelia's death is eroticized and associated with female gendered nature; even her drowning 'has associations with the feminine and the irrational, since water is the organic symbol of woman's fluidity: blood, milk, tears'.[114] As in Desdemona's story of Barbary, Ophelia is described as singing as she dies:

> Her clothes spread wide,
> And mermaid-like a while they bore her up;
> Which time she chanted snatches of old tunes,
> As one incapable of her own distress,

[111] Culpeper, *Directory*, 67–8. Quoted by Peterson, 'Fluid Economies', 39.
[112] Paré, *Workes of the Famous Chirugion*, 634. Quoted by Veith, *Hysteria: The History*, 115.
[113] Peterson, 'Fluid Economies', 47.   [114] Showalter, *Female Malady*, 11.

> Or like a creature native and endued
> Unto that element. But long it could not be
> Till that her garments, heavy with their drink,
> Pulled the poor wretch from her melodious lay
> To muddy death.
>
> (IV.vii.175–83)

Gertrude's description of the 'mermaid-like' Ophelia, wrapped in flowers, singing herself to a watery grave, invokes symbols of the feminine to portray her death as alluringly and unknowingly sexual; not merely immersed in water, she is 'like a creature native and endued | Unto that element'. The eroticism of her death is continued at her burial, in which the grave is presented as a substitute for the marriage bed. 'I thought thy bride-bed to have decked' Gertrude laments, 'and not t'have strewed thy grave' (V.i.241–2). As in the river, Ophelia is wrapped in flowers and garlands in the grave, 'her virgin rites' and 'maiden strewments' being the only ceremonies allowed her after suicide (V.i.226–7). Laertes adopts this floral imagery, once again imagining her body as the site where fecundity and decay meet: 'from her fair and unpolluted flesh | May violets spring', he comments (V.i.234–5).

The representation of Ophelia's madness exerts a powerful influence on later stage representations, one example of which can be found in the depiction of the Jailer's Daughter in Shakespeare and Fletcher's *Two Noble Kinsmen*. John Fletcher, who is believed to be mostly responsible for the subplot in which the Jailer's Daughter appears, is clearly drawing on Shakespeare, with whom he collaborated; scenes from *Hamlet* are echoed and extended, and the Jailer's Daughter's illness (as is characteristic of Fletcher) is subjected to more detailed medical diagnosis.[115] In addition, the play broadens its exploration of virginity by depicting not one but two pubescent virgins, who have strikingly different reactions to heterosexual love; unlike the Jailer's Daughter, who is eager to consummate her love for Palamon, Emilia wishes to remain a virgin and prefers same-sex friendships. Even more than *Hamlet*, *Two Noble Kinsmen* thus focuses on the threshold moment of a woman's sexual

---

[115] Fletcher is generally thought to have written seven of the nine scenes in which the Jailer's Daughter appears (II.iv; II.vi; III.ii; III.iv; III.v; IV.i; and V.ii); the other two are probably by Shakespeare (II.i and IV.iii). For a summary of the debate surrounding the authorship question and the various positions scholars have taken see Hamlin, 'Bibliographical Guide', 186–216.

maturity, illuminating the medical dangers of virginity and the complex social and economic transactions involved in love and marriage.

A TALE OF TWO VIRGINS: SHAKESPEARE AND FLETCHER'S *THE TWO NOBLE KINSMEN*

The lovesick behaviour of the Jailer's Daughter in Shakespeare and Fletcher's *The Two Noble Kinsmen* draws upon the tropes surrounding Ophelia's madness, making the affiliation between female lovesickness and uterine disorders explicit. Carol Neely argues that the representation of her distemper corresponds to a new typology of female melancholy, later described by Burton as 'Maid's, Nun's and Widow's Melancholy' in the 1628 edition of his *The Anatomy of Melancholy*.[116] However, it is also true to say that her illness draws on the stereotypical features of both green sickness and uterine fury: it is aligned with the onset of puberty, and is closely related to both her menstrual cycle and her physical need for sex. Moreover, Burton's description of 'Maid's, Nun's and Widow's Melancholy' itself draws on descriptions of green sickness.[117] Thus if the Jailer's Daughter's madness represents a new form of melancholy, it is one that derives from pre-existing medical categories. There are significant differences between the madness of the Jailer's Daughter and Ophelia. Ophelia's heightened sexuality, although powerful, is nevertheless depicted as sweet and delicate, whereas the erotic desires of the Jailer's Daughter are given more explicit expression. The two characters also come to different ends: Ophelia's madness results in death, as befits tragedy, while the Jailer's Daughter is cured via a tragicomic consummation.

[116] Neely, *Distracted Subjects*, Ch. 3.

[117] Although Veith claims this section is referring to hysteria (*Hysteria: A History*, 127–8), Burton categorically states that 'Maid's, Nun's and Widow's Melancholy' merely *resembles* hysteria: '*fauces siccitate præcluduntur, ut difficulter posit ab uteri strangulatione decerne*, like fits of the mother' [The throat closes up with dryness, so that it is difficult to distinguish from hysteria] (*Anatomy*, i.415; trans. v.57). The malady more closely resembles green sickness, with its emphasis on virginity and abstinence and with symptoms that include 'a beating about the backe . . . skin [that] is many times rough, squalid . . . the heart it selfe beats . . . pain in their heads' (i.414–16). King treats Burton's three primary sources—Luis Mercado's *Operum tomus primus* (1620–9), his *De mulieribus affectionibus* (1587), and Rodrigues de Castro's chapter 'De melancholia virginum et viduarum' from his *De universa mulierum medicina* (1603)—as discussions of green sickness (*Disease of Virgins*, 2, 6, 15, 144).

Some of the divergences between the lovesickness of Ophelia and the Jailer's Daughter reflect wider artistic differences between Shakespeare and Fletcher. Shakespeare demonstrates an understanding of early modern medical ideas; moreover, his dramatic representations of psychological distress frequently explode the medical categories of its day, creating new vocabularies and patterns for mental illness that are more sophisticated than, and have outlasted, the cultural models that they reinvent and challenge. Indeed, doctors do not frequently feature in his plays, and when they do, they rarely provide the solution that will allow the play to end happily. In *Macbeth* (1606), for example, the doctor is strikingly sympathetic, not for his medical knowledge, but for his acknowledgement of its limitations; the doctor sees Lady Macbeth's anxious sleepwalking as outside his professional capabilities, telling her gentlewoman, 'This disease is beyond my practice' (V.i.56). Fletcher, on the other hand, appears to be an avid reader of the medical lore of his day, directly importing the vocabulary and cures from contemporary medical texts. Plays in which he has had a hand frequently contain either doctors or individuals who have an understanding of medicine, who diagnose and cure characters and are crucial for the tragicomic resolution.[118] The subplot of *The Two Noble Kinsmen* follows this pattern: much more attention is given to the diagnosis of the malady of the Jailer's Daughter, who is cured near the end of the play by a doctor.

The Two Noble Kinsmen dramatizes the story from Chaucer's *The Knight's Tale* of Arcite and Palamon and their love for Emilia, who is the sister of Hippolyta, Queen of the Amazons. The play opens with the wedding procession of Theseus and Hippolyta, which is interrupted by three queens in mourning for their husbands. The women entreat Theseus to make war on Creon in order that they may bury their husbands' bodies, and Theseus eventually agrees to delay his wedding in order to comply with the queens. Theseus defeats Creon, after which he discovers the wounded bodies of Palamon and Arcite, who have fought valiantly for Creon, and are near death. Palamon and Arcite are put in

---

[118] See my discussion of Fletcher's *The Mad Lover*, Fletcher and Massinger's *A Very Woman*, and Fletcher and Middleton's *The Nice Valour*. Other plays that fit this paradigm include Beaumont and Fletcher's *Cupid's Revenge* (1615), Fletcher's *The Humorous Lieutenant* (*c*.1619), Fletcher and Massinger's *The Custom of the Country* (1619), and Fletcher's *The Noble Gentleman* (1624–5).

prison, where they recover from their injuries; their friendship, however, turns into rivalry when they see Emilia in the garden outside their prison cell, and fall in love with her. Palamon and Arcite are freed from prison (Arcite is banished from Athens, and Palamon escapes with the help of the Jailer's Daughter) and the two men meet and prepare to fight. Before they come to blows, however, they are interrupted by Theseus, who pardons the men and declares that a trial of strength will decide their fate: the winner will be granted Emilia's hand in marriage, and the loser and his followers will be beheaded. Arcite wins the competition, but before he can marry Emilia, he is thrown off his horse to his death. As a result, Palamon is saved from execution and weds Emilia in Arcite's place. Just as the play opens with funerals and weddings, it ends with the uneasy combination of love and death.

The subplot focuses on another love triangle, this time between the Jailer's Daughter, the Wooer (her fiancé), and Palamon. Unlike Emilia, who is not interested in marrying either of the knights, the Jailer's Daughter falls hopelessly in love with Palamon, whom she frees from prison—an action she believes will cost her father his life. The Jailer's Daughter follows Palamon into the woods where she becomes mad and almost drowns. Eventually she is treated by a doctor, who suggests that she will be cured of her madness if the Wooer has sex with her. The Wooer disguises himself as Palamon, convinces the Jailer's Daughter that he is her beloved, and the two leave the stage, presumably to have sex. At the end of the play her father suggests that his daughter has recovered her wits and is soon to be married. The last-minute swapping of lovers in the main plot (in which Palamon takes Arcite's place) is thus echoed in the subplot through the bed trick, which cures the Jailer's Daughter of her madness.

The Jailer's Daughter is not in any of the sources; her appearance in *The Two Nobel Kinsmen* suggests both the popularity of mad characters on the early modern stage and an interest in the medical dangers and marriage choices (or lack of them) of young pubescent women. Whereas Ophelia's insanity develops offstage, the audience watches the Jailer's Daughter progress through various stages of lovesickness before descending into madness. Palamon's affect on her is powerful and immediate; she recalls how 'First I saw him ... Next, I pitied him ... Then, I lov'd him' (II.iv.7–14). Frustrated by her recognition of the social gap between them, she recognizes the fruitlessness of her love:

> He never will affect me. I am base,
> My father the mean keeper of his prison,
> And he a prince. To marry him is hopeless,
> To be his whore is witless. Out upon't,
> What pushes are we wenches driven to
> When fifteen once has found us? . . .
>
> .   .   .   .
>
> What should I do to make him know I love him?
> For I would fain enjoy him.
>
> (II.iv.2–7, 29–30)

Palamon's social elevation exacerbates the Jailer's Daughter's sense of her own unworthiness, and she is torn between two equally non-viable alternatives: her lowly status precludes marriage and her scruples prevent her from becoming 'his whore'. As in green sickness, her lovesickness springs from her burgeoning sexuality, and the sexual drives which emerge at the onset of puberty.

The Jailer's Daughter's love for Palamon leads her to free him from prison, risking her father's and her own life. She loves him 'beyond reason | Or wit or safety', imagining that if she is executed for her actions 'Some honest-hearted maids, will sing my dirge | And tell to memory my death was noble, | Dying almost a martyr' (II.vi.11–12, 15–17). Tired and alone, the Jailer's Daughter wanders through the woods searching for Palamon without success. Rather than recognizing that he has abandoned her, she imagines that he has been killed by a wolf and longs for an end to her pain:

> I am moped—
> Food took I none these two days,
> Sipped some water. I have not closed mine eyes
> Save when my lips scoured off their brine. Alas,
> Dissolve, my life; let not my sense unsettle,
> Lest I should drown or stab or hang myself.
> O state of nature, fail together in me,
> Since thy best props are warped. So which way now?
> The best way is the next way to a grave.
>
> (III.ii.25–33)

The Jailer's Daughter's senses are increasingly unsettled from her lack of food and sleep, and she characterizes herself as 'moped', the lower-class equivalent to melancholy in early modern England.[119] She wishes, 'O for a prick now, like a nightingale, | To put my breast against. I shall sleep like a top else' (III.iv.25–6). No longer simply imagining her martyrdom, she portrays herself as actively seeking her death—the 'prick' she longs for ambiguously promising both consummation and annihilation.

As in Ophelia's madness, the distemper of the Jailer's Daughter fits into paradigms of gender and illness, which suggest that female lovesickness is sexual, irrational, and self-destructive. The sexuality of the Jailer's Daughter's becomes more pronounced as she loses her sanity and she follows the conventional pattern for female madness on the early modern stage: her hair is loose, her speech is childlike and lyrical, and she sings bawdy folk songs, which associate her burgeoning sexuality with the natural rites of spring and the fecundity of nature (III.v.134–58). Whereas Ophelia's sexualized language remains oblique and enigmatic, the Jailer's Daughter expresses her sexual desires openly, a distinction which is in part due to her lower social class.[120] She loves Palamon as much as any 'young wench . . . That ever dreamed or vowed her maidenhead | To a young handsome man', and would 'fain enjoy him' (II.iv.12–14, 30). She asks for her wedding gown, exclaiming 'For I must lose my maidenhead by cocklight' (IV.i.112). Yet like Ophelia, the Jailer's Daughter's madness is aesthetically appealing and performative. When the Jailer's Daughter stumbles across a group of countrymen planning a Morris Dance, they immediately want her to participate in their entertainment, assuming that her insanity will enhance her performance and that as 'a dainty madwoman' she will 'do the rarest gambols' (III.v.73, 76).

The Jailer's Daughter's eagerness to lose her maidenhead is contrasted with Emilia's devotion to a single life, and initially it seems as if the differences between these women offer two opposing perspectives on virginity: while Emilia embodies the 'clear virginity' of elevated Neoplatonic traditions, the Jailer's Daughter portrays its diseased, pathological form (I.i.31). Unlike the Jailer's Daughter, Emilia is adamant that she wishes to remain a virgin. She rejects heterosexual bonds in favour of same-sex friendship, a preference that is founded on her lost Amazonian

[119] MacDonald, *Mystical Bedlam*, 160–4.
[120] Bruster, 'Madwomen's Language', 282.

past and on her devotion to Flavina, a childhood friend who died when the pair were both eleven.[121] Asserting that 'the true love 'tween maid and maid may be | More than in sex dividual' (I.iii.81–2), Emilia offers an idealistic image of her friendship with Flavina, in which the two are second selves to one another, mirroring each other in their affections and tastes: 'What she liked | Was then of me approved; what not, condemned'; when Emilia would pluck a flower and put it between her breasts, 'she would long | Till she had such another' (I.iii.64–5, 68–9).

Emilia's friendship with Flavina provides one instance of how women in Shakespeare take up an idealized discourse of same-sex friendship (more frequently associated with men in early modern literature), and recalls Helena's poignant remembrance of her days of 'childhood innocence' with Hermia in *A Midsummer Night's Dream* (1601), when they would sew and sing together 'As if our hands, our sides, voices, and minds | Had been incorporate' (III.ii.203, 208–9). However, such same-sex partnerships are frequently confined in Shakespeare to a time before the onset of sexual maturity. Indeed, Theseus and Pirithous's friendship is noteworthy in that it has managed to outlast this period. More typical in Shakespeare is the depiction of the two knights of *The Two Noble Kinsmen*, Palamon and Arcite, whose pledges to be 'one another's wife, ever begetting | New births of love' quickly transform to threats of violence the minute they find themselves competitors for Emilia's affection (II.ii.80–1). Although such erotic rivalry is ultimately the result and sign of their close affection and identification, it simultaneously acts to belittle their idealized conception of their friendship and themselves.

Although in *The Two Noble Kinsmen* Flavina is dead and thus her friendship with Emilia is not subject to the same explicit critique, there are hints that their relationship would have been beset by similar problems had it been allowed to mature. Emilia and Flavina's intimacy is, after all, expressed through their imitation of one another, in which they long to possess the same things, be they flowers, clothing, or songs. Desire is thus constructed as imitative and displaced, so that

---

[121] For a discussion of Emilia's Amazonian identity see Roberts, 'Male Self-Definition'; for same sex friendship see Weller, 'Friendship Tradition'.

it matters less what the object is, than that it is loved by the friend; this quality renders erotic rivalry inevitable had their friendship continued into adulthood, and also provides a rationale for Emilia's inability to articulate a preference for either Palamon and Arcite, who both love her.

Emilia's elevated celebration of same-sex friendship is also undermined by Hippolyta, who hints that Emilia's attitude is merely the product of her pubescent, virginal state. Likening her distaste for heterosexual love to a 'sickly appetite | That loathes even as it longs', Hippolyta reinterprets such scorn as the symptom of an underlying desire, associating it with the disorderly appetites of the green-sick girl (I.iii.90–1). Hippolyta, on the point of marriage and thus past the moment of queasy readiness the green-sick girl embodies, tells Emilia she is no longer '*ripe* for [her] persuasion' (I.iii.92, emphasis added). When next we see Emilia, picking flowers with her maid, she seems in part to justify her sister's characterization of her contradictory desires. She talks repeatedly about men and erotic love, whilst simultaneously suggesting her adherence to her virginity by praising the rose, 'the very emblem of a maid', which 'like chastity . . . locks her beauties in her bud' (II.ii.137, 141–2).

However, Palamon and Arcite's love for Emilia means that she will not ultimately remain a maid: the victor in a competition of arms will gain her hand in marriage, while the loser will forfeit his life. Emilia is understandably horrified that a man will die because of love for her, and wonders how she has come to deserve such a fate:

> What sins have I committed, chaste Diana,
> That my unspotted youth must now be soiled
> With blood of princes, and my chastity
> Be made the altar where the lives of lovers
>
> .   .   .   .
>
>   must be the sacrifice
> To my unhappy beauty?
>
>   (IV.ii.58–61, 63–4)

Although Emilia is ostensibly describing herself as an altar on which one of the knights must be sacrificed, her description of her 'unspotted youth' which 'must be soiled | With blood of princes' also conjures up an image of violent defloration, in which blood can refer both to male semen and hymeneal blood.

The association between blood and sex is further reinforced when Emilia goes to the altar of Diana on the eve of the knights' competition in order to pray either that the man who loves her best will 'Take off my wheaten garland' or that she may 'Continue in thy band', preserving her virginity (V.iii.24, 26). Here, Diana is the 'cold, and constant queen...who to thy female knights | Allow'st no more blood than will make a blush, | Which is their order's robe' (V.iii.1, 4–6). As blood can suggest the physical source of passion, the refined blood of male seed, and the blood of menstruation, Diana's disciples here are cold, chaste, and possibly even green sick, an interpretation reinforced by the reference to the goddess' 'rare green eye' (V.iii.8). However, despite Emilia's appeal to Diana to remain a virgin, her entrance in this scene—with '*her hair about her shoulders*' and '*stuck with flowers*'— suggests that she is destined for other things. Calling to mind both the stereotypical appearance of the sexually frustrated mad woman and the iconography of Chloris/Flora, Emilia's appearance implicitly suggests that far from being the bloodless servant of Diana, she inhabits the flourishing state of the green-sick girl and is therefore ripe to lose her virginity. Diana answers Emilia's request with a vision that confirms this:

> See what our general of ebbs and flows
> Out of the bowels of her holy altar,
> With sacred act, advances—but one rose!
> If well inspired, this battle shall confound
> Both these brave knights, and I a virgin flower,
> Must grow alone, unplucked.
>
> (V.iii.27–32)

Although Emilia takes heart from this promising image, which seems to indicate that she will be able to remain an 'unplucked' virgin, the vision of the single rose on a tree does not last. Instead, it is immediately followed by '*a sudden twang of instruments, and the rose falls from the tree*'. 'Thou here dischargest me', Emilia concludes, 'I shall be gathered' (V.iii.34). Gordon McMullan argues that the flower that appears before Emilia can be read as 'a symbolic palimpsest: at once a symbol of virginity, menstruation and defloration'.[122] This conjunction of meanings is particularly apt for the green-sick virgin, for whom the blood of defloration and that of menstruation are closely related and may even be mingled: as we have seen earlier, the sexual intercourse that deflowers the woman simultaneously opens up the veins of her womb, releasing her menses (her 'flowers') and trapped seed. Within this context, the 'ebbs and flows' attributed to Diana, the goddess of the moon, can here suggest the ebbs and flows of menstruation and their relation to the lunar cycle, a reading which is reinforced by the image of the rose emerging 'out from the bowels'. By being 'discharged' of Diana's service, Emilia is thus entering the world of passion, consummation, and menstruation.

The representation of Emilia's virginity creates a subtext for reading the madness of the Jailer's Daughter, reinforcing its relation to menstruation and suggesting the two characters' interrelation. Indeed, the appearance of Emilia at the altar of Diana with '*her hair about her shoulders*' and '*stuck with flowers*' links the two characters visually. Like Emilia, the Jailer's Daughter is also described as gathering flowers, an activity linked both to her mourning (she believes her father will be executed because of Palamon's escape from prison) and her lovesickness (she comments, 'We maids that have our livers perished, cracked to pieces with love, we shall come there and do nothing all day long but pick flowers with Proserpine') (IV.iii.21–4). By dramatizing two very different responses to heterosexuality and pubescence, the play emphasizes the unhappy fate of female desire in a patriarchal world, where a woman's filial obligations always outweigh her own erotic preferences. Despite the women's very different wishes, both Emilia and the Jailer's Daughter will be trafficked in marriage by men, who (no matter how kindly their intents) ensure that neither of the women get what they want. Maidenheads may have an ethical worth, but they also have a market value; like 'New plays', they are 'Much followed' and can fetch a high price 'If they stand sound and well' (Prologue, 1–3).

The Jailer's Daughter almost meets a watery end like Ophelia. The Wooer's narration of this moment echoes Gertrude's description of Ophelia's death, drawing on stock images of lovesickness. As with

---

[122] McMullan, 'Rose for Emilia', 143.

Ophelia, the Jailer's Daughter's thoughts oscillate between filial anxieties and lovesick self-laceration. The Wooer tells the Jailer:

> she talked of you, sir—
> That you must lose your head tomorrow morning,
> And she must gather flowers to bury you,
> And see the house made handsome. Then she sung
> Nothing but 'willow, willow, willow', and between
> Ever was 'Palamon, fair Palamon',
> And 'Palamon was a tall young man'. The place
> Was knee-deep where she sat; her careless tresses
> A wreath of bull-rush rounded; about her stuck
> Thousand freshwater flowers of several colors—
> That she appeared, methought, like the fair nymph
> That feeds the lake with waters, or as Iris
> Newly dropped down from heaven. Rings she made
> Of rushes that grew by and to 'em spoke
> The prettiest posies—'Thus our true love's tied',
> 'This you may lose, not me', and many a one.
> And then she wept, and sung again, and sighed—
> And with the same breath smiled, and kissed her hand.
>
> (IV.i.76–93)

In the Wooer's chaotic recollection, the Jailer's Daughter is newly aestheticized: she sits by a lake, her hair loose, covered in colourful flowers that she weaves into true-love knots. There is a surreal or fairy-tale quality to the Wooer's description, as though the madness of the Jailer's Daughter has infused her with mythical qualities. No longer an ordinary woman, she looks like a 'fair nymph' who has either fallen from heaven or sprung from the flower-filled water which half immerses her.

The doctor, who attributes the Jailer's Daughter's 'perturbed mind' to 'a thick and profound melancholy', clearly assumes that her madness is related to menstruation (IV.iii.46–7, 56).[123] He asks her father if her 'distraction is more at some time of the moon than at some other' and assumes that sexual intercourse will cure her (IV.iii.1–2). The Wooer, who is contracted to her in marriage, is happy to lend a hand in this scheme; in the Doctor's view, 'It is a falsehood she is in, which is with falsehood to be combated' (IV.iii.90–1). Under the doctor's instruction,

---

[123] Neely, *Distracted Subjects*, 86.

the Wooer adopts the behaviour and mannerisms of Palamon, singing the Jailer's Daughter 'green songs of love' and appearing decked in 'sweet flowers' so that she is 'half-persuaded' that he is Palamon (V.vi.4). Urging the Wooer to have sex with the Jailer's Daughter, the Doctor reassures him that 'there the cure lies mainly'; he tells the Wooer:

> Please her appetite,
> And do it home—it cures her *ipso facto*,
> The melancholy humor that infects her.
>
> (V.iv.9, 36–8)

As the doctor predicts, the Jailer's Daughter seems eager to consummate her passion: 'We'll to bed then', she tells the Wooer, adding 'We shall have many children' (V.iv.87, 94). Nonetheless, as the two walk offstage together her final words are poignant: 'But you shall not hurt me', she tells the Wooer, 'If you do, love, I'll cry' (V.iv.112–13). Her words reinforce the play's 'pervasive sense of disenchantment and loss', contributing to the sense, hinted at in the main plot, that the achievement of erotic satisfaction is also the moment of its loss.[124]

The cure of the Jailer's Daughter offers an extreme instance of how erotic objects are phantasmic dreams of the imagination: the Jailer's Daughter loves not the real Palamon, but her ideal, internalized image of him. In many respects, however, this is not so different from the depiction of desire we are given in the main plot. Palamon and Arcite's love for Emilia—based upon a fleeting glance through prison bars—seems equally fabricated, more the product of their love for one another than any actual understanding of the woman they are pursuing. In this respect Emilia appears as the conduit through whom the men express their passion, rather than its true aim. Palamon seems to realize this as he watches Arcite die, lamenting 'That we should things desire, which do cost us | The loss of our desire! That nought could buy | Dear love, but loss of dear love!' (V.iv.110–12); these words both express what gaining Emilia has cost him (Arcite), and also suggest the illusionary nature of all desire, whose end is satisfaction. Thus, if neither of the two women gets what she really wants, then the same can be said of the men, who are equally 'brutalized by love, compulsory heterosexuality, and arranged

---

[124] Wickham, '*Two Noble Kinsmen* or *A Midsummer Night's Dream*', 186; quoted by Neely, *Distracted Subjects*, 90.

marriages'.[125] The Jailer's Daughter may awaken to discover that the prince she has bedded is really a frog, but this seems an apt image for the delusional nature of erotic love itself, illustrating the uneasy compromises of both tragicomedy and erotic satisfaction.

Despite her eventual death or cure, the insane, liminal state of the lovesick woman is presented in *Hamlet* and *The Two Noble Kinsmen* as powerfully exotic and erotic, inspiring fear and desire in her onlookers. The mad woman's bawdy words and sensual behaviour are circumscribed by her vulnerability, and her madness suggests how dependent she is upon masculine reason, as well as the male organ, to restore her to sexual and psychological health. The imagery of water, flowers, and dishevelled hair associates the madwoman with sensuality and the female body, confirming the claim that 'Beliefs about gender and sexuality influenced conceptions of madness in sixteenth- and seventeenth-century England'.[126] However, although the representation of Ophelia and the Jailer's Daughter supports the argument that Elizabethan and Jacobean literature tends 'to pathologize, to make diseased, female desire', seeing it as an affliction of the womb, alternative models of gender and illness recur in early modern literature that are quite distinct from the Ophelia paradigm.[127] Although depictions of madness tend to be gendered, and are related to hysteria, green sickness, and uterine fury, other models of female lovesickness are less straightforward. As the next chapter will make clear, even in the case of characters seemingly modelled on Ophelia, important differences emerge that challenge and reinvent conventions of female lovesickness.

---

[125] Neely, *Distracted Subjects*, 90 n. 27.
[126] MacDonald, 'Women and Madness', 280.
[127] Peterson, 'Fluid Economies', 38.

3

Beyond Ophelia: The Anatomy
of Female Melancholy

In Shakespeare's *Twelfth Night* (1601), Orsino muses over the differences between the love felt by men and that experienced by women; the duke tells the disguised Viola:

> There is no woman's sides
> Can bide the beating of so strong a passion
> As love doth give my heart; no woman's heart
> So big, to hold so much. They lack retention.
> Alas, their love may be called appetite,
> No motion of the liver, but the palate,
> That suffer surfeit, cloyment, and revolt.
> But mine is all as hungry as the sea,
> And can digest as much.
>
> (II.iv.92–100)

According to Orsino, men experience a passion which is not only more intense but also of a superior quality; unlike his own desire, which is 'as hungry as the sea', women's feelings are transitory, weak, and easily satisfied. Women's emotional deficiencies are linked both to their physical frailty (their sides are too weak to bear a strong passion, their hearts are small and 'lack retention') and to the distinct physiological origin of female desire. Whereas male love is seen as arising from the liver, the seat of passion and the organ responsible for erotic melancholy, female affection is said to spring from the palate, and is thus a superficial bodily 'appetite'. As Orsino tells Viola, 'Make no compare | Between that love a woman can bear me | And that I owe Olivia' (II.iv.100–2).

Orsino's assumption that men are ennobled by desire while women fall prey to base bodily appetites appears vindicated by contemporary critics, who frequently regard male and female lovesickness as distinct maladies with different physiological origins. Seen principally as a disorder of the womb, female lovesickness is thought to be of a lower order (physically, emotionally, and culturally) than its masculine counterpart, indicating not an elevated emotional state but a bodily need for sex. This model of gender and illness, implicit across a wide range of scholarship, is summed up neatly by Laurinda Dixon in *Perilous Chastity*. Although Dixon's concern is with the study of lovesick maidens found in seventeenth-century Dutch genre painting, rather than medical history, her comment serves to encapsulate a widespread paradigm of the relationship between gender and illness in relation to lovesickness:

Male lovesickness…was considered a type of heroic melancholia— 'erotomania'—induced by the hot passion of love igniting the bodily humors and leaving smoky black remains to settle in the spleen or liver. The cause in women was the troublesome womb or 'mother', which inflamed by the hot passions by abstinence, affected the rest of the body by corroding organs, exhaling poisonous vapors, or creating sympathetic reactions, depending on whose theory one followed. The word *love*, when applied to women, did not carry the same idealistic, Neoplatonic, chivalric connotations as when applied to men. Since hysteria was considered an illness with a purely physical origin in the uterus, physicians spoke of love, when discussing women, as a thinly disguised euphemism for sexual intercourse.[1]

Dixon's account sounds remarkably similar to that of Orsino: whereas men's melancholy arises from the liver and has idealistic connotations, the female version is the exact equivalent of hysteria.[2] The dissemination of this gendered paradigm of illness can be found in a number of critical works. Elaine Showalter examines changing constructions of female sexuality and madness through the figure of Ophelia, suggesting that 'Whereas for Hamlet madness is metaphysical, linked with culture, for Ophelia it is a product of the female body and female nature'.[3] In *The Gendering of Melancholia*, Juliana Schiesari similarly argues that while male melancholy is 'a privileged state of inspired genius', women's

---

[1] Dixon, *Perilous Chastity*, 109.
[2] As King rightly points out, by merging medical conditions which early modern writers chose to distinguish, Dixon 'fails to understand the rich range of ways in which medicine has historically claimed to hold the keys to the health of women of all ages and social classes' ('Green Sickness', 373 n. 3).
[3] Skultans, *English Madness*, 81; Showalter, 'Representing Ophelia', 80–1.

sorrow is always 'expressed by less flattering allusions to widow's weeds, inarticulate weeping, and other signs of ritualistic (but intellectually and artistically unaccredited) mourning'.[4] And George Rousseau articulates these ideas in explicitly literary terms: 'The Hamlets and Lears are noble, strong, active and mad...in contrast to the female condition of lingering low spirits.'[5] Whereas lovesickness in men is defined as a form of melancholia, in women it is associated with diseases of the reproductive tract: women's illnesses are thus constructed as bodily and passionate rather than intellectual and creative.

In this chapter I challenge this model of gender and illness, arguing that the representation of female melancholy cannot be reduced to a single pattern that classifies the form of melancholy according to the gender of the sufferer. Contrary to common critical opinion, Renaissance women are often represented, both by themselves and others, as suffering from intellectual melancholy. Female lovesickness, moreover, is not the equivalent of green sickness or hysteria; it is a species of melancholy which can be depicted, not only as a passionate illness which degenerates into madness, but also as a spiritual and cerebral affliction. In *Twelfth Night* it is Viola, cross-dressed as Cesario, who is able to defend women's emotions. Asserting that she knows 'Too well what love women to men may owe. | In faith, they are as true of heart as we', Viola invents a narrative describing how her 'father had a daughter loved a man' whose history was a 'blank' (II.iv.105–6, 107, 110). This daughter

>   never told her love,
> But let concealment, like a worm i'th'bud,
> Feed on her damask cheek. She pined in thought,
> And with a green and yellow melancholy
> She sat like patience on a monument,
> Smiling at grief.
>
>   (II.iv.110–15)

In contrast to Orsino's pejorative definition of women's affections as purely physical appetites, Viola describes the lovesickness of her 'sister' as a mental suffering that leads to a 'green and yellow melancholy';

---

[4] Schiesari, *Gendering of Melancholia*, 14.
[5] Rousseau, 'Depression's Forgotten Genealogy', 85.

she internalizes her suffering, pining 'in thought' while simultaneously 'smiling at grief'.

This chapter will explore this alternative model of female lovesickness, identifying further examples of women pining 'in thought'. In literature, women can be portrayed as possessing the rational resources to overcome their affliction, or they can be shown to employ it to fashion a public self, or simply to indulge in the bittersweet pleasure of their distemper. The opening section gives an overview of women suffering from erotic and intellectual melancholy in order to dispute the notion that women were barred from more cerebral and philosophical maladies. I offer examples of early modern Englishwomen who fashioned themselves as melancholy in their diaries, portraits, and letters, and outline the many ways that melancholy and lovesick women appear in literature. The following two sections, ordered chronologically, provide more detailed examinations of specific literary texts, namely Beaumont and Fletcher's *The Maid's Tragedy* (*c.*1610) and Ford's *The Broken Heart* (1633). Although both Aspatia and Penthea are influenced by the figure of Ophelia, the somatic effects of their affliction and their ability to suppress or redirect its virulence differentiate them from Shakespeare's heroine. Where Aspatia is far more knowing and manipulative in fashioning and employing her melancholy, Penthea is driven mad by her absolute self-control, a sign not of her subservience to her passions but of her self-destructive mastery of them.

HISTORICAL AND LITERARY EXAMPLES OF MELANCHOLIC WOMEN

The Renaissance is a time of renewed interest in the figure of the lovesick woman in literature and art. The humanist revival of ancient literature brought a number of lovesick women to the fore (such as Sappho, Phaedra, and Medea),[6] and female-voiced complaint poems also became increasingly popular genre during this time.[7] The shift in the artistic depiction of Mary Magdalen also reflects this interest; whereas earlier paintings and sculptures frequently depict her in relation to her saintly life (as an Apostle of Christ, or as Christ's companion),

---

[6] Wack, *Lovesickness*, 176.   [7] See Kerrigan, *Motives of Woe*.

the most pervasive image of Mary Magdalen during the sixteenth and seventeenth centuries represents her as the lovesick weeper, lamenting Christ's death.[8] The developing artistic interest in the figure of the lovesick woman was accompanied by a shift in the medical construction of lovesickness as a physiological disorder. A new aetiology posited an excess of seed as a possible cause of lovesickness, making it a disease of the genitals, as well as one of the liver and mind. Seed (or sperm) was thought to be produced by both men and women, but was of particular importance in women's physiology. As Wack writes, 'Once connected directly to pathology of the sexual organs, lovesickness may have then become "visible" as a disease of women, since women's ailments received special notice insofar as they were related to sexual physiology.'[9] Illnesses of the female reproductive tract, such as green sickness and the suffocation of the mother (or hysteria), were already well known, and once they shared an aetiology, aspects of these could be employed to explain female lovesickness. However, lovesickness's shared aetiology with green sickness and hysteria has encouraged the critical fallacy that female lovesickness is a purely physiological disorder, either because all three diseases are perceived to be synonymous, or because their common medical cause is thought to imply the same dominant characteristics; it has also contributed to the belief that the discourse of melancholy excludes women.

A number of studies have either stated or implied that women almost never suffered from melancholy, reinforcing the idea that male and female lovesickness are separate illnesses with distinct aetiologies and cultural meanings. Vieda Skultans writes that cerebral melancholy 'curiously bypassed women', while in her analysis of melancholy and its role in the formation of masculine identity, Lynn Enterline consistently takes the male gender of the melancholic sufferer for granted.[10] Even Elaine

---

[8] Haskins, *Magdalen*, 229–96. Burton treats religious melancholy in the third partition of his *Anatomy*, regarding it as a species of lovesickness. Some of the spiritual, ennobling aspects of early modern female lovesickness are clearly influenced by the medieval tradition of the female mystic, whose yearning for Christ is expressed through the language of love in a manner that is highly erotic. Voaden argues that during this liminal moment, the female mystic 'has achieved a position of power in a culture which habitually denies power to women ... she is watched, she is listened to, she exploits her significance' ('Medieval Erotic Vision', 80). See also see Bynum, *Holy Feast*.

[9] Wack, *Lovesickness*, 175.

[10] Skultans, *English Madness*, 81; Enterline, *Narcissus*, 7.

Showalter, who rightly identifies the existence of female melancholy in the period, nonetheless supports the view that Renaissance women were excluded from the forms of melancholy associated with intellectual and imaginative genius, arguing that 'Women's melancholy was seen instead as biological, and emotional in origins'.[11] And Juliana Schiesari, in her influential study *The Gendering of Melancholia*, regards the melancholy tradition, from Ficino to Freud, as a specific representational form of male creativity, which converts feelings of disempowerment into a privileged artefact; in the 'rare cases' when women suffer from melancholy, she writes, 'they appear more affected by its negative or pathological effects'.[12] However, while Schiesari is right to point out the gender asymmetry in the *discourse* of melancholia, it is important not to confuse textual discourse with historical practice since '[f]ew prescriptions of behaviour, including those organized by gender ideology, enforce absolute conformity or even obtain universal assent'.[13] The androcentric discourse of melancholy was readily appropriated by early modern women eager to enjoy the positive social and cultural connotations that attached to melancholic display.

Historical examples demonstrate that melancholy was not an exclusively male domain. The dress, language, and posture associated with melancholy were available to women both as a form of expression and a means of self-fashioning. Nor were women confined to purely negative or pathological forms of melancholy; rather, women could self-consciously fashion themselves as melancholic to exhibit their elevated social status and intellectual disposition. The medical notes of Dr Richard Napier suggest that social rank, rather than gender, was the most distinguishing aspect of melancholy in early modern England.[14] Napier's notes also affirm that women were susceptible to the type of melancholy believed to be the direct result of excessive study; Napier lists at least twelve women whose melancholy was caused by 'overmuch

[11] Showalter, 'Representing Ophelia', 81.
[12] Schiesari, *Gendering of Melancholia*, 14. Schiesari argues that 'the discourse of melancholy legitimates that neurosis as culturally acceptable for particular men, whose eros is then defined in terms of a literary production based on the appropriation of sense of lack, while the viability of such appropriation seems systematically to elude women'. In contrast to melancholy, Schiesari posits mourning as the neglected, and less narcissistic, form of female grief (pp. 2–3, 14–15).
[13] Lamb, *Gender and Authorship*, 4.
[14] MacDonald, *Mystical Bedlam*, 152–3, 243.

learning'.[15] Further examples from the period are not difficult to find. Elizabeth of Bohemia is described in complimentary terms by the French ambassador as being 'very gentle, rather melancholy than gay', and Lucy Hutchinson explains how her scholarly absorption in books engendered in her a 'melancholly negligence both of her selfe and others'.[16] Lady Anne Clifford describes herself and her aunt, the Countess of Warwick, as melancholy in her diaries.[17] And poems or songs could be dedicated to women as expressions of, or means of alleviating, their melancholy; Robert Tofte, for example, dedicates his 'Laura' to Lucy Percy in 1597, urging her to accept his poems in order to drive away 'That selfe-pleasing, yet ill easing humour of never glad melancholie'.[18] Moreover, women writers could employ melancholy as a means of legitimating their entry into print. Helen Hackett has shown how Mary Wroth appropriates a discourse of heroic melancholy usually thought to be male; in *Urania*, 'Pamphilia's melancholy is of the heroic kind more usually attributed to men', which is used to stress 'her self-control in adversity and its fruits in writing and self-certainty'.[19] And Margaret Hannay has shown how Mary Sidney used her position as the melancholic mourner for her brother to authorize much of her literary work.[20]

For high-ranking women, melancholy provided a compelling discourse of interiority, through which they could express feelings of lovesickness, loneliness, or alienation. Often when such aristocratic women reveal their melancholy, they do so in a way that simultaneously advertises their learning and their understanding of elite cultural codes. Queen Elizabeth, for example, describes herself as melancholic to Francis Duke of Anjou during their courtship. In a letter dated 4 May 1582, she displays her scholarly knowledge of the forms and effects of the disease, cataloguing some of the more fanciful effects of melancholy as listed in Laurentius' *A Discourse of the Preservation of the Sight*, whilst suggesting that the Duke's absence makes her feel 'not of this world'.[21] Whereas Elizabeth positions her own sense

[15] Ibid. 186. See also King, 'Learned Women', in *Women of the Renaissance*, 194–218.
[16] Marshall, *Winter Queen*, 23; Hutchinson, *Memoirs,* 31.
[17] Clifford, *Diaries*, ed. Clifford, 27, 59, 76.
[18] Tofte, 'Laura', in *Poetry of Robert Tofte*, ed. Nelson, 3.
[19] Hackett, 'Mary Wroth's *Urania*', 68, 83.   [20] See Hannay, *Philip's Phoenix*.
[21] *Letters of Queen Elizabeth I*, ed. Harrison, 152. Also see Doran, *Monarchy and Matrimony*.

of emotional detachment within a medical context, Dorothy Osborne (1627–95) draws upon the strand of melancholy popularized by Petrarchan poetry when depicting herself as melancholic in her letters to her future husband, Sir William Temple. In 'Letter 24' written in 1653, she depicts herself in the posture typical of a melancholic lover: 'When I have supped, I go into the garden, and so to the side of a small river that runs by it, where I sit down and wish you with me … I sit there sometimes till I am lost with thinking.'[22] And in her *True Relation of my Birth, Breeding and Life*, Margaret Cavendish, first Duchess of Newcastle (1623–73), differentiates being 'crabbed or peevishly melancholy' from her own intellectual form of the distemper, which she classifies as 'solitary and contemplating melancholy':

For I being addicted from my childhood to contemplation rather than conversation, to solitariness rather than society, to melancholy rather than mirth, to write with the pen then to work with the needle, passing my time with harmless fancies (their company being pleasing, their conversation innocent), in which I take such pleasure as I neglect my health.[23]

For Cavendish, who wrote prolifically and 'expected the world to take her writings seriously', melancholy is part of a wider discourse of establishing herself as an intelligent woman and a writer associated with her introspective nature and bookishness: it is born from her love of contemplation and goes hand in hand with 'elevated thoughts'.[24]

The portrait of Lucy Harrington, Countess of Bedford at Woburn Abbey, by Honthorst (Fig. 4), depicts Bedford in the classic pose of the melancholic, dressed in black, and seated with her head resting gently on her hand. Her posture can be compared to the image of *Democritus* on the 1632 frontispiece of *The Anatomy of Melancholy* (Fig. 5); Burton describes how

Albertus Durer paints melancholy, like a sad woman leaning on her arme with fixed lookes, neglected habit &c. … of a deepe reach, excellent apprehension, judicious, wise and witty: for I am of that Noblemans mind, *Melancholy advanceth mens conceits, more then any humour whatsoever*, improves their meditations more then any strong drinke or sacke.[25]

---

[22] Osborne, *Letters of Dorothy Osborne*, 69, 102. See also pp. 49, 68, 141–2, 146, 175.
[23] Cavendish, *True Relation*, 94–6.
[24] Graham *et al.* (eds.), *Her Own Life*, 87; Cavendish, *True Relation*, 95–6.
[25] Burton, *Anatomy*, i.391.

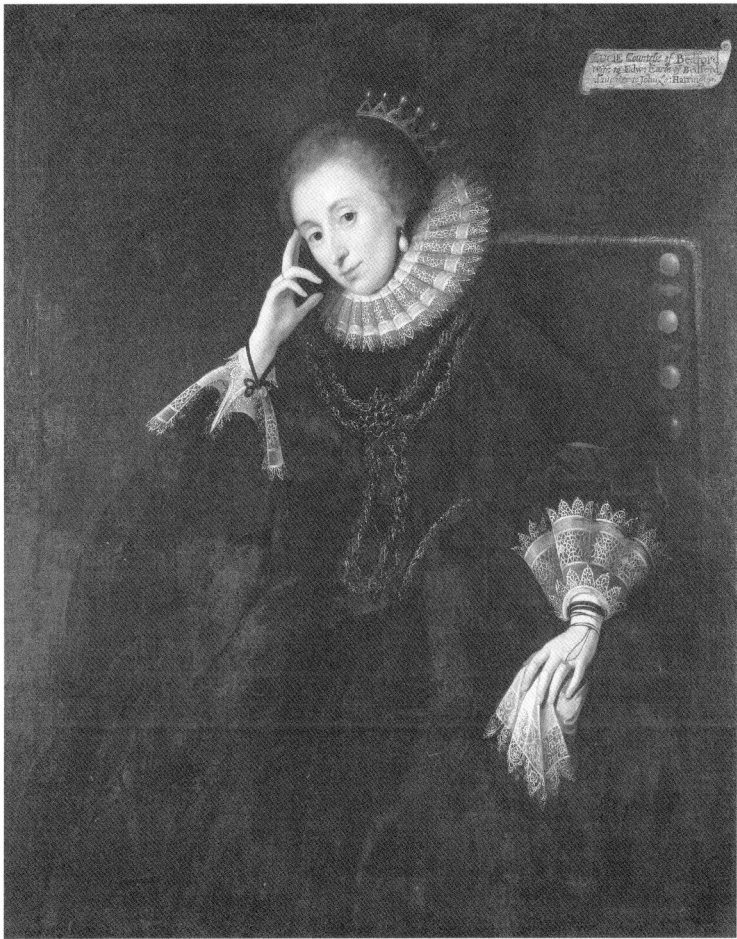

Fig. 4. Gerard van Honthorst, *Lucy Harrington, 3rd Countess of Bedford* (*c*.1620).

Burton associates Bedford's pose with intelligence and contemplation, a posture that would be appropriate for an educated woman, indicating her elite social status and her literary pretensions.[26] Clearly, Bedford's identity as a woman neither precluded her from participating in melancholic self-fashioning, nor prevented her from enjoying the

---

[26] See Lewalski, 'Lucy', 60–1.

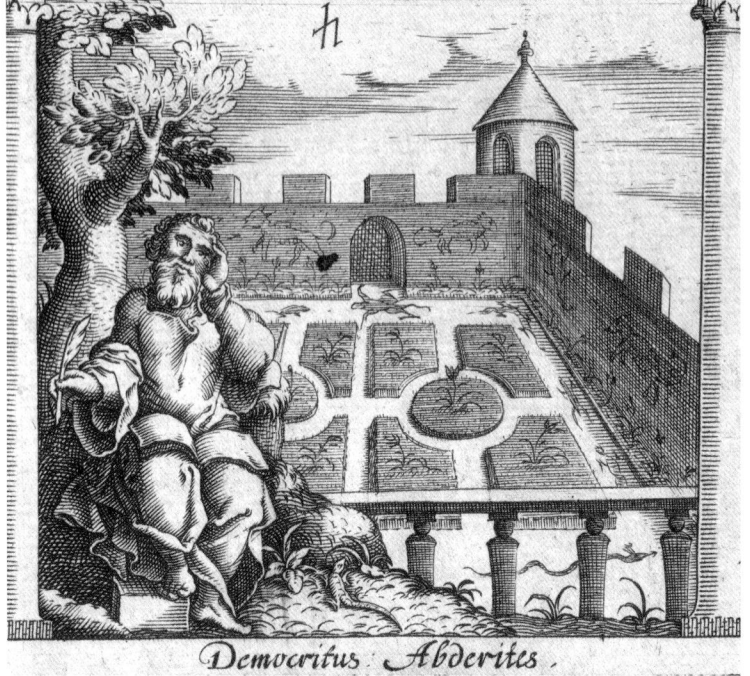

Fig. 5. *Democritus*, detail from the frontispiece of Robert Burton's *The Anatomy of Melancholy* (1628).

positive social and cultural connotations attached to such display. John Dowland, perhaps recognizing Bedford's melancholic self-fashioning, dedicates to her his *Second Booke of Songes or Ayres* (1600), music which takes melancholy as its subject.[27] Paintings of lovesick women could also employ images associated with melancholic contemplation. The genre painting, *Elegantly Dressed Young Woman* (Fig. 6) attributed to Simon Kick from the 1630s depicts a woman dressed in black, her head gently resting on her right hand, while her left hand holds a lemon. The painting in the background, of a boat in a storm, indicates her tempest-tossed mind, but her posture is composed and her expression serene. The lemon the woman holds in her hand hints at the cause of

---

[27] Holman, *Dowland: Lachrimae*, 50–2. See also Poulton, *John Dowland*, 76–8.

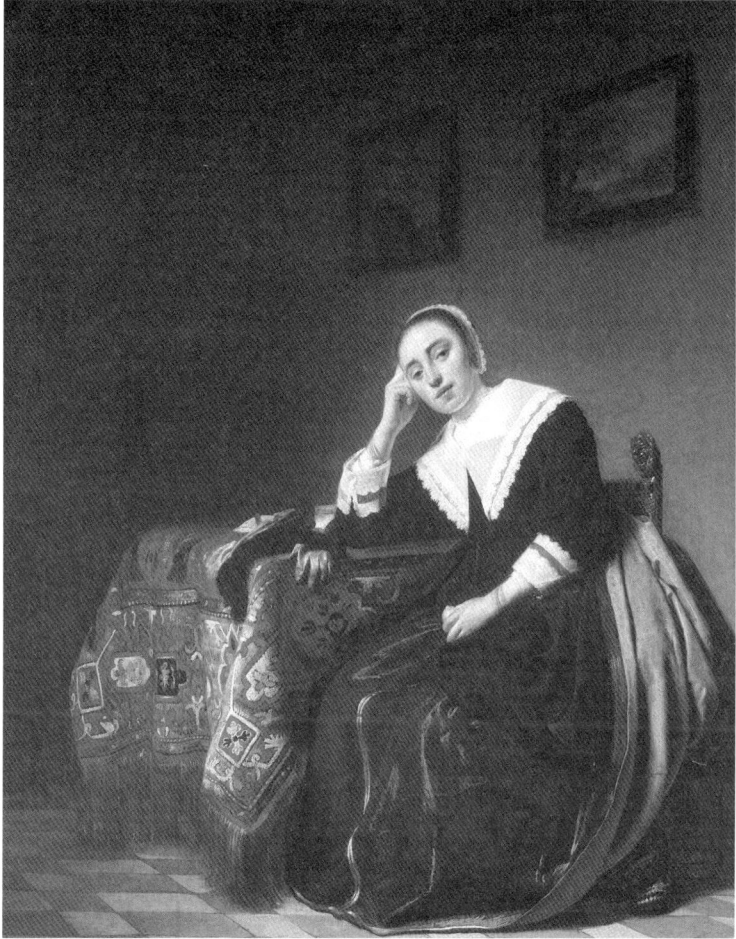

Fig. 6. Attributed to Simon Kick, *Lady Seated at a Table* (*c*.1630).

her distemper. Lemons could represent 'God's blessing' or 'false friend-ship', but the best-known interpretation for them was found in Alciati's *Emblemaa cum commentariis* (1621): 'These golden fruits belong to Venus: the sweet bitterness | Tells us that. Even so is love *glukupikros* [bitter-sweet] for the Greeks'.[28]

---

[28] Alciati, *Emblemata*, 221.

In early modern literary texts female characters are represented as melancholic in a variety of ways, challenging the widespread critical view that melancholy 'curiously bypassed women' in the Renaissance.[29] At the negative end of the spectrum, women's melancholy is sometimes depicted as a debilitating, bodily illness, suggesting that a woman is irrational, malicious, or hypocritical. In Marmion's *Hollands Leaguer* (1631), for example, Triplaena's melancholy is depicted as a case of spiteful bad temper, and in John Marston's *The Dutch Courtesan* (1605) Franchischina's malady is associated with her malevolence.[30] However, such depictions are not exclusive to women, nor is this the primary way in which female melancholic characters are represented. Most literary texts represent female melancholy as having an emotional and cerebral basis, and in some cases the tendency to equate melancholy with green sickness is exposed as reductive. In Chapman's *Monsieur D'Olive* (1606), for example, Euryone's 'maiden melancholy' originates 'in [her] minde', and in Brome's *The Sparagus Garden* (1635) Annabell is 'in bodily health . . . but very sad and much disconsolate' while melancholy.[31] Alternatively, Shirley's *St. Patrick for Ireland* (1640) derides the propensity to assign an erotic origin to all female complaints. Emeria, who has been raped by Prince Corybreus, experiences a virulent melancholy that

[29] Skultans, *English Madness*, 81. There are a number of melancholic female characters in early modern literary texts. Among those who are described as melancholy, but are not discussed in this study are: Julia and Silvia in Shakespeare's *The Two Gentlemen of Verona* (*c.*1588); Bel-imperia in Kyd's *The Spanish Tragedy* (1592); Dido in Marlowe's *Dido Queene of Carthage* (1594); Florila in Chapman's *A Humerous Dayes Myrth* (1597); Fallace in Jonson's *Every Man Out of his Humour* (1599); Olivia in Shakespeare's *Twelfth Night* (*c.*1601); Isabella in *The Wit of a Woman* (1604); Constantia in Barry's *Ram-Alley* (1610); Leonora in Webster's *The Devils Law-Case* (*c.*1610); Leucothoe in May's *The Heire* (*c.*1620); Pecunia in Jonson's *The Staple of Newes* (1626); Sophia in Massinger's *The Picture a Tragae Comaedie* (1629); Cleona in Shirley's *The Gratefull Servant* (1629); Lady Frampul in Jonson's *The New Inne* (1631); Carintha in Shirley's *The Humorous Courtier* (*c.*1631); Sybill in Knevet's *Rhodon and Iris* (1631); Eubella in Shirley's *Loves Crueltie* (1631); Constantina in Hausted's *The Rivall Friends* (1632); Valeria in Marmion's *A Fine Companion* (1632); Luce in Heywood's *The Wise-woman of Hogsdon* (*c.*1632); Rosomond in Shirley's *The Ball* (1632); Gynecia in Shirley's *The Arcadia* (*c.*1632); Horner's Neece in Shirley's *The Constant Maid* (*c.*1632–40); Julia in Ford's *Love's Sacrifice* (1633); Eugenia in Shirley's *The Bird in a Cage* (1633); Leonora and Violante in Shirley's *The Gamester* (1633); Rosinda in Shirley's *The Young Admirall* (1633); Aretina in Shirley's *The Lady of Pleasure* (1635); Aglaura in Suckling's *Aglaura* (1637); and the Bride in Nabbes's *The Bride* (1638).

[30] See also Brome's *Northern Lasse* (1632) where the widow Fitchow employs melancholy to achieve a position of dominance in her marriage (sigs. C2ʳ–C2ᵛ).

[31] Chapman, *Monsieur D'Olive*, sig. C2ʳ; Brome, *The Sparagus Garden*, sig. Hʳ.

the Bard assumes to be the consequence of sexual frustration.[32] However, far from signalling a need for sex, Emeria's discontent indicates her resistance to the lustful Prince whom she eventually kills in retribution.

The representation of lovesickness as a destructive malady with sexual origins is not exclusive to women: men's melancholy could also be depicted, in medical texts and literature, as a passionate affliction arising from sexual frustration. Nor is it true, as Rousseau claims, that men's disappointments in love were 'rarely, if ever, linked to pathology of the sexual organs'.[33] Pent-up seed was believed to be a cause of lovesickness in men and also women, and sex was prescribed as a cure for both.[34] Men's melancholy could also have derogatory associations, conveying effeminacy, machiavellianism, madness, or the spiritual disquiet which arises from a guilty conscience. Melancholic men are sometimes accused of being emasculated by their passions, but the distemper is more frequently depicted as being the natural consequence of sin. In Kyd's *The Spanish Tragedy* (1592), for example, Hieronimo describes melancholy as an essential ingredient of the psychological make-up of the murderer, who travels from a 'guilty conscience' through 'melancholy thoughts' to 'dispaire and death'.[35] Following Kyd's example, malcontents such as Don John in Shakespeare's *Much Ado About Nothing* (1598–9), Flamineo in Webster's *The White Devil* (*c*.1611), and Orestes in Goffe's *The Tragedy of Orestes* (1632) are all described as melancholic. And in Thomas Nabbes's *Microcosmus: A Morall Maske* (1637) the character Melancholy is predisposed to vindictive machinations: 'I could hatch a conspiracy', he boasts, that would 'cause posterity attribute all Matchiavillianisme to Melancholy'.[36]

Far from being ennobled by their malaise, many male characters are beset by a destructive form of erotic melancholy, thought by critics to typify the female version of the illness, in which they weep, rave, and babble incoherently. For example, in Harding's *Sicily and Naples* (1640) the King becomes irrational and incoherent when lovesick; Piero observes, 'I have seen him weep | Like a fond mother o'er her

---

[32] Shirley, *St. Patrick*, IV.i.57–74.   [33] Rousseau, 'Strange Pathology', 113–14.
[34] See Chs. 1 and 5.   [35] Kyd, *The Spanish Tragedy*, III.xi.14, 17, 19.
[36] Nabbes, *Microcosmus*, D[r]. At times characters in plays misinterpret an individual's melancholy as a sign of his or her guilt. See, for example, S.S.'s *Honest Lawyer* (1616) in which Griffen incorrectly assumes that Benjamin's 'ghastly melancholy points him out for the murderer' (sig. H1[r]).

tender babe…Then rave, and curse, talk as he wanted reason | To guide his speech's organ'.[37] And in Massinger's *The Emperour of the East* Thedosius' 'melancholy fit' is described by Chrysapius in similar terms:

> wee might heare him gnash
> His teeth in rage, which opend, hollow grones
> And murmurs issu'd from his lippes, like windes
> Imprison'd in the cavernes of the earth
> Striving for liberty; and sometimes throwing
> His body on his bed, then on the ground,
> And with such violence, that wee more then fear'd
> And still doe, if the tempest of his passions
> By your wisdome bee not lay'd, hee will commit
> Some outrage on himselfe.[38]

Far from being cerebral or contemplative, Thedosius' melancholy resembles a hysterical fit: he groans, gnashes his teeth, has difficulty breathing and speaking, and moves in a violent, uncontrollable manner.

Just as representations of melancholic men can fall into a paradigm of behaviour usually associated by modern critics with female forms of the distemper, female characters are often depicted as suffering from types of melancholy that are often thought to be exclusively male. In Ford's *The Lover's Melancholy*, for example, Eroclea adopts many of the features of melancholic self-fashioning found in Nicholas Hilliard's portrait of the *Man Among the Flowers* while cross-dressed as 'Parthenophill': she seeks isolation in 'silent groves' with only a lute.[39] Similarly, in Peaps's *Love, In it's Extasie* (1649), Desdonella stays 'in a Cave' with her 'melancholy Lute' during her feigned death.[40] And in Knevet's *Rhodon and Iris* Eglantine is 'A perfect Map of mellancholy': 'shee's out of love with all society', playing 'melancholly notes' on her lute in order 'to slake | Those furious flames that scorch [her] tender heart'.[41] Such behaviour became a recognizable code that women could employ to express their lovesickness; so that when Eudora retires 'into her orchard' in Chapman's *The Widow's Teares* (1612), it is interpreted as 'A pregnant badge of love'

---

[37] Harding, *Sicily and Naples*, 62. See also Martino in Beaumont and Fletcher's *A Very Woman* and the Passionate Lord in Beaumont and Fletcher's *The Nice Valour*.
[38] Massinger, *Emperour of the East*, in *The Plays and Poems of Philip Massinger*, ed. Philip Edwards and Colin A. Gibson, 5 vols. (Oxford, 1976), vol. iii, V.ii.11–20.
[39] Ford, *Lover's Melancholy*, I.i.105.
[40] [Peaps], *Love in it's Extasie*, sig. [B4ᵛ].   [41] Knevet, *Rhodon and Iris*, sig. [B4ᵛ].

suggesting that 'shee's melancholy'.[42] Similarly, in Manuche's *The Loyal Lovers* (1652) Apfia is able to read Letesia's emotional state through her stance: 'This is the third time | I have taken you alone in melancholy postures', she tells her, 'Venus grant you are not in love'.[43]

Sabina, in Chamberlain's *The Swaggering Damsell* (1640), enjoys the bittersweet pleasure of her malady. 'Love', Sabina tells her maid Betty, is 'a pretty pleasant vexation'. The exchange between the two women clarifies the extent to which Sabina cultivates, and relishes, her 'extreame melancholy':

SABINA: Prethee *Betty* helpe me to cosen the time a little with some pretty love Song.
BETTY: That will but make yee the more melancholy forsooth.
SABINA: Though it doe, yet me thinkes I love it dearely.
BETTY: Me thought yee said ye were afraid of being melancholy but now forsooth?
SABINA: I did so, and so I am, and yet I love it.
BETTY: I had heard 'em say forsooth, that melancholy people are like Spaniells.
SABINA: Why prethee?
BETTY: They say a Spaniell, the more a man beates him the more he fawnes upon him; so melancholy people, me thinkes, the more the humor torments 'em the more they love it.
SABINA: Tis very true, come reach me my Lute.[44]

Betty articulates the paradoxical nature of melancholy that is both an illness to be shunned and a refined state of contemplation to be cultivated; Sabina is both 'afraid of being melancholy' and 'love[s] it dearly', singing 'some pretty love Song' to prolong her malaise. Here, melancholy is given a class distinction rather than one based on gender: it is Sabina who cultivates the distemper and her lady servant who is baffled by it.

A woman's melancholy can also be described as a sign of her reason and self-possession, as in the depiction of Calantha's melancholy in Harding's *Sicily and Naples*. Calantha, who becomes melancholic after her father is killed and her troops are vanquished, is able to command 'the people of her breast' as well as of her country. Piero describes her melancholy in positive terms:

[42] Chap[man], *The Widow's Tears*, II.iii.35–6.
[43] Manuche, *Loyal Lovers*, 10, 9.
[44] C[hamberlain], *Swaggering Damsell*, sigs. D2ʳ, D2ᵛ.

> she talks so prettily
> Clothes griefs in such a sad and pious garb,
> So void of any rudeness, that we see
> Composedness in distraction, reason in madness.[45]

Calantha's madness is described as 'pretty', but unlike Ophelia's insanity, her aesthetic appeal cannot be linked to sexualized language or behaviour. Instead she 'clothes griefs in . . . a sad and pious garb', a description that suggests that she appears not with loose hair and dishevelled clothing, but wearing the traditional black clothing of the melancholic as befits her 'reason in madness'. Roberts believes that she is similar to Ford's Calantha in *The Broken Heart*, arguing that both 'embody an ideal of strength, and more particularly, of reason'.[46]

Women's melancholy could also be represented as spiritually gratifying. In Jonson's *The Case is Altered* (1609), for example, Phoenixella suggests that her melancholy is not without its rewards:

> Although perhaps unto a general eye
> I may appear most wedded to my griefs,
> Yet my mid forsake no taste of pleasure,
> I mean that happy pleasure of the soul,
> Devine and sacred contemplation.[47]

And in Heywood's pastoral play *Amphrisa, or the Forsaken Shepheardesse* (1597), a woman's melancholy is associated with her artistic skill. Amphrisa, 'the wisest shepheardesse | That lives in . . . Arcadia', becomes melancholic after she is abandoned by her lover. Alope presents her with a willow wreath to alleviate her suffering, explaining that if 'this charm'd circle' is worn, 'All th' Arcadian Swains & Nymphs . . . Will take note of his falshood, and your faith'. Here, the adoption of standard emblems of the forsaken lover allows Amphrisa to articulate her plight visually: the willow wreath signals her abandonment, suggesting her 'innocence, and his inconstancie', and enables her to regain control over her emotions; 'from this houre,' she declares, 'Hearts griefe nor heads pain shall of me have power. | I now have chac'd hence sorrow'.[48] The Queen, who has

---

[45] Harding, *Sicily and Naples*, 62–3.
[46] Roberts, 'Introduction', in Harding, *Sicily and Naples*, 14.
[47] Jonson, *Case is Altered*, in *Complete Plays*, vol. i, II.iv.35–6. See also I.ix.45–8.
[48] Heywood, *Amphrisa*, *Dramatic Works*, vol. vi. 298, 299, 303, 304.

been eavesdropping on the shepherdess, commends her for her lyrical words and self-possession. 'Faire Virgin', she tells Amphrisa,

> I could wish
> Your Willow were a Lawrel. Nay so 'tis:
> Because all such may be styl'd Conquerors,
> That can subdue their passions.[49]

The Queen's desire to transform Amphrisa's willow into a laurel (given both to poets and to conquerors) is evocative, in that it unites Amphrisa's melancholic suffering with her poetic skill; Amphrisa's melancholy is associated with her creativity and her ability to subdue her passion. Melancholy, far from being a destructive malaise, is aligned with Amphrisa's poetic inspiration and self-control.

Literary depictions of women could draw on Neoplatonic and Petrarchan traditions, either to suggest that women possess the rational resource to govern their passions, or alternatively, to depict their lovesick passion as the celestial vision that inspires them to a heroic quest. Spenser's 'Hymn to Beauty' from *Fowre Hymnes* celebrates this construction of women; Petrarchan poetry often represents women as restraining their lovers through their chastity and rational self-control. Sidney's *Astrophil and Stella* 'depicts the man's desire controlled by the woman's reason' and in the *Canzoniere* Laura similarly resists and controls Petrarch not out of amorous indifference, but out of a desire to protect the honour of her lover and herself.[50] In the *Trionfo della Morte*, Laura's spirit returns after her death to explain to Petrarch how her aloof behaviour was the strategy she employed to temper her lover's desire. Mary Sidney Herbert translates the passage:

> Thow saw'est what was without, not what within.
> And as the brake the wanton steede doeth tame,
> So this did thee from thy disorders winne.
> A thousand times wrath in my face did flame,
> My heart meane-while with love did inlie burne,
> But never will; my reason overcame.[51]

---

[49] Ibid. vi. 304.
[50] *Collected Works of Mary Sidney Herbert*, ed. Hannay, Kinnamon, and Brennan, i.266.
[51] Herbert, *Triumph of Death* (*c*.1600), in *Collected Works*, i. 280.

Like a skilful rider Laura is able to 'brake' and 'tame' her fiery passions as well as those of her lover; her chilly exterior does not signify her indifference, but is rather the result of her moral fortitude. John Lyly's *Sappho and Phao* similarly features a woman who is able to control her passions, offering an example of womanhood which refutes the misogynistic belief, often echoed in the play, that 'women's hearts are such stones, which, warmed by affection, cannot be cooled by wisdom'.[52] Sappho conquers not only her love for Phao, but also love itself, an accomplishment given symbolic significance in Act V when Cupid adopts Sappho as his new 'mother' (V.ii.16–17). Finding herself 'rid of the disease', Sappho proclaims: 'I myself will be the queen of love. I will direct these arrows with better aim and conquer mine own affections with greater modesty' (V.ii.28–30). By rejecting her amorous impulses Sappho establishes her rational superiority to Phao, which befits her social superiority and justifies her rule: Sappho, highly skilled in self-government, is perfectly suited to govern others.[53]

Many of the positive aspects of female melancholy are present in Cavendish and Brackley's *The Concealed Fancies* (*c*.1645), which depicts melancholy as a form of female self-authorship, signifying a woman's refined intellect and indicating her independence and power in romantic relationships. Composed around 1645 by the sisters Jane Cavendish and Elizabeth Brackley (daughters of William Cavendish, Duke of Newcastle, and stepdaughters to the prolific author Margaret Cavendish), the play is 'densely metatheatrical, full of references not only to the playing of parts in general but to particular and specific Renaissance plays'.[54] Luceny and Tattiney, the two female protagonists, also take up and transform conventional romantic languages 'in a bid

---

[52] Lyly, *Sappho and Phao*, IV.iii.98–100. Lyly's portrait of Sappho was intended as a compliment to Queen Elizabeth, before whom the play was presented. Berry, *Chastity*, 1–2.

[53] Lyly's flattering portrait of Sappho as a rational woman skilled in self-government reverses Ovid's account of Sappho found in Epistle XV of his *Heroides*, in which 'wanton' Sappho, overcome by her passions, longs not to conquer her desires but to have them fulfilled. Ovid's Phao does not reciprocate Sappho's love but rather flees to Sicily's Mount Etna in order to escape Sappho's passion, a rejection which causes Sappho to throw herself off the cliff at Leucadia. Where in Ovid's account Sappho's suffering results from Phao's refusal of her love, Lyly's Sappho is distressed by the eruption of her own passionate impulses: it is not Phao that Lyly's Sappho wishes to conquer, but herself.

[54] Hopkins, 'Judith', 399.

for self-determination'; as Dorothy Stephens argues, Cavendish and Brackley 'do not want to jettison the Petrarch tradition but . . . to woo its very confusions'.[55] In this context, melancholy is repeatedly associated with the women's attempts to gain the upper hand in their relationships, signifying both their inwardness and their sophisticated handling of discursive and social forms.

Luceny and Tattiney, both fashion themselves as melancholic. Luceny tells her sister, 'I dressed myself in a slight way of carelessness which becomes as well, if not better than a set dress', and she is quick to explicate her suitor's lovesick behaviour as a manipulative form of social posturing.[56] Even as he acts his part, Luceny unravels the social conventions of Courtley's conduct, mocking and undermining his attempts at seduction. She asks Courtley: 'Now, will not your next posture be to stand with folded arms? But that posture now grows much out of fashion. That's altered to a serious look of admiration, as if your face was so terrible as to turn men to statues' (I.iv.67–71). Tattiney similarly interrogates the sincerity of Presumption's lovesick posturing, asking him: 'Now, do you think the pulling down your hat and looking sad, shall make me believe your speech for truth?' (II.ii.20–2). Luceny and Tattiney's playful verbal sparring with their lovers hints at the power games underlying flirtation, and their fears about the ways marriage might change their lives. Luceny maintains that she will accept no 'governor' over her behaviour except her father, turning to the Bible to insist that 'man and wife should draw equally in a yoke' (II.iii.34, 37–8). She fears, however, that this will not be the case. 'My destruction', she tells her sister, 'is that when I marry Courtley I shall be condemned to look upon my nose whenever I walk' (II.iii.47–9). Luceny's solution is to remain in perpetual courtship even after marriage, making permanent the transitory phase when women are granted the upper hand (II.iii.52). Her sister feels likewise. Answering her sister's observation that 'Presumption doth throw his cloak as if he intended to govern you', Tattiney insists that marriage will not curtail her authority in her relationship with Presumption (II.iii.106–7). 'He is my servant,' she tells Luceny, 'for I intend to

---

[55] Stephens, *Limits*, 144–5, 164.
[56] Cavendish and Brackley, 'Concealed Fancies', in Cerasano and Wynne-Davies (eds.), *Drama by Women*, I.iv.6–8; all quotations taken from this edition.

be his mistress' (II.iii.112–13). Significantly, the arrangement is not reciprocal. While Tattiney expects to continue as her husband's mistress, she tells her sister that after marriage 'I hope to continue my own' (II.iii.108).

Melancholy functions within the play as the instrument and sign of a woman's self-empowerment, contributing to the discourse of sexual–political struggle that informs the romantic plot. Even after marriage, Tattiney is determined to remain 'always in my careless garb' (II.iii.148–9), imitating the habit of the melancholy scholar, whose appearance functions as a sign of his refined subjectivity and self-absorption. Presumption seems aware of just such implications, listing dress as one area which he intends to regulate after marriage. He tells Courtley, 'I mean to follify her all I can, and let her know that garb, that doth best become her, is most ill-favoured. So she shall neither look, walk, or speak, but I will be her perpetual vexation' (III.iii.10–14). Tellingly, Presumption's objection to Tattiney's chosen dress is not aesthetic, but concerns what it signifies about her intellectual and emotional independence.

After their cousin's castle, Ballamo, is besieged Luceny's and Tattiney's melancholic posturing takes on a more serious aspect. The authored stage direction, 'Enter *Luceny* and *Tattiney*, melancholy' (III.ii), suggests that they wear the traditional black apparel of the melancholic, clothing that enables the sisters to protest indirectly against their compromised political position. Their melancholy also takes on a religious dimension during this time. Luceny and Tattiney become 'nuns in melancholy', sublimating their distemper into a heightened spiritual state (III.v.22). Luceny describes the silent and lonely pleasures of her sadness:

> When I in sadness am and then do think,
> I'm lulled asleep in melancholy wink;
> Each chamber ceiling doth create true sad,
> Yet tempered so as I am quiet, glad.
> Then when I walk nuns' gallery round,
> My thoughts tell me I'm falling in a swoon,
> And when that flowers fine I have,
> Then sure I'm decked for my grave.
> So if each one will have a fine-loved death,
> Enter your self in sadness, sweeter earth;
> Then, when my quiet soul desires to walk,

The gardens do revive my tongue to talk.
So in white sheet of innocence I pray,
Each one that wishes me to see,
For ghosts do love to have their own delights
When others think they have designs of frights.
So even as they, I wish no fear to none,
But on my friends contemplate alone.

(V.ii.1–18)

Luceny describes a saddened, but peaceful state of introspection. Her soliloquy draws on general, 'masculine' traditions of melancholy (she is solitary, given to contemplation, and drawn to the garden) while also incorporating specifically female traditions (she covers herself with 'flowers fine' as if 'decked for my grave'). Despite her grief, however, Luceny is 'tempered' in her sadness, a control that transforms mere sadness to something paradoxically 'glad' and meaningful.

Eventually, the castle is liberated. Tattiney and Luceny discard their nun's clothes and embrace their lovers. Presumption, who originally thought he would be able to govern Tattiney's behaviour and dress, has long since learned that this would never earn him her hand. Suspecting his 'rigid thoughts' she rejects him, only to find that when faced with losing her he transforms himself (III.iii.113). He gives 'her leave for to be free', declaring that 'when married, my soul shall not think of wife, | For she shall be my mistress, joy of life' (III.iii.115, 118–19). The couple thus achieve, in Tattiney's words, 'an equal marriage', reinforcing Margaret Ezell's claim that 'the ideal of marriage in this drama is a companionate one, with equal respect between parties' (Epilogue, 85).[57] Cavendish and Brackley's *The Concealed Fancies* thus offers an almost straightforward example of how female melancholy could be portrayed in a positive light; for social as well as intellectual reasons, Luceny and Tattiney revel in their melancholy, finding in it their 'truer soul of glad' (V.ii.27–8). Less obviously positive, however, is the representation of Aspatia's erotic melancholy in Beaumont and Fletcher's *The Maid's Tragedy*. Although Aspatia's affliction seems to fall into the same acutely gendered category of illness as Ophelia', on closer inspection her suffering reveals itself to be far more disruptive and manipulative.

[57] Ezell, 'Pen', 290.

MASOCHISM AND REVENGE IN BEAUMONT AND FLETCHER'S *THE MAID'S TRAGEDY*

In *The Maid's Tragedy*, Beaumont and Fletcher radically recast the role of the lovesick woman. Unlike Ophelia and the Jailer's Daughter, both of whom are overwhelmed by their madness, Aspatia is conscious of her lovesickness, actively employing it to articulate her suffering and manipulate those around her. Not simply a victim of her feelings, Aspatia is aware of the tradition into which her suffering fits. Since she is restrained from other ways of enacting revenge, lovesickness furnishes her with a vocabulary through which she can express herself: it becomes a fraught form of empowerment, even as it expresses her powerlessness and leads to her death. Like Shakespeare and Fletcher's Jailer's Daughter, Aspatia resembles Shakespeare's Ophelia. However, unlike *The Two Noble Kinsmen*, *The Maid's Tragedy* involves a much more sophisticated handling of its literary precursor. In Beaumont and Fletcher's play, Aspatia is both a lovesick victim and a melancholic revenger (fusing the role of Ophelia with that of Hamlet), a position made possible because of her knowing and 'artificial' assumption of her melancholic role.[58] Acting as 'a surrogate artist', she learns to 'manipulate a fluid and contingent world with a dramatist's inventiveness and authority'.[59]

At the opening of the play, Aspatia's lovesickness is presented in conventional terms. Formerly betrothed to Amintor, Aspatia is abandoned by him when the King persuades him to marry Evadne instead. Amintor complies with the King's order, not knowing that the King has suggested the marriage to hide his own secret liaison with Evadne. Meanwhile Aspatia, abandoned and outcast, is struck with a deep melancholy; Lysippus' description of her behaviour reads like a catalogue of symptoms of lovesickness:

> this lady
> Walks discontented, with her wat'ry eyes
> Bent on the earth. The unfrequented woods

---

[58] Critics have long recognized the fact that *The Maid's Tragedy* is modelled on *Hamlet*. See e.g. Davies, 'Beaumont and Fletcher's *Hamlet*'.
[59] Kerrigan, *Revenge Tragedy*, 17.

Are her delight, and when she sees a bank
Stuck full of flowers she with a sigh will tell
Her servants what a pretty place it were
To bury lovers in, and make her maids
Pluck 'em and strow her over like a corse.
She carries with her an infectious grief,
That strikes all her beholders; she will sing
The mournfull'st things that ever ear hath heard,
And sigh, and sing again.[60]

Aspatia is here the very picture of unrequited love: she wanders through the solitary woods, with lowered, tear-filled eyes, sighing and singing mournful songs. Like Ophelia, she is drawn to the water's edge where she covers herself in flowers, transforming the flowery bank where lovers embrace into the imagined site of her own burial. However, unlike Ophelia, who actually drowns herself, Aspatia goes to the riverbank to enact a *fictional* representation of her death. Carefully crafting the scene, she selects the 'pretty place' for her burial and instructs her servants in their parts. Aspatia's staging of her own funeral is the first indication of her awareness of, and control over, her sickness; this in turn suggests a more complex relationship between her suffering and her behaviour as a lovesick woman. Her masochistic behaviour is not merely an unconscious internalization of her social and emotional powerless, but is rather part of a deliberate role she takes up in order to expose her beloved's betrayal. Aspatia self-consciously plays the part of the lovesick woman with 'an infectious grief | That strikes all her beholders'.

Aspatia's 'infectious grief' works with dramatic effect when she prepares Evadne, her rival in love, for what was originally to be her own bridal bed. In an intimate scene, which seems designed to recall the unpinning scene in *Othello* (*c.*1604), Aspatia helps Evadne undress, and sings a willow song that recounts a man's faithlessness in love. However, unlike Desdemona's willow song which ends with the woman's approval of her own abandonment—'Let nobody blame him, his scorn I approve' (IV.iii.50)—Aspatia's song lays the guilt firmly on the man's shoulders, declairing 'I dièd true. | My love was false, but I was firm, | From my hour of birth' (II.i.75–7). And where Desdemona denies Othello's guilt,

---

[60] Beaumont and Fletcher, *The Maid's Tragedy*, I.i.89–100.

attributing responsibility for her death to 'Nobody, I myself' (V.ii.133), Aspatia insists upon the wrong done to her; she asks Amintor if he will go and 'see the virgins weep, | When I am laid in earth, though you yourself | Can know no pity?' (II.i.117–19). Her melancholic words have their desired effect: Amintor feels 'Her grief shoot suddenly through all my veins' and his 'eyes run' (II.i.128, 129).

Aspatia's self-conscious manipulation of her melancholy enables her to teach others how to take up the garland of lost love. She tells Evadne:

> May no discontent
> Grow 'twixt your love and you! But if there do,
> Inquire of me and I will guide your moan,
> And teach you an artificial way to grieve,
> To keep your sorrow waking.
>
> (II.i.92–6)

Aspatia's ability to 'guide your moan' reinforces the sense that she controls her melancholy, manipulating the traditional tropes of lovesickness in order to perpetuate her sorrow; 'Thus I wind myself | Into this willow garland', she tells Amintor (II.i.119–20). By perpetuating her grief in this way, Aspatia imitates the self-destructive behaviour of the revenger, who dwells upon the wrongs done to him or her to resist the natural process through which pain fades and wounds heal. As Francis Bacon observes, 'a Man that studieth *Revenge*, keepes his owne Wounds greene, which otherwise would heale and doe well'. Bacon regards this as a pointless and self-destructive exercise: 'That which is past is gone, and irrevocable; and wise men have enough to do with things present and to come; therefore they do but trifle with themselves, that labour in past matter.'[61] Freud, on the other hand, suggests that such a 'compulsion to repeat' can have subtle psychological benefits; like children who master frightening experiences by repeating them in games, so too do revengers re-enact a painful moment of loss as a means of rewriting it (in which they move from being victims of crimes to their perpetrators).[62] Like Bacon's revenger, Aspatia pours salt into her emotional wounds, keeping a painful past alive by recollecting and repeating it. Her grief is thus 'artificial', not in the sense that it is false or insincere, but rather because

---

[61] Bacon, 'Of Revenge', in *Essayes*, 17.
[62] Freud, 'Mourning and Melancholia', in *Complete Psychological Works*, xiv. 244–53.

it is aesthetically inventive and deliberately fostered; it is something that is 'made by ... art', 'brought about by constructive skill'.[63] She expresses her sorrow, not to purge her grief, but to 'keep ... sorrow waking'.[64]

Aspatia's artistic continuation of her grief is depicted when she teaches the art of lovesickness to her gentlewomen, Olympias and the appropriately named Antiphila. Like a tutor in a school for melancholy, Aspatia directs her women to perform their melancholy in their posture and expression, commending Olympias's 'downcast ... eye' which 'Shows a fine sorrow' and likening her to Oenone and Dido (II.ii.28, 29). Aspatia also directs Antiphila in a piece of needlework that represents Ariadne, who was abandoned by Theseus on the island of Naxos after she had helped him find his way out of the Cretan labyrinth. Her action recalls the trope whereby a rejected or violated woman turns to an artistic representation as a means of expressing pain or achieving consolation, generally through sympathetic identification and ecphrasis. Like Lucrece in Shakespeare's *The Rape of Lucrece* (1594), who gazes upon the painting of Troy to 'Los[e] her woes in shows of discontent', Aspatia reads her pain in this embroidery as well as in her servants' performance of her grief. Nevertheless, Aspatia's relation to the embroidery once again suggests her self-conscious artistry. Unlike Lucrece who looks at the image of Hecuba 'And shapes her sorrow to the beldame's woes', Aspatia instead sees herself as the paradigm of lovesickness, the model that all other literary representations must follow.[65]

Aspatia tells Antiphila that she is 'much mistaken' in her representation of Ariadne (II.ii.62):

> These colours are not dull and pale enough
> To show a soul so full of misery
> As this sad Ladies was. Do it by me;
> Doe it again by me, the lost Aspatia,
> And you shall find all true but the wild island.
> And think I stand upon the sea-beach now,

---

[63] *Oxford English Dictionary* (Oxford, 1987).

[64] Her behaviour differentiates her from a writer like Robert Burton whose study of melancholy acts as a form of therapy, as he admits: 'I write of Melancholy ... to avoid Melancholy'. Burton, 'Democritus to the Reader', in *Anatomy*, i.6.

[65] Shakespeare, *Rape of Lucrece*, ll. 1580, 1458.

> Mine arms thus, and mine hair blown with the wind,
> Wilde as that desert . . .
>
> .   .   .   .
>
>   —Look, look, wenches,
> A miserable life of this poor picture!
>
>   (II.ii.63–70, 77–8)

Aspatia draws attention to her confident mastery of the look and posture of erotic melancholy. Her arms, we assume, are crossed in the traditional lovesick posture, and her wild hair, which might at first reflect her lack of control, is instead revealed to be yet another aspect of her melancholic self-fashioning. Aspatia also rewrites the embroidered depiction of Theseus. As in her willow song, she resists traditional paradigms that allow men to escape retribution for their faithlessness. Learning that Theseus was able to navigate his ship to safety successfully after deserting Ariadne, Aspatia warns the embroidered Theseus 'you shall not go so', instructing Antiphila to add to her needlework the image of 'a quicksand, | And over it a shallow smiling water | And his ship ploughing it' (II.ii.53, 54–5). ''Twill wrong the story', Antiphila protests. ''Twill make the story', Aspatia asserts, since it has been 'wronged by wanton Poets' (II.ii.56, 57). She demands that the embroidery be changed, transforming 'her safe, feminine, domestic craft – weaving – into art as a new means of resistance'.[66]

Aspatia is thus not only instructing women in the art of melancholy, but is also teaching them 'The truth of maids and perjuries of men' (II.i.107). Melancholy, rather than being linked to helplessness, functions, as Ronald Huebert argues, as 'a cry of protest against a social order and a masculine world that expects and condones only stereotypical female behaviour'.[67] Aspatia instructs her women to 'credit anything the light gives life to | Before a man' and to become 'new married' to their grief, resisting the notion that women are simply passive objects who receive their identity from men (II.ii.16–17, 3). Thus, when Aspatia challenges Olympias that 'thou hast an easy temper, fit for stamp', she is challenging her gentlewoman to harden herself, and her heart, against the sexual and psychological imprint of a man (II.ii.12). Aspatia

---

[66] Klindienst makes this comment about Philomela. See 'Voice of the Shuttle is Ours', 26.

[67] Huebert, 'An Artificial Way to Grieve', 601.

longs to look like 'sorrow's monument' and will stand 'till some more pitying god | Turn[s] her to marble' (II.ii.74, 38–9). Her fixed sorrow emphasizes the firmness of her love in relation to men's affections, which are depicted in the play as turning easily from one love to the next, reversing the cultural cliché, expressed in *The Rape of Lucrece*, that 'men have marble, women waxen minds, | And therefore are they formed as marble will'.[68]

Aspatia's lovesick complaints also have a wider political significance within the play, as her personal unhappiness is the direct result of the King's tyrannous behaviour and sexual misconduct; as Sandra Clark observes, 'the ruler's attempts to enforce absolutist principles are expressed in sexual terms'.[69] Although Amintor was not compelled to break off his engagement with Aspatia (he himself admits 'It was the King first moved me to't, but he | Has not my will in keeping'), he does so at the request of the King, who wants him to marry Evadne so that his own affair with her will remain hidden (II.i.130–1). Amintor's betrayal of Aspatia thus reflects a larger crisis at court, and his rejected lover's subsequent melancholy simultaneously signals her political dissatisfaction, reminding the court not only of Amintor's bad behaviour but also of the King's (and thus fuelling the wider political sedition). Certainly Calianax's disillusionment with his monarch springs from his anger at his daughter's mistreatment, and he eventually aids the rebellion against the King.

Aspatia's control of her malady, her role as a revenger and 'surrogate artist', and her resistance to the process of time that might heal her wounds are all brought to a climax in her carefully crafted death. Intent on finding 'Some yet unpractised way to grieve and die', Aspatia goes to Amintor disguised as her own brother and challenges him to fight (II.i.124). Aspatia's suicide is transformed into a perverse form of erotic fulfilment: 'love, the symbol of regeneration, becomes inextricably linked with destruction, as death becomes the consummation of love.'[70] Aspatia's erotic desires are redirected into masochistic urges; she spreads her arms, welcoming Amintor's blows as if they were caresses (V.iii.102). And despite her claim that 'Those threats I brought with me sought

---

[68] Shakespeare, *Rape of Lucrece*, 1240–1.
[69] Sandra Clark, *Sexual Themes*, 103.
[70] Norland, 'Introduction', in Beaumont and Fletcher, *Maid's Tragedy*, ed. Norland, p. xvii.

not revenge, | But came to fetch this blessing from thy hand', Aspatia is nevertheless successful in achieving a perverse form of retribution (V.iii.205–6). She effectively reminds Amintor of the 'baseness of the injuries you did Aspatia', and prompts him to kill her, an action which contributes to his suicide (V.iii.56). Aspatia lives to hear Amintor repent his betrayal of her, and dies in his arms.

Beaumont and Fletcher's *The Maid's Tragedy* offers just one example of how representations of lovesickness in early modern literature are more complex than has been suggested by conventional critical paradigms of gender and illness. Aspatia's ability to exert a degree of control over the symptoms of her malady differentiates her from Ophelia, and subtly renegotiates the interplay of gender, authority, and sickness apparent in Shakespeare's text. Lovesickness provides Aspatia with a subtle vocabulary of complaint, enabling her to criticize her lover and the monarch while simultaneously conforming to a highly conventional female role: she is both the faithful, devoted mistress and the angry avenger. Her artistic reworkings provide a proto-feminist commentary on the misogynistic cultural tradition from which she derives, revealing how lovesickness can operate as a complex strategy for self-assertion.

'DIVORCE BETWIXT MY BODY AND MY HEART': STARVATION IN FORD'S *THE BROKEN HEART*

Beaumont and Fletcher's portrayal of Aspatia suggests that, in certain circumstances, the lovesick woman is able to control and even exploit her malady. This sense of wilful manipulation is reinforced in John Ford's *The Broken Heart*, where Penthea's madness is caused, not by an ungovernable passion, but by her mastery over her appetites and desires. *The Broken Heart*, as the title suggests, is concerned with the consequences of thwarted love. Before the play begins, Ithocles has forced his sister Penthea to marry Bassanes, a jealous older man, rather than her beloved Orgilus, with whom she had a precontract of marriage. Penthea and Orgilus would have married had not Thrasus, Penthea's father, died, and Ithocles taken control of his sister's marriage in order to further his own ambition. The result is that all three are miserable: Penthea is trapped in an unhappy marriage, Orgilus is in love with Penthea (whom he still considers his wife), and Bassanes is consumed with jealousy, believing that Penthea will eventually have an affair with her former betrothed. Orgilus, whose 'griefs are violent', thus asks for his father's consent to leave Sparta and go to Athens on a 'voluntary exile' to 'take off the cares | Of jealous Bassanes . . . To free Penthea from a hell on earth . . . Lastly, to lose the memory of something | Her presence makes to live in me afresh' (I.i.71, 77, 78–82). Despite this, however, Orgilus does not go to Athens, but disguises himself as a scholar, Aplotes, in order to watch over his former lover.

Orgilus' first meeting with Penthea since her marriage emphasizes the different ways that the pair are handling their unhappy situation. Despite Orgilus' claim that he does not wish to 'steal again into her favours, | And undermine her virtues', he nevertheless attempts to do just this (I.i.74–5). He entreats Penthea:

> Turn those eyes,
> The arrows of pure love, upon that fire
> Which once rose to a flame, perfumed with vows
> As sweetly scented as the incense smoking
> On Vesta's alters; virgin tears, like
> The holiest odours, sprinkled dews to feed 'em
> And to increase their fervour.
>
> (II.iii.27–33)

Although Orgilus attempts to depict his sensual desires as pure and holy, the recurring image of fire highlights the inflamed nature of his passions. Penthea, on the other hand, seeks to temper Orgilus' feelings as well as her own: 'Rash man' she chastises him,

> thou layest
> A blemish on mine honour, with the hazard
> Of thy too desperate life. Yet I profess,
> By all the laws of ceremonious wedlock,
> I have not given admittance to one thought
> Of female change, since cruelty enforced
> Divorce betwixt my body and my heart.
>
> (II.iii.51–7)

Even as Penthea chastises Orgilus, she admits her continued love for him, finding that his speech 'ripens a knowledge in me of affliction | Above all sufferance' (II.iii.44–5). Her emotions, however, are circumscribed by her virtuous self-mastery.[71] Penthea's advice to her former lover is kind but firm: 'live happy | Happy in thy next choice, that thou mayst people | This barren age with virtues in thy issue!' (II.iii.90–1). Nonetheless, Orgilus continues to urge Penthea to sleep with him: 'I would possess my wife', he tells her (II.iii.71).

Penthea's self-restrained and dignified response to Orgilus epitomizes her behaviour throughout the play: she resists Orgilus' advances, is patient and kind to her jealous husband, forgives her brother, Itho-cles, and even attempts to aid him in his amorous suit. By Act III, however, she longs for death, asking her brother, 'Pray kill me, | Rid me from living with a jealous husband' (III.ii.64–5). Having been betrothed to Orgilus before consummating her marriage to Bassanes, she comes to see her marriage as a form of adultery and resolves to starve herself:

> To all memory
> Penthea's, poor Penthea's name is strumpeted.
> But since her blood was seasoned, by the forfeit
> Of noble shame, with mixtures of pollution,
> Her blood—'tis just—be henceforth never heightened
> With taste of sustenance. Starve. Let that fullness
> Whose plurisy hath severed faith and modesty—
> Forgive me. O I faint!
>
> (IV.ii.147–54)

Penthea associates eating with erotic desire (both produce an excess of blood, a 'plurisy', that engenders lust), so that her refusal of food corresponds to (and helps to foster) her rigid suppression of her sexual impulses. Her madness and death are thus not the products of her ungoverned passion, but result instead from her perverse self-mastery. Even the form of her death—self-starvation—is achieved by an effort of will, demonstrating an absolute control over her body and 'appetites'. A related depiction of suicide can be found in Heywood's *A Woman Killed with Kindness*, in which Anne engages in an adulterous relationship, and

---

[71] Her behaviour is appropriate to the play's prominent Spartan setting (the Spartans were known both for their 'powers of endurance and self-restraint' and for 'the chastity and moral strength of their women'). Spenser, 'Introduction', in Ford, *Broken Heart*, ed. Spenser, 21.

then starves herself in order to punish and to purify her body.[72] Anne's decision to refuse food suggests that she has gained a new discipline over her desires, and her wilful and dangerous asceticism offers a physical correlation to her starved emotional state. Penthea is similarly starved of affection. Beseeching Penthea for her love, Orgilus describes the emotional hunger that they both feel:

> All pleasures are but mere imagination,
> Feeding the hungry appetite with steam
> And sights of banquet, whilst the body pines,
> Not relishing the real taste of food.
> Such is the leanness of a heart divided
> From intercourse of troth-contracted loves.
> No horror should deface that precious figure
> Sealed with the lively stamp of equal souls.
>
> (II.iii.34–41)

Orgilus describes his and Penthea's state as a kind of emotional starvation, in which the 'hungry appetite' is only met with 'steam' and 'sights of banquets'. Unlike the conventional model that suggests that all women's distempers arise from bodily needs, Penthea suffers from an appetite that is spiritual and emotional, rather than sexual. Sex does not satisfy her, but merely proves an empty, unnourishing act that aggravates, rather than alleviates, her desires. Her 'body pines' for the 'real taste of food': reciprocated love between two 'equal souls'.

Penthea's rejection of all forms of emotional and physical nourishment dramatizes the point at which her self-abnegation transforms into a renunciation of life itself; no longer content merely to moderate her appetites, she starves herself completely. Ithocles finds his sister's behaviour inhuman, remarking 'Nature | Will call her daughter, monster', but this view neglects the affinity between her behaviour and other acts of stoical self-mastery within the play, which are similarly self-destructive (IV.ii.155–6). As Michael Neill points out, all of the central characters

---

[72] Heywood's *Woman Killed with Kindness* also depicts starvation as a form of physical and ethical cleansing. When Anne is near the point of death she asks her brother, Sir Charles, 'Can you not read my fault writ in my cheek?' He replies, 'Alas, good mistress, sickness hath not left you | Blood in your face enough to make you blush', playing on the associations between blood and sexual passion (Scene xvii. 56, 58–9). For discussions of female starvation see Bynum, *Holy Feast*; Gutierrez, *Shall She Famish*; and Bell, *Holy Anorexia*.

in *The Broken Heart* take dramatic charge of their deaths in order to preserve their good name; 'it is as if the characters themselves can already discern, in the carefully ritualized spectacles through which they fashion their own ends, the lineaments of that "high-tuned poem" through which their heroic endurance will be preserved for all posterity.'[73] Penthea's food refusal thus conforms to the culturally admired principles of self-restraint, whilst simultaneously suggesting stoicism's more nihilistic aspect. If stoicism strives for the freedom from emotional disturbance (*ataraxia*), then Ford's play hints darkly that true tranquillity of the soul is only found in death. However, if to live well requires that one expect, and even orchestrate, one's death, then living without love is figured as a kind of death-in-life.[74] Penthea is 'buried in a bride-bed', her love for Orgilus 'buried in an everlasting silence' (II.ii.38; II.iii.69). If death parts the soul and body, Penthea's unhappy marriage divides her physical self and her emotions; as Orgilus explains to his father, Penthea has been 'Compelled to yield her virgin freedom up | To him who never can usurp her heart' (I.i.51–5). Penthea's enforced marriage divides sexual intercourse from love—her body from her heart.

Ironically, however, in attempting to eradicate her sexual desires, Penthea chooses a form of death that replicates traditional symptoms of erotic melancholy. Her refusal to eat, drink, or sleep in order to extinguish the 'plurisy' in her blood both mimics the behaviour of the lovesick individual and has the contrary effect of driving her into a physiological state of lovesickness. Like Ophelia, she appears on stage with her hair loose, giving frenzied expression both to her suppressed love for Orgilus and to her anger towards her brother. Penthea's madness can thus be seen to be superficially similar to Ophelia, but for entirely different reasons: it is Penthea's self-conscious imitation of the symptoms of erotic melancholy, used to conquer her passion for Orgilus, which leads to her madness and effects her self-destruction.[75] During her madness she tells Orgilus, 'We had been happy' and then points at Ithocles, a signal that Orgilus interprets as an incitement to revenge

[73] Neill, *Issues of Death*, 335.
[74] Ford suggests in his stoical tract, *A Line of Life*, that 'men as indeavor to live well, live with an expectation of death' (*The Nondramatic Works*, 303).
[75] Paradoxes such as these are a central feature of *The Broken Heart*. See Barton, 'Oxymoron'.

(IV.ii.114). This gesture has cost Penthea the sympathy of some early critics. Despite the fact that it is Orgilus who interprets this signal and carries out Ithocles' murder, critics censure Penthea for directing Orgilus' revenge. Gifford finds 'a spice of selfishness in her grief', and Clifford Leech maintains that although she is 'in appearance the most pathetic of seventeenth-century stage women, Penthea is simultaneously the most ruthless'.[76]

That critics find Penthea the most to blame for Ithocles' murder suggests that for Penthea to be anything other than a passive victim renders her selfish and malicious. Like Ophelia, Penthea is torn between brother and lover, between feelings of love and thoughts of revenge, and like her she indirectly instigates a revenge plot. In fact, Penthea's only real contribution to Ithocles' murder occurs during a bout of madness, after she has forgiven her brother, but this does not moderate the view of those critics who misinterpret her actions as simply a manipulative plan for revenge. She insists that wrong has been done to her, an insistence that according to Leech transforms her from the 'victim of others' into 'the most active figure in the play'.[77] Such criticism of Penthea can be seen to replicate an early modern expectation that women should be self-effacing and passive. Any action in contravention of the woman's role as 'victim' is constructed as inappropriate and immoral. The persistence of the gendered model of acceptable female behaviour in early modern England illuminates why so many angry and frustrated women are represented in the drama as turning their violent impulses upon themselves: their bodies are the only sphere over which they have absolute control and which they can harm without feelings of guilt or social retribution. Inscribing their emotional wounds onto their bodies, heroines such as Aspatia and Penthea rely upon self-inflicted injuries to articulate their anger, so that they 'succeed, by the circuitous path of self-punishment, in taking revenge on the original object'.[78] Channelling their frustration into their own deaths, they simultaneously elevate themselves into 'Love's martyrs' (IV.iv.153).

Thus, if critics like Gifford and Leech are excessive in their condemnation of Penthea, they are nonetheless right to recognize that she is more than just a passive victim, or rather that she exploits her status

[76] Gifford, *Works of John Ford*, i. 293; Leech, *John Ford*, 27.
[77] Leech, *John Ford*, 24.
[78] Freud, 'Mourning and Melancholia', in *Complete Psychological Works*, xiv.251.

as a victim for her own ends. Penthea's self-starvation communicates, in frighteningly physical terms, her lack of emotional nourishment (she denies herself any 'taste of sustenance' just as she refuses her beloved's longed-for advances), making Ithocles and Bassianus acutely conscious of how they have mistreated her. As Maud Ellmann suggests, 'Self-starvation is above all a performance. Like Hamlet's mouse-trap, it is staged to trick the conscience of its viewers, forcing them to recognize that they are implicated in the spectacle that they behold'.[79] In Girard's words: 'The masochist . . . does not want to crush the wicked so much as to *prove* to them their wickedness and his own virtue; he wants to cover them with shame by making them look at the victims of their own infamy'.[80] Nowhere is this more evident than in Penthea's carefully crafted death. Like Aspatia, Penthea exhibits a self-conscious theatricality in her final moments:

> PHILEMA: She called for music
> And begged some gentle voice to tune a farewell
> To life and griefs. Chrystalla touched the lute.
> I wept the funeral song.
> CHRYSTALLA: Which scarce was ended,
> But her last breath sealed up these hollow sounds:
> 'O cruel Ithocles, and injured Orgilus!'
> So down she drew her veil; so died.
>
> (IV.iv.4–10)

Penthea's dignified end suggests that she is aware of the tradition into which her suffering fits, and is able to control aspects of its appearance in order to communicate her distress and her brother's culpability: her song emphasizes that for her 'Love is dead', while her final words emphasize her brother's betrayal (IV.iii.148). And just as critics debate the extent to which Penthea is an active revenger or passive victim, she offers two related but contradictory accounts of her fall: she is either the siren luring men to their destruction, or the faithful turtledove who mourns her lost beloved. These contrary roles are evident in one of her mad speeches:

---

[79] Ellmann, *Hunger Artists*, 17.
[80] Girard, *Deceit*, 188. As Hamilton argues, Penthea's masochism and 'pathos have an aggressive and vengeful side' ('Divided Mind', 184).

> Sure, if we were all sirens, we should sing pitifully.
> And 'twere a comely music, when in parts
> One sung another's knell. The turtle sighs
> When he hath lost his mate; and yet some say
> 'A must be dead first.
>
> (IV.ii.69–73)

The image of the siren links Penthea's madness to powerful forces of female destruction. Like the mythical mermaid, Penthea's own mad 'song' draws her lover and brother to their destruction, prompting Orgilus to carry out his revenge. Orgilus' staging of Ithocles' murder again places Penthea in the role of the siren: her funeral dirge provides the sad music that lures Ithocles to the trick chair where he is murdered.

However, despite the way in which Penthea is depicted as playing an essential role in the deaths of lover and brother, it is important to note that she does not actually call herself a siren, but rather seems to recognize the category into which her madness will be cast. She offers instead another metaphor for her madness: that of the faithful turtledove that sings its mournful song after losing its mate. However, unlike the turtledove, whose partner 'must be dead' before it sings its dirge, Penthea mourns a lost love who is alive and standing beside her. Similarly, Orgilus refers to Penthea as a faithful turtledove, casting himself instead as the siren who lures Ithocles to the trick chair in order 'To sacrifice a tyrant to a turtle' (IV.iv.29). These two metaphors suggest different levels of culpability: the siren indicates an active, destructive role, where the turtle dove suggests passive grief. Nevertheless, both emphasize the tragic nature of the love between Orgilus and Penthea, who can only be united in death. As in the case of Calantha and Ithocles, Orgilus and Penthea also depict how 'the lifeless trunk shall wed the broken heart', suggesting that in the transitory, earthly realm 'Love only reigns in death' (V.iii.93, 100). Ford's depiction of characters shifting between cultural roles offers a challenge to the traditional paradigm associating women with passion and men with reason; in fact, one could argue that in *The Broken Heart* it is the women who represent reason and the men who represent passion. Ford distinguishes between women's emotions and their need to express those feelings: sexual desire does not necessarily lead to carnality, nor does grief lead to tears. Penthea's madness, which may initially seem to follow traditional depictions of female insanity, actually indicates her control over her body and desires. Similarly, Calantha dies through an effort of self-will, breaking her own heart in order to join Ithocles. Despite the fact that Bassanes ascribes such self-control to a 'masculine spirit', Ford nevertheless gestures towards a more complex pattern of gender and behaviour, in which individuals can act 'Without distinction betwixt sex and sex' (V.ii.95, 98).

Penthea's ability to achieve a rigid control over her desires follows the stoical principles espoused in Ford's *A Line of Life* (1620) that 'the first branch of resolution is to know, feele, and moderate affections, which like traitors, and disturbers of peace, rise up to alter and quite change the Laws of reason' (p. 307). However, while Ford's non-dramatic works advance a fairly conventional Neo-Stoic position, *The Broken Heart* offers a much more complex depiction of the relationship between passion and self-restraint, dramatizing the point at which the discourse of rational self-mastery becomes self-destructive and masochistic. Thus while some critics maintain that the play is celebrating the 'iron principles' of a 'state devoted to the cultivation of the masculine virtues of Endurance, Restraint and Honour', the play seems instead to be questioning them, as Hawkins claims.[81] Nowhere is this more evident than in Penthea's destructive self-control. Critics like Burbridge are correct to suggest that Penthea pursues 'a morbid intensification of her own tragic fate', but it is not the case that she starves herself 'for no really compelling reason': Penthea, like Aspatia, is able to communicate through her suffering, achieving a grim, self-destructive revenge.[82]

---

[81] Morris, 'Introduction', in Ford, *Broken Heart*, ed. Morris, p. xix; quoted by Hawkins, 'Mortality', 131.

[82] Burbridge, 'Moral Vision', 398, 403.

4

Lovesickness and Neoplatonism

In Book III Canto ii of Spenser's *The Faerie Queene* (1590–6), Britomart sees an image of Aretegall in Merlin's mirror, and is struck by all of the pathological symptoms of lovesickness—she sighs, weeps, is 'full of fancies fraile', and complains that her passion 'suckes the bloud, which from my hart doth bleed'.[1] Britomart, highly aware of the destructive consequences of excessive passion, is, however, initially distrustful of her vision. Glauce, her nurse, attempts to reassure her, by suggesting that her passion in no way resembles the 'shamefull lusts' of Biblis for her twin brother, Caune, or Pasiphaë's passion for a bull; but Britomart maintains that while her love may be less unnatural than that of these women, it lacks a real presence in whom to seek satisfaction (III.ii.41). Worried that her vision is just an invented fantasy, sprung from her own mind, she tells Glauce that her desires 'can have no end', but rather

> ...feed on shadowes, whiles I die for food,
> And like a shadow wexe, whiles with entire
> Affection, I doe languish and expire.
> I fonder, than *Cephisus* foolish child,
> Who having viewed in a fountain shere
> His face, was with the love thereof beguild;
> I fonder love a shade, the bodie farre exiled.
>
> (III.ii.44)

Britomart compares herself to Narcissus, but believes herself doubly beguiled: where Narcissus falls in love with his watery reflection believing it to have real substance, she loves an image, knowing all the while that it is a mere 'shade'. Like the youth in Shakespeare's Sonnet 1 who, 'contracted to thine own bright eyes', rejects sexual reproduction for

---

[1] Spenser, *The Faerie Queene*, III.ii.27, 37. Walker suggests that Spenser's portrait of the lovesick Britomart recalls Virgil's Dido ('Spenser's Elizabeth Portrait', 182).

self-reflection, Narcissus' fruitless longing suggests the psyche's ability
to be its own object of desire.[2] He is the 'wretched boy', who, according
to Glauce,

> Was of himselfe the idle Paramoure;
> Both love and lover, without hope of ioy,
> For which he faded to a watry flowre.

(III.ii.45)

Narcissus dotes on his own watery image, and Britomart fears that her
desires are similarly self-enclosed and non-generative; she believes that
she has fallen in love with 'the shadow of a warlike knight', rendering
her, like the mythical youth, 'both love and lover' (III.ii.45).

Britomart's worries prove to be groundless, however. Her amorous
affection is Platonic, not narcissistic, rendering the image that Britomart
sees a revelatory vision rather than a solipsistic illusion. Indeed, Spenser
has fused separate traditions of lovesickness in order to transform what
initially appears to be an illicit, disorderly passion, into something
ennobling and heroic.[3] Merlin's 'glassie globe' where Britomart first
beholds her love thus recalls not the story of Narcissus but rather
Plato's description of the lover in *Phaedrus*: 'the lover is his mirror in
whom he is beholding himself, but he is not aware of this' (III.ii.21).[4]
In this context, 'the shadow of a warlike knight' that Britomart loves
represents the image of the ideal lover that the real Artegall shadows and
embodies. As Glauce suggests, Britomart's affection is not some 'filthy
lust, contarie unto kind', but is 'the semblant pleasing most your mind'
(III.ii.40). Spenser in this way invokes the myth of Narcissus in order
to reconfigure it positively: whereas Narcissus wastes away, transfixed
by his own image, Britomart dresses herself as a knight in order to
pursue her vision, refashioning herself into a mirror image of the knight
she loves, in a quest for reciprocal, procreative affection. The loving
process, dramatized by her cross-dressing, does not diminish her, but

---

[2] Shakespeare, Sonnet 1, in *Sonnets*, 5.
[3] Although Wells differs from me in regarding Britomart's Lovesickness as a form of
hysteria, we agree that her malady has a positive meaning. Wells argues: 'Britomart's quest
necessitates a reevaluation of female love-melancholy that implicitly revises misogynist
contemporary accounts of the female body as a dangerous and even maddening influence
on the mind' (*Secret Wound*, 221).
[4] Plato, *Phaedrus*, in *Collected Dialogues*, trans. Jowett, 157.

rather allows her to embody the Neoplatonic notion of androgynous wholeness.[5]

Britomart's confusion with regard to her passion illustrates the difficulty in distinguishing between the love which is, in Spenser's words, a 'sacred fire...ykindled first above, | Emongst th'enternal spheres' and the 'filthy lust' which 'base affections move' (III.iii.i). Robert Burton in *The Anatomy of Melancholy* suggests the difference between Platonic love and love that is an illness: whereas Platonic love is 'a voluntary affection, and desire to injoy that which is good', which 'stirres us up to the contemplation of that divine beauty', lovesickness, also known as heroical love, is 'a frequent cause of melancholy, and deserves much rather to bee called burning lust, then by such an honourable title';[6] The first, noble love

inflames our soules with a divine heat, and being so inflamed purgeth, and so purged, elevates to God, makes an attonement, and reconciles us unto him. That other love infects the soule of man, this cleanseth; that depresses, this erares; that causeth cares and troubles, this quietnesse of minde; this informes, that deformes our life.   (iii.32)

However, despite the fact that Burton insists upon a binary classification of love, clearly distinguishing ennobling forms of love from those that are merely an illness, the two traditions are not mutually exclusive, but are often understood through, and mediated by, one another, sharing a common terminology, an association with melancholy, and an interest in the interpretation of extreme states of consciousness.[7] Robert Burton predicates his physiological explanation of desire upon an analysis of love drawn principally from the writings of Neoplatonic philosophers, and other writers who treat love as an illness incorporate the ideas, allegories, and theories of Platonic love.[8] Similarly, philosophical treatises

---

[5] Perry, *Erotic Spirituality*, 3. See also Wind, *Pagan Mysteries*, 212–15; Schwartz, 'Aspects of Androgyny', 121–31.

[6] Burton, *Anatomy*, iii.11, 12, and 51.

[7] The early modern term 'heroical', for example, carried two distinct meanings. Whereas Burton's use of 'heroical' derives from the medical tradition, in which the term is a synonym for lovesickness, other writers use the term in its Neoplatonic sense to describe elevated, non-corporeal love. For the complex derivation of the term 'heroical' and its association with erotic melancholy see Lowes, 'Loveres Maladye of Heroes'. For an example of 'heroical' used in a Neoplatonic context, see Jonson and Jones, *Loves Triumph*, in *Selected Masques*, ed. Orgel, 296–303.

[8] Burton, *Anatomy*, iii.9–13. See also Beecher and Ciavolella, 'Ferrand', 3–4.

on Platonic love integrate physiological explanations of desire within a Neoplatonic framework. Plato directly compares the experience of falling in love to becoming ill, and in Speech Seven of his *Commentary on Plato's Symposium on Love*, Ficino diverges from a metaphysical and theological viewpoint to address love as an illness, establishing the concept of *fascination*.[9] Literary texts also fuse these two traditions in unexpected ways. Britomart's lovesickness is a fitting example. Although struck by all of the pathological symptoms of lovesickness, her illness is nevertheless a revelatory vision.

Importantly, Britomart is a woman, and in this she illustrates a change in the discourse of Neoplatonism, which was originally constructed to refer exclusively to the affection between men. When Platonic love is reformulated by writers to apply to heterosexual love, it prompts a reconsideration of the female beloved, who is increasingly imagined as the naturally chaste and cerebral gender. Spenser is a strong participant in this new formulation, not only employing Platonic love in this new heterosexual context, but also making Britomart's ultimate aim procreative marriage, another change to the way that Platonic love was originally envisaged. Neoplatonic love as described by Ficino promotes a strict hierarchy of ascent from the physical to spiritual realm, in which heterosexual physical reproduction, while honourable, is inferior to the homoerotic replication of souls. The fact that for Spenser a Platonic, celestial impulse can have marital procreation as its goal not only dissolves the opposition between the corporeal and spiritual, but also reverses the hierarchy between procreative and sublimated passion: in *The Faerie Queene*, it is not disorderly, sexual passion that acts as a contrast to non-consummated passion, but rather generative love which is set against the inertia and 'paralysis in appetite' of non-generative desire, epitomized by the Bower of Bliss.[10] In this Britomart truly is the opposite of Narcissus, who for many early modern thinkers 'was a figure for stasis, for listlessness and withdrawal from public "business"', or, in Francis Bacon's words, for 'anything that yields no fruit'.[11]

---

[9] Ficino, *Commentary on Plato's Symposium on Love*, speech vii. chs. iv–v.
[10] Lewis, *Allegory of Love*, 339.
[11] Gregerson, *Reformation of the Subject*, 75. Bacon, 'Narcissus: or Philautia [Self-Love]', in *Of the Wisdom of the Ancients*, in *Works*, xiii.90; quoted by Gregerson, *Reformation of the Subject*, 75.

This chapter explores in more detail the complex relationship between medical ideas about love and those derived from Neoplatonism, outlining important differences between love as an illness and love as an ennobling passion, and suggesting points at which the two philosophies overlap or are in conflict. I begin with a brief outline of the construction of love according to Neoplatonism, before turning to an examination of two plays written during the Caroline period, when the cult of Platonic love was at its height. In John Ford's *'Tis Pity She's a Whore* (probably written between 1626 and 1631) and William Davenant's *The Platonic Lovers* (performed at Court and at the Blackfriars in the season of 1635–6), the figure of the lovesick subject can be read as a reaction to the growing influence of Neoplatonism at the Caroline court. Ford interrogates philosophical ideas about love in psychological terms, representing Giovanni's incestuous love for his sister as a type of Neoplatonic mirroring which is also a form of narcissism. Davenant, on the other hand, by reminding his audience of the hazardous physical symptoms of lovesickness, aims to challenge the Neoplatonic construction of love, promoting a notion of heterosexual desire that is physiological and sexual, rather than abstract and spiritual. Whereas in *'Tis Pity* the discourse of Platonic love coexists with the language of erotic melancholy, in *The Platonic Lovers* these two constructions of love are placed in opposition.

NEOPLATONIC INTERPRETATIONS OF LOVE AND THE FEMALE BELOVED

Neoplatonism is a term applied to the philosophical and religious writings of a heterogeneous group of thinkers who attempted to expand and synthesize the metaphysical writings of Plato. Its main proponents were Italian: Marsilio Ficino (1433–99), Giovanni Pico della Mirandola (1469–1533), Pietro Bembo (1470–1547), and Giordano Bruno (1548–1600). Their writings, although diverse, can be characterized by an opposition between the corporeal and spiritual realms, based upon Plato's dualist distinction between the 'idea' and its material manifestation. In their attempt to fuse classical ideas with Christianity, the Florentine Academy of the Italian Renaissance maintained that although humans live in the transitory world, they nonetheless have souls that are capable of comprehending the forms or ideals, the non-temporal reality, behind their shadowy material manifestations. According to this theory, the cosmos consists of a hierarchy extending from the unity of God to the multiplicity of the physical world: all things, spiritual and material, emanate from the 'One', which is the source of all truth, beauty, and goodness. Through the agency of love, the human soul desires to advance to the level above it in an ascending return to God, rising from the sensual appreciation of physical beauty to a divine, spiritual rapture.[12]

Neoplatonism suggests that love is a spiritual impulse, which edifies and completes the lover. The lover is attracted to the amorous object because their souls are complementary. This idea draws on the myth recounted by Aristophanes in the *Symposium*, in which humans were originally spherical in shape (consisting of two pairs of arms, legs, and genitals) before being divided by Zeus into two halves. According to this myth, in looking for a partner, we are looking for our missing other half, so that 'Love is just the name we give to the desire for and pursuit of wholeness'.[13] In Neoplatonism, the lover recognizes a more perfect image of the self that is mirrored in the amorous object; as Ficino writes: 'the soul of the lover becomes a mirror in which the image of the beloved is reflected . . . when the beloved recognizes himself in the lover, he is forced to love him.'[14] When affection is reciprocated, the lovers' souls begin to mingle to form a perfect and complete self. The lover thus yearns, not merely for the beloved, but for the lost pieces of the self that the latter embodies. This process is often illustrated by describing what happens to a lover when s/he gazes into the eyes of the beloved and finds there a miniature of his or her self reflected in the pupils of the beloved (often called 'making babies' by early modern authors): just as the lover finds an image of the self in the eyes of the beloved, so too does s/he discover a spiritual resemblance within, and is thus able to achieve a greater degree of self-knowledge.[15] Ficino constructs love as a spiritual appetite that can neither be entirely consumed by, nor

---

[12] See Armstrong, *St Augustine*; Allen, *Platonism of Marsilio Ficino*; Nelson, *Theory of Love*.

[13] Plato, *Phaedrus*, i.26.

[14] Ficino, *Commentary on Plato's Symposium on Love*, II.xiii. In 'De l'amitié' Montaigne writes of his friend, La Boëtie, 'he *is* me' ('On Affectionate Relationships', 215).

[15] Burton, *Anatomy*, iii.243. See Davenant, *Platonick Lovers*, sig. C1ᵛ; and Donne, 'The Ecstasy', in *John Donne*, 11–12.

contained within, the beloved. Love precedes and exceeds the amorous object, who is merely a medium through which the lover desires and gains knowledge of more abstract ideals. Love is not dependent upon the physical presence of the beloved, but rather springs from the lover's idea of him or her: indeed, the physical presence of the beloved can actually impede the amorous process, limiting the lover to the finite and material manifestations of the beloved.[16] Absence allows the lover to engage with the true aspect of desire, which is a contemplation of love itself. Whilst the fulfilment of love requires presence, desire—the appetite which draws the lover to a contemplation of the beautiful and good—is predicated on a lack. It is in this solitary, contemplative state that the lover is drawn closer to God and experiences spiritual ecstasy.

The complex history of Neoplatonism's transmission, translation, and adaptation rendered it open to a wide variety of interpretations.[17] The various forms of Neoplatonism were introduced into England by two principal means: by the importation of books from the Continent, the most influential of which was Castiglione's *The Courtier*, which came into in England in 1531 and was translated into English in 1561; and by visits to and from England by several of Neoplatonism's leading exponents, such as John Colet, Desiderius Erasmus, and Giordano Bruno.[18] During the European Renaissance, 'the philosophy of Plato was read and valued more than at any other time since the closure of the Athenian Academy'.[19] However, unlike in France and Italy, the influence of Plato in England was not widespread. Some sense of this discrepancy between the Continent and England can be seen in the dissemination of Platonic texts. As Sears Jayne has noted, between 1485 and 1578 there were more than a hundred editions of various works of Plato in France, whereas in England during the same period, there was not one.[20] Nonetheless, there were a variety of cultural exchanges through which ideas of Neoplatonism entered England indirectly, such

---

[16] There are interesting correspondences between the Neoplatonic idea of the beloved and the medical idea of the beloved as a phantasm. See Chs. 1 and 5.

[17] My account of the transmission of Neoplatonism is based on Hutton, 'Introduction to the Renaissance', 67–75. See also Jayne, 'Introduction to *Marsilio Ficino's Commentary*', 19–20; and Hart, *Art and Magic*.

[18] Hart, *Art and Magic*, 4.   [19] Hutton, 'Introduction to the Renaissance', 67.

[20] Jayne, 'Introduction to *Marsilio Ficino's Commentary*', 21.

as through masques, paintings, royal iconography, and poetry.[21] The popularity of Neoplatonism in England grew during the early seventeenth century until it reached its zenith in the Caroline period with Henrietta Maria's cult of Platonic love, and with the Cambridge School of Neoplatonism, which reinstitutionalized the philosophy as a subject for academic study.[22]

The most important and popular aspect of Neoplatonism in the Renaissance was the doctrine of Platonic love, which became an important medium for compliment in courtly circles.[23] It found its fullest expression in the poetry of the period, especially Petrarchan poetry, where it functioned as an essential element of the language of courtly love.[24] In Neoplatonism, an overtly Christian philosophy was synthesized with the language of romantic love, so that the beloved functioned simultaneously as the object of passionate desire and as the instrument through which sexual desire could be sublimated in order to achieve spiritual transcendence. The beloved in this way acquired a new metaphysical and theological significance: as the lover passed from loving the body to loving the soul, and finally to loving God, he achieved mystical rapture.

The concept of love formulated by Plato refers exclusively to the affection between men, and before Ficino's reformulation of the philosophy Platonic love was primarily associated with homosexuality.[25] This connection appears to have prohibited proper scholarly investigation prior to the publication of Ficino's *Commentary on Plato's Symposium on Love*, prompting medieval theologians to remove references to Platonic love from their larger discussions of Platonism. Jill Kraye points out several examples of this, such as the Camaldulensian monk Ambrogio Traversari, who deleted the homosexual love poems attributed to Plato

---

[21] Gatti, 'Stuart Court Masque', 809–42; Hart, *Art and Magic*, 5.

[22] See Patrides, *Cambridge Platonists*; and Cassirer, *Platonic Renaissance*.

[23] Jayne, 'Introduction to *Marsilio Ficino's Commentary*', 19. See also Giudici, 'De l'amour courtois à l'amour sacré'.

[24] French sources, such as DuBellay and the Pléiades, probably affected the Platonism of English poetry even more than the Italian sources; other courtly texts also helped to popularize ideas of Platonic love, especially Castiglione's *The Courtier*. See Hutton, 'Introduction to the Renaissance', 72.

[25] My discussion of the way in which Neoplatonism changes from being an exclusively male discourse to a heterosexual one is based on Kraye, 'The Transformation of Platonic Love', 76–81.

from his Latin version of Diogenes Laertius' *Lives of the Philosophers* in 1433, and George of Trebizond whose comparison of Aristotle and Plato in 1458 attempted to save Christendom from the perceived homosexual and pederastic orientation of Platonic love. Even Cardinal Bessarion, who defends Plato's attachment to young men as chaste in his *In calumniatorem Platonis*, nevertheless asserts that the lustful poems were not actually by Plato. Ficino, on the other hand, accepts the notion of Platonic love, but interprets its homosexual aspect allegorically, asserting that the divinely inspired amatory fury of Platonic love involved a chaste relationship between men. Pico della Mirandola attributed this to the fact that Platonic love was directed at the soul or intellect, which was much more beautiful in men than in women. But while Ficino, Pico, and Bessarion 'expunged any taint of carnal homosexuality from Platonic love, they did not question its homoerotic nature, nor its relegation of heterosexual love to an inferior status on the grounds that love between the sexes resulted in physical procreation, whereas love between men led to spiritual perfection'.[26]

The circulation of Ficino's formulation of Platonic love is demonstrated in the notes to Spenser's *The Shepheardes Calender* of 1579. E. K. glosses the reference to Hobbinol, describing him as Colin Clout's 'very speciall and most familiar freend, whom he entirely and extraordinarily beloved'.[27] E. K. then goes on to defend the chaste nature of the men's relationship, and compares it to heterosexual and homosexual passion; whereas platonic love is directed at the soul, heterosexual and homosexual passion are both associated with an immoderate desire for the body:

In thys place seemeth to be some savour of disorderly love, which the learned call pæderastice: but it is gathered beside his meaning. For who that hath red Plato his dialogue called Alcybiades, Xenophon, and Maximus Tyrius of Socrates opinions, may easily perceive, that such love is muche to be alowed and liked of, specially so meant, as Socrates used it: who sayth, that in deede he loved Alcybiades extremely, yet not Alcybiades person, but hys soule, which is Alcybiades owne selfe. As so is pæderastice much to be præferred before gynerastice, that is the love whiche enflameth men with lust toward woman

---

[26] Kraye, 'The Transformation of Platonic Love', 80–1.
[27] Spenser, *Shepheardes Calender*, in *Shorter Poems*, 33. See also Montaigne, 'On Affectionate Relationships', 208–9.

kind. But yet let no man thinke, that herein I stand with Lucian or hys develish disciple Unico Aretino, in defence of execrable and horrible sinnes of forbidden and unlawful fleshlinesse. Whose abominable errour is fully confuted of Perionius, and others.   (pp. 33–4)

Although much of the poetry in *The Shepheardes Calender* celebrates heterosexual love, the gloss offered by E.K. on Platonism reiterates the traditional hierarchy that associates the *quality of love* with the *gender of the object*, denigrating sexual love as incompatible with spiritual affection.[28] Ficino, while not disparaging heterosexual love, also prioritizes male-male, non-corporeal friendship, suggesting that physical reproduction is inferior to spiritual propagation. While always affirming the importance of love, Neoplatonism thus privileges the love of a male over that of a female. Unsurprisingly, then, when a woman assumes the role of the male Platonic beloved there is an attempt to elide or efface her real corporeal presence, and in doing so, to give her the same rarefied status as the male Platonic lover. The apology offered by Ficino for the homocentricity of Platonic love, redefining the relationship between lover and beloved as chaste rather than carnal, thereby extends to heterosexual love, creating a new paradigm in which the female beloved incites *spiritual* desire.

This new heterosexual version of Platonic love thus celebrates the female mistress while simultaneously denigrating sexual intercourse and physicality. Ficino's hierarchical categorization of love, elevating the spiritual over the physical, is, for example, turned by Bruno into an expression of outright hostility towards the Petrarchan obsession with the female body.[29] In his dedication to Sir Philip Sidney in *The Heroic Frenzies* (1585), Bruno laments the 'base, ugly and contaminated wit that is constantly occupied and curiously obsessed with the beauty of a female body'. Whereas true, inner beauty and goodness enable the lover to achieve spiritual transcendence, physical beauty has the potential to trap the lover in the transitory realm of the flesh (which

[28] Many of these tensions can be traced back to early periods, especially the ideas concerning spiritual friendship between men in the Middle Ages and the courtly love tradition from the twelfth century. As Jaeger points out, although both of these traditions were initially premised on the idea that 'any love that incorporated and included sex was not ennobling', there was an attempt to reconcile ideas about virtue with sexuality (and thus ennobling love with heterosexual desire) 'from the end of the eleventh century on, when women emerged in the discourse of ennobling love' (*Ennobling Love*, 7).

[29] See Nelson, *Theory of Love*, 170–1.

upon closer inspection is actually repellent). Bruno moves in a mocking tone from the woman's lips, hair, and dress to 'That scourge, that disgust, that stink, that tomb, that latrine, that menstruum, that carrion, that quartan ague, that excessive injury and distortion of nature, which with surface appearance, and shadow, a phantasm, a dream, a Circean enchantment put to the service of generation, deceives us as a species of beauty'.[30] Neoplatonism, as well as allowing men to achieve spiritual transcendence, is a means of escape from the materiality and repulsiveness of women's flesh.

Despite the implicit hostility towards women and women's bodies embedded in Neoplatonic theory, the discourse of Platonic love did serve to reaffirm the nobility and importance of women, defending 'woman as worthy of love and of loving because she, like man, is rational, and reason is the source of love.'[31] In Castiglione's *The Courtier*, the discussion about Neoplatonism at the end of Book IV contributes to a defence of women and is reformulated to include marriage as a goal.[32] Moreover, as Ann Rosalind Jones shows, 'Women poets in coteries found a highly usable set of conventions in Neoplatonism...which stressed the equality of the lovers and the mutual refinement they stimulated.'[33] Platonic love was also good for women in more practical ways; as well as affording women an elevated and ennobled position in the amorous process, it also justified a prolonged period of courtship, the time at which the woman was traditionally able to dominate her partner by withholding both physical and emotional favour.[34] The consequent elevation of women finds reflection in the early modern English discourse of Platonic love, in which the intensity of the suitor's love is expressed through professions of loyalty and servitude to a confident and commanding mistress.

---

[30] Bruno, 'Argument', in *Heroic Frenzies*, 60. Bruno's words are in line with a well-known cure for lovesickness; see Ch. 6.

[31] Jordan, *Renaissance Feminism*, 75. Jordan discusses several Neoplatonic writers who affirm the virtue and rationality of women, including Mario Equicola in his *Libro di natura d'amore* (1526) and Girolamo Ruscelli in his *Lettura ove ... si pruvova la soma perfettione delle donne* (1552).

[32] Castiglione, *Book of the Courtier*, 349.   [33] Jones, *Currency*, 34–5.

[34] This inversion of the gender hierarchy during the period of courtship was strengthened by the position of women at the Stuart courts, where the traditional female virtues of silence and modesty were replaced by those of wit and learning. See Hobby, *Virtue of Necessity*, 4.

The importance of the discourse of Platonic love to many of the English masques and plays of the Caroline period can be attributed to the influence of Queen Henrietta Maria. As a young woman at the French court, the queen had witnessed the attempts of the Marquise de Rambouillet to refine the manners and sexual mores of the French royal circle. The salon founded by Rambouillet inspired Henrietta Maria to attempt a similar programme of refinement at the English court, where she established Platonic love as a fashionable cult and court game.[35] The popularity of the discourse at the English court was first noted by the newswriter James Howell in 1634:

The Court affords little News at present, but that there is a love call'd Platonick Love, which much sways there of late; it is a Love abstracted from all corporeal gross impressions and sensual Appetite, but consists in Contemplations and Ideas of the Mind, not in any carnal fruition. This love sets the Wits of the Town on Work; and they say there will be a Mask shortly of it, whereof her Majesty and her Maids of Honour will be part.[36]

The interest of Queen Henrietta Maria in the language of Neoplatonism had a strong influence upon poets and playwrights keen to signal their attachment to the values of the Caroline court, while also furnishing writers with a language to engage with and criticize contemporary political issues.[37]

Caroline writers reacted in a variety of ways to the new fashion; some of them praised Platonic love while others expressed outright derision.[38] Positive depictions describe love as a celestial, spiritual impulse that ennobles the lover.[39] Love in these instances is not merely a 'toy' or 'sport but for the Idle Boy' but rather an emotion that can 'entertain | Our serious thoughts' when directed at a virtuous 'perfect Virgin'.[40] Platonic love is represented as the opposite of lust, and its

[35] Barton, *Ben Jonson*, 264.   [36] In Howell, *Epistolae*, ed. Jacobs, 317.
[37] As Sharpe has argued: 'love was the metaphor, the medium, though which political comment and criticism were articulated in Caroline England' (*Criticism and Compliment*, 24). See also Orgel and Strong, who show how 'Neoplatonism underscores the idealization of the monarchy' (*Inigo Jones*, i.55).
[38] For a discussion of the treatment of Platonic love in Caroline plays see Stavig, *Traditional Moral Order*, 36–43. See also Leech, *Shakespeare's Tragedies*, 195–9.
[39] Nabbes, *Springs Glorie*, sig. C3ʳ.
[40] Herbert, 'Platonick Love' ['Madam, believe't], and 'Platonick Love' ['Disconsolate and sad'], 72, 82; Robert Heath, 'On the Report of Clarastella's death', in *Clarastella*, 54.

advocates emphasize that physical desire must either be eschewed or sublimated in order for souls and minds to unite in an affection that is based on admiration, friendship, and equality; such lovers do not share their 'ignobler selves' but 'like those above | Unmatter'd forms' unite spiritually.[41] The philosophy thus promotes friendship and equality between lovers, who are united in their thoughts and souls rather than their bodies. Unlike traditional depictions of marriage, which place the man in the dominant position, Platonic love is portrayed in such a way as to erase the gender divide or even to afford the woman an elevated position.[42]

However, while many literary works celebrate Platonic love, an even greater number attack the philosophy as an unnatural and artificial doctrine.[43] Many works challenge the idea that physical love is inherently sinful, suggesting that complete love results from both a spiritual and a bodily union.[44] Whereas virginity is aligned to illness in these poems, lovesickness is, paradoxically, depicted as a natural and integral aspect of affection.[45] In other places, the adherents of Platonic love are criticized for being hypocritical; they are depicted as employing the idealized discourse of Neoplatonism either as a seduction technique, or as a means of covering up sexual liaisons,[46] and in some instances, writers associate Platonic love with the hypocrisy of the court.[47] Finally, some writers assert that the philosophy's emphasis on chastity emasculates the male lover, rendering him passive.[48] While the supporters of Platonic love

---

[41] Hall, 'Platonick Love', in *Poems*, 30. See also Lawes, 'To his Platonick Mistris', in *Ayres, and Dialogues*, 9, and 'Affection for a Lady he Never Saw', in Hall, *Ayres, and Dialogues*, 11; and Cavendish, 'Love's Sole's Conversation', in *The Phanseys*, 23.

[42] Hall, 'Platonick Love', in *Poems*, 30.

[43] Cokain suggests that Platonic love must concern friendship rather than romantic relationships, citing Jonson's *The New Inn* as having proved that love is 'Desire of union with the belov'd' ('To my Especial Friend Mr. Henry Thimbleby', in *Small Poems*, 175–6).

[44] See Cokain, 'The Fifth Song' [It is an offence to love], in *Small Poems*, 154; Cowley, 'Platonick Love', in *Collected Works*, ii.37, 31–2; H[ookes], 'Against Platonick Court-Love', in *Amanda*, 6, 7, 8, 9.

[45] Cleveland, 'The Antiplatonick', in *Poems with Additions*, 20; See also Cokain, 'To My Friend and Kinsman Mr. George Giffard', in *Small Poems*, 84.

[46] See Lawes, 'Falshood Discovered', in *Ayres, and Dialogues*, 18; Davenant, *Platonick Lovers*, sig. I3ᵛ; [Mayne], *Citye Match*, 44; Shirley, *Lady of Pleasure*, V.iii.52–62.

[47] See H[ookes], 'Against Platonick Court-Love', in *Amanda*, 6–9; Lawes, 'Platonick Love', *Treasury of Musick*, 34.

[48] H[ookes], 'Against Platonick Court-Love', in *Amanda*, 7.

suggest that the philosophy promotes a just equality between lovers, those who attack it often suggest that non-corporeal affection places women in an unnatural position of dominance.[49]

SEEING DOUBLE: NEOPLATONISM AND NARCISSISM IN JOHN FORD'S *'TIS PITY SHE'S A WHORE*

A number of critics examine John Ford's *'Tis Pity She's a Whore* in relation to the Neoplatonic theory of love. George Sensabaugh suggests that Ford's adherence to Platonic love leads him to regard love as 'the sole guide to virtue', a position that enabled him to adopt an 'unbridled individualism in matters of marriage and love'.[50] Tucker Orbison, on the other hand, maintains that Ford always places ideas about Platonic love within a wider ethical framework, in which individuals must restrain their passionate impulses; for Orbison then, Ford is critical of Giovanni's brand of Platonism, and most critics following Orbison agree with this view. Mark Stavig, for example, argues that 'Giovanni is simply not a good Platonist' and Ford is 'satirizing the perverted arguments that he uses', and Dorothy Farr feels that Ford demonstrates a 'dislike of the pretension of current neo-Platonism'.[51] Other critics have explored the way in which Giovanni's love for his sister is ultimately a form of *self*-love. R. J. Kaufmann suggests that by the end of the play Giovanni's love for his sister has 'become an abstract self-oriented thing' amounting to a kind of 'psychological autointoxication'.[52] Lois Bueler argues that 'brother and sister been locked into an intolerably claustrophobic solipsism'.[53] Similarly, Charles Forker regards Giovanni as 'the narcissist

---

[49] Carew, 'To Ben Jonson upon Occasion of his Ode to Himself', in Jonson, *The New Inn*, 219.

[50] Sensabaugh, *Tragic Muse*, 173.

[51] Stavig, *Traditional Moral Order*, 97, 102; Farr, *John Ford and the Caroline Theatre*, 153–4. Other studies of Ford and Platonic love include: Ure, 'Cult and Initiates', 298–306; Sensabaugh, *Tragic Muse*, and 'Platonic Love in the Court'; Sutton, 'Platonic Love in Ford's *The Fancies*', 299–309; and Kessel, 'Allegorical Reading'. See also Champion, 'Jacobean Tragic Perspective', 82; and Sensabaugh, who discusses Ford's interest in Platonic love in relation to his understanding of Burton and Renaissance psychology ('Ford Revisited').

[52] Kaufman, 'Ford's Tragic Perspective', 369, 370.

[53] Bueler, 'Role-Splitting', 329.

par excellence': 'What may look from inside the temple of narcissism like religious mystery and sacrificial rite is seen by the sane who live outside as madness, depravity, [and] monstrous egotism.'[54] However, what seems to be overlooked in both of these strands of literary criticism is the interrelation between these two discourses, in which Giovanni's narcissism is intimately related to his Platonism.[55]

In *'Tis Pity*, Ford fuses Platonic and narcissistic love, offering not a satirical caricature of misused Neoplatonic theory, but a complex vision of the way in which these two discourses intertwine. Like Britomart, who looks in a mirror and falls in love with a 'shadow' who is a reflection of the self and a creation of her own imagination, Giovanni also sees his beloved as his elevated mirror, but in Ford's play Annabella is *both* Giovanni's Platonic mirror and his narcissistic twin.[56] Ford thus dissolves Spenser's opposition between Neoplatonic and narcissistic love, depicting a pair of lovers who evoke sympathy as well as condemnation (as the title of the play instructs). Ford has long been recognized as an avid reader of Burton; here he reimagines the esoteric philosophy of Neoplatonism in psychological terms, in which the fervour of Platonic ecstasy re-emerges in Giovanni as its sister state, that of pathological madness.

Ford was not alone in recognizing that Neoplatonism's emphasis upon a spiritual resemblance between lovers allowed for the narcissistic mirroring of the lover in the ennobled object of desire. For other Renaissance writers as well, Neoplatonism's emphasis upon the internal experience of the lover, whose end is ultimately private and self-regarding, lay it open to charges of being narcissistic. Abraham Cowley in his poem 'Platonick Love', for example, challenges the notion that

---

[54] Bueler, 'Structural Uses of Incest', 140; Forker, *Fancy's Images*, 167. See also Finke, 'Painting Women', 368.

[55] An exception to this is Forker, who points out that 'the idea of incest as narcissistic twinship was of course already implicit in Plato's Symposium' (*Fancy's Images*, 165).

[56] Other critics have argued that there is a less clear distinction between Platonic love and that which is narcissistic or incestuous. Stephens argues that because Spenser frequently uses the word 'semblant' to mean 'apparent double', 'the "semblant" so pleasing to pleasing to Britomart's mind is not only a likeness of Artegall wavering in the crystal ball but a projected image that resembles Britomart herself insofar as it bodies forth her most private desires' (*Limits*, 76). Moreover, both David Lee Miller and James Nohrnberg regard the sexuality in Book III of *The Faerie Queen* as inherently incestuous. See Miller, *Poem's Two Bodies*, 278–81; and Nohrnberg, *Analogy of* The Faerie Queene, 436.

it is the similarity between lovers that forms the basis of attraction, suggesting that this form of love can be compared to 'When a fair *woman* courts her *glass*'.[57] Cowley suggests that although 'When *Souls* mix, 'tis an *Happiness*', nevertheless the loving process is not 'compleat till *Bodies* too do joyne' (ii.2–3). Here, physical union mirrors, rather than prohibits, the spiritual union of lovers:

> In thy immortal part
> *Man*, as well as I, thou art.
> But something 'tis that differs *Thee* and *Me*;
> And we must *one* even in that *difference* be.
> I Thee, both as a *man*, and *woman* prize;
> For a perfect *Love* implies
> Love in *all Capacities*.
>
> (ll. 8–17)

Although Cowley supports the Neoplatonic construction of the soul as an androgynous entity that contains and reflects the lover, he nevertheless challenges the notion that it is only this similarity that is the basis of love: it is the union of souls *and bodies* which constitutes 'perfect love', and this physical union is only possible because of the anatomical difference between lovers. This idea is summed up in Donne's 'The Cannonization': 'The phoenix riddle hath more wit | By us; we two being one, are it. So, to one neutral thing both sexes fit'; sex is here the physical enactment of the spiritual union between lovers, in which the couple briefly comes to resemble a hermaphroditic whole (symbolized through the Phoenix).[58] Because individuals who only love the soul only love their likeness, Neoplatonism ultimately promotes self-love; as Cowley writes: 'For he whose *soul* nought but a *Soul* can move, | Does a new *Narcissus* prove, | And his own *Image* love' (ii.19–20).

In many respects it seems fitting that the affiliation between Neoplatonism and narcissism finds its dramatic realization in a play about the incestuous love between siblings, in which the very features of resemblance and consanguinity, normally meant to prohibit sexual union, instead become the source of erotic desire. Susan Wiseman argues that 'the idea of incest constitutes what we might call the absent centre in Giovanni's discourse, the hidden precondition of his Platonic language',

---

[57] Cowley, 'Platonick Love', in *Collected Works*, ii.16.
[58] Donne, 'The Cannonization', in *John Donne*, 23–5.

and this is true not least because in both incest and Platonic love the erotic object is also an uncanny double of the self.[59] In incest, this doubling is destructive, allowing roles within the family to overlap and become confused; rather than reaching outward in a regenerative manner, the incestuous family turns inward, feeding off itself in a manner that is frequently imagined as a kind of cannibalism. In Shakespeare's *Pericles*, for example, Antiochus' incestuous relationship with his daughter renders her 'mother, wife, and yet his child', so that, in the words of the riddle, 'I am no viper, yet I feed | On mother's flesh, which did me breed'; and in some ancient and mythic stories, incestuous individuals are punished by being tricked into eating their own children (Scene i, ll. 107–8).[60] In economic terms, incest also amounts to a kind of greedy self-consumption, violating the expected cultural practice, outlined by Claude Lévi-Strauss, by which women are exchanged as marriage partners, forging new kinship systems and facilitating the exchange of wealth.[61] In the words of Livia in Middleton's *Women Beware Women*, incest is 'ill husbandry ... That spares free means, and spends of his own stock'.[62] In Neoplatonism, on the other hand, loving one's double is regenerative, signifying self-completion rather than self-consumption. In this context, sibling incest is an aspect of 'the human urge toward wholeness, or androgyny, of which sexual union is a symbol'.[63]

The opening scene of *'Tis Pity* reveals how Giovanni's Neoplatonic mystification of his erotic impulses is ultimately a form of narcissism; as A. P. Hogan suggests, Giovanni feels a love which is 'even more incestuous than it may at first appear, since its origin and object are

---

[59] Wiseman, 'Incestuous Body', 215.

[60] This is the case in the story told by the mythographers Parthenius and Hyginus of Clymenus who, having raped his daughter, is later punished by having his son (the product of the incest) served to him in a meal (Forker, *Fancy's Images*, 143). Tereus is similarly avenged, although in this instance the child who is eaten is the product of his legal, non-incestuous union, rather than of the rape of his wife's sister, Philomela.

[61] As Bueler argues, incestuous individuals in early modern plays frequently display 'the evil of an aggravated selfishness', demonstrating 'Levi-Strauss's central thesis about the attraction and the taboo of incest', in which one might ' "gain without losing, enjoy without sharing" ' ('Structural Uses of Incest', 127, 143).

[62] Middleton, *Women Beware Women*, II.i.13, 16. Bueler uses this quotation in a similar manner ('Structural Uses of Incest', 137).

[63] Heilbrun makes this point about Byron's *Manfred*. See *Recognition of Androgyny*, 38.

essentially the self'.[64] Giovanni tells the Friar that incest is not a 'leprosy of lust', but is rather a mere 'customary form, from man to man':

> Say that we had one father, say one womb
> (Curse to my joys!) gave both us life and birth:
> Are we not therefore each to other bound
> So much the more by nature, by the links
> Of blood, of reason (nay, if you will have't,
> Even of religion), to be ever one,
> One soul, one flesh, one love, one heart, one all?[65]

Giovanni follows the Neoplatonic idea that 'likeness generates love' to its logical conclusion, extending Ficino's list of likeness of complexion, nourishment, education, habit, and opinion, to include that of 'one womb'.[66] Montaigne recognized the possibility of such a response, arguing that familial affection might deepen, rather than thwart, romantic love; incest should thus be avoided because of the danger it poses to one's psyche: 'the love a man beareth to such a woman may be immoderate; for if the wedlocke, or husband-like affection be sound and perfect, as it ought to be, and also surcharged with that a man oweth to alliance and kindred, there is no doubt, but that surcease may easily transport a husband beyond the bounds of reason.'[67] For Giovanni too, the ties of blood deepen his desires to the point of a dangerous obsession. More than just becoming one, Giovanni loves his sister because he perceives them to be one already, sharing the same beauty, background, and biology.

Despite the Friar's warning that 'death waits on thy lust', Giovanni reveals his love to Annabella, suggesting to her that the Church approves (I.i.59). Annabella returns his love, admitting 'Thou hast won | The field, and never fought' (I.ii.239–40). In fact, the play hints that Annabella's desire for her brother is equally narcissistic. As David Bergeron observes, Giovanni 'is a mirror by which and through which she perceives her love for him: each reflects the other'.[68] This is hinted at

---

[64] Hogan, 'Overall Design', 310.

[65] Ford, *'Tis Pity*, ed. Wiggins, I.i.74, 25, 28–34; all quotations from the text are taken from this edition.

[66] Ficino, *Commentary on Plato's Symposium on Love*, II.iix.

[67] Montaigne, *Essays*, i.211, quoted by McCabe, who makes this point with regards to *'Tis Pity* (*Incest*, 230–1).

[68] Bergeron, 'Brother–Sister Incest', 212.

when Annabella sees Giovanni from a distance and feels drawn to him, not knowing that it is her brother. This moment recalls of an alternative version of the Narcissus myth, in which the youth dies in mourning for his twin sister, who he believes he sees in his reflection. Like Narcissus, Annabella's love springs from a moment of (mis)recognition, in which the real object of desire is the refracted image of the self.[69] Angela Carter picks up on this aspect of the lovers in her short story 'John Ford's *'Tis Pity She's a Whore*', a rewriting of the play that combines John Ford the early modern dramatist with John Ford the American film-maker. Strikingly, in the scene in which the siblings' incestuous desire emerges, brother and sister bend down to pick up a shattered mirror: 'In the fragments of the mirror, they kneel to see their round, blond, innocent faces that, superimposed upon one another, would fit at every feature, their faces, all at once the same face, the face that never existed until now.'[70] In Ford's play, as in Carter's story, Giovanni and Annabella's love springs from their sense of their sameness; as Giovanni argues, 'Wise nature first in your creation meant | To make you mine; else't had been sin and foul | To share one beauty to a double soul' (I.ii.231–3). In their carefully mirrored vows of affection, Ford emphasizes the lovers as reflections of the self. 'She is like me, and I like her', Giovanni tells the Friar. Annabella is responsive to the language of amorous similitude. When Sorenzo calls upon her to ask for her hand in marriage, she adopts the trope of the mirror as a means of rejecting him, suggesting that as well as being no beauty, he lacks the ability to reflect her adequately; 'You are no looking-glass', she tells him (III.ii.41).

Although Giovanni's description of beauty as a justification for love, and his elevation of Annabella as a goddess deserving worship suggests his adherence to the cult of Platonic love, his own brand of the philosophy does not repudiate the physical realm, but rather invests sensual pleasure with a transcendent meaning. He knows his Neoplatonic philosophy, and can argue:

---

[69] Wiseman argues: 'This moment of recognition of "something secretly familiar" is reminiscent of the repeated moments of recognition in the story of the Sand-man retold by Freud in his essay on the uncanny and also recalls Plato's description of the lover as a mirror' ('Incestuous Body', 217).

[70] Carter, 'John Ford's *'Tis Pity*', 24.

> the frame
> And composition of the mind doth follow
> The frame and composition of the body;
> So where the body's furniture is beauty,
> The mind's must needs be virtue; which allowed,
> Virtue itself is reason but refined,
> And love the quintessence of that; this proves
> My sister's beauty, being rarely fair,
> Is rarely virtuous; chiefly in her love,
> And chiefly in that love, her love to me.
> If hers to me, then so is mine to her;
> Since in like causes are effects alike.
>
> (II.v.15–26)

Nevertheless for Giovanni beauty functions not as a conduit to divine rapture, but as an end in and of itself. It is not Anabella's mind, virtue, or soul on which Giovanni dwells on time and time again, but her lips, breath, eyes, hair, and those 'unnamed' parts that are for 'pleasure framed' (II.v.52–3, 57–8). Whilst a desire to integrate the body and soul is not unusual in early modern texts,[71] Giovanni ultimately abandons the spiritual for the sensual, a perversion of Neoplatonism which goes hand in hand with his dangerous atheism, as he proclaims 'Let poring bookmen dream of other worlds: | My world and all of happiness is here, | And I'd not change it for the best to come' (V.iii.13–15). Annabella thus does not trigger an ascending return to God, but replaces God in a heaven which is reconfigured as an imitation of the earthy; it is the place where the lovers can 'kiss one another, prate or laugh, | Or do as we do here' (V.v.40–1).

However, as the play progresses Giovanni's idealized discourse of romantic love gives way to that of patriarchal authority and possession. Giovanni increasingly imagines his sister's body as a realm to rule and a commodity to enjoy, cataloguing her features as if they were his private 'world of variety' (II.v.50). He tells Annabella, 'I envy not the mightiest man alive, | But hold myself, in being king of thee, | More great than were I king of the world' (II.i.18–20). Similarly, the vocabulary of erotic reflection, initially Platonic, comes to resemble a

---

[71] Huebert shows how in a great deal of early modern literature 'spiritual urges of the soul are consummated in tactile and erotic sensations' (*Baroque English Dramatist*, 38).

different sort of mirroring: namely, that found in early modern conduct books. Burton summarizes this tradition, in which wives are instructed to act as their husband's mirrors, reflecting their every mood and whim:

a good wife . . . should be as a looking-glasse, to represent her husbands face and passion: If he be pleasant, she should be marry: if hee laugh, she should smile; if hee looke sad, shee should participate of his sorrow, and beare a part with him, and so they should continue in mutuall love one towards another.[72]

'Mutual love' is ensured via a woman's absolute emotional subservience, so that, from one point of view, a successful marriage looks like a man's union with himself. This is certainly what Giovanni seems to desire; as Laurie A. Finke suggests, 'Through incest, Giovanni quite self-consciously attempts to achieve a union with himself by "annihilating the otherness—the autonomy—of his sister" '.[73] However, whilst 'the mirror emblem totally suppresses any autonomy in the wife', it simultaneously uncovers the radical instability of masculine identity, which seeks a confirmation of the self outside the self.[74] Giovanni may be sublimely arrogant in his claim that he 'could command the course | Of time's eternal motion', but the clause which immediately follows, 'hadst thou been | One thought more steady than an ebbing sea', reveals how this Marlovian posture is ultimately dependent on Annabella's compliance (V.v.12–14).[75] This, perhaps, more than sexual jealousy, explains Giovanni's need to murder his sister once she renounces their incestuous relationship.

The shift in Giovanni's treatment of his sister springs in part from his rivalry with Sorenzo, Annabella's suitor. Although Annabella initially rejects Sorenzo, she eventually marries him after she discovers that she is pregnant with Giovanni's baby and becomes convinced that marriage is the only way for her to save her soul and that of her brother. At first, Giovanni's childlike single-minded devotion to his sister makes him appear utterly unlike Sorenzo, who is a sophisticated womanizer adept at using the language of love to his own ends.[76] However, the two

---

[72] Burton, *Anatomy*, iii.53.   [73] Finke, 'Painting Women', 368.
[74] Jones, *Currency*, 27.   [75] McCabe, *Incest*, 232.
[76] When Sorenzo wishes to be rid of Hippolita, his former lover, he rejects her in the language of Christian repentance: 'The vows I made, if you remember well, | Were

men have more in common than first appears. Like Sorenzo, Giovanni manipulates ethical discourses for selfish purposes; he uses Platonic love to justify his incestuous relationship with his sister, but will also take up a more conventional stance when it suits him, as when he argues against his sister marrying, as this 'would be to damn her' proving her 'greedy of variety of lust' (II.v.41–2). By the end of the play, Giovanni and Sorenzo seem to mirror rather than oppose one another, competing first for sexual possession of Annabella and later to kill her. In this context, Giovanni's last violent act is less his own glorious achievement than the perverse realization of Sorenzo's carefully scripted murder; Sorenzo, after all, has devised the scene in which Annabella will be killed, gathering an appropriate audience, and dressing her in her wedding gown; what he fails to foresee is that Giovanni will take the role of central actor, usurping Sorenzo's part at the bloody banquet, as he had previously in the bedroom. Sorenzo threatens Annabella, 'I'll rip up thy heart'; Giovanni does just this (IV.iii.53).

Giovanni's emergence in the final scene carrying his sister's heart on a dagger recalls emblematic depictions of 'Cruel Love', allowing the Petrarchan conceit of possessing a loved one's heart to be made shockingly literal.[77] In this vivid stage picture, emblematic conventions of lovesickness coexist with its construction as a corporeal disease, fusing the image of the Platonic lover with that of the love-sick madman. Returning to the banquet, Giovanni uses the language of 'food and feast' to reveal his sexual relationship with his sister:[78]

> You came to feast, my lords, with dainty fare.
> I came to feast too, but I digged for food
> In a much richer mine than gold or stone
> Of any value balanced. 'Tis a heart,
> A heart, my lords, in which is mine entombed.
>
> (V.vi.23–7)

Giovanni's description of Annabella's heart as 'food' offers a disturbingly literal picture of incest as a kind of cannibalism. Conceptualized as

---

wicked and unlawful' he tells her, 'twere more sin | To keep them than to break them' (II.ii.85–7).

[77] See Neill, 'Strange Riddle'.
[78] Anderson, 'The Heart and the Banquet', 211.

a territory to be possessed or a food to be consumed, Giovanni's metaphors for his sister's body suggest his desire for complete possession of her. In this Giovanni demonstrates the 'melancholy cannibalism' outlined by Kristeva, in which an individual attempts to possess 'the intolerable other' whilst simultaneously repudiating its loss'; 'Better fragmented, torn, cut up, swallowed, digested . . . than lost'.[79] Like other revengers, Giovanni is triumphant: 'now survives | None of our house but I, gilt in the blood | Of a fair sister and a hapless father' (V.vi.66–8). The line offers a striking aural pun on 'gilt'—Giovanni is both gilded in blood (or as he puts it, 'trimmed in reeking blood') and guilty of incest—his aesthetic achievement is also his ethical undoing (V.vi.10).[80] Nevertheless, Giovanni glories in his sister's death, finding in this 'rape of life and beauty' his 'last and greatest part' (V.vi.19; V.v.107). His dying words describe his hopes for the afterlife; it is the place wherein he can 'enjoy this grace, | Freely to view my Annabella's face' (V.vi.106–7). As Richard McCabe notes 'even in death the possessive pronoun persists'.[81]

Giovanni's murder of his sister suggests the extent to which Giovanni's struggle with his rival has replaced his concern for his sister; love has given way to competition. It also provides an apt image of the self-defeating nature of revenge, in which stratagems misfire, trapping their creators instead; as Macbeth comments, 'This even-handed justice | Commends th'ingredience of our poisoned chalice | To our own lips' (I.vii.10–12). Hippolyta acts out this metaphor of course (drinking from the poisoned cup intended for Sorenzo), but it is in Giovanni that the self-consuming circularity of revenge meets that of incest; even more than most revengers, Giovanni finds the conclusion of revenge in its origins: 'The hapless fruit | That in her womb received its life from me, | Hath had from me a cradle and a grave' (V.v.95–7). In Giovanni's 'unkind' murder of his sister, Ford thus telescopes the perverse logic of vengeance into a single act (V.v.93). Giovanni's murder of Annabella is a form of psychological suicide: as well as losing his beloved mistress, he has lost his beloved self.

---

[79] Kristeva, *Black Sun*, 12.
[80] Ford discusses the gap between aesthetic beauty and its moral meaning in *Line of Life*, observing 'how easy it is to guild a rotten post' (p. 308).
[81] McCabe, *Incest*, 239.

'NEW SECTS OF LOVE': WILLIAM
DAVENANT'S *THE TEMPLE OF LOVE* AND
THE PLATONICK LOVERS

Unlike Ford's play, which exposes the uncanny interconnection between Platonic love and pathological forms of desire, Davenant's masque *The Temple of Love* (1635) and his play *The Platonick Lovers* (1636) juxtapose the language of Platonic love with an examination of physical appetites: whereas Davenant's masque suggests that the idealized discourse of affection must not deny the importance of fecundity, particularly within the royal marriage of Charles I and Henrietta Maria, *The Platonick Lovers* exploits the comic potential of Platonic love, suggesting that the artificial philosophy must eventually give way to a 'natural', sexual relationship which reinstates 'husband's government' (H3^r). In these two works, the cause and consequence of affection is shown to be physiological and sexual, not just abstract and spiritual. Perfect love is achieved, not through the rejection of all sensory pleasure, but through the union of both bodies and souls.

Davenant's works also suggest how the discourse of lovesickness within Caroline drama carries with it sexual-political implications. Although the philosophy of Neoplatonism was originally constructed around homoerotic relations, its vocabulary of hierarchy and subservience is soon applied to heterosexual love. This appropriation effected a change in the traditional gender hierarchy, in that it both granted the beloved a new metaphysical and theological significance as well as enabled her to occupy a dominant position in her relationship with a male suitor. Importantly, the emphasis within Neoplatonic philosophy upon the need to avoid sexual intercourse meant that women were able to extend the time of their courtship, the liminal period during which they exercised control over their suitors. The hostility of male dramatists, such as Davenant, to this protracted inversion of the traditional gender hierarchy informs their portrayal of Platonic love as an emasculating force. Within the teleology of the drama, the civil solution of marriage effects a double remedy, offering a cure for the physical suffering of the lovesick male patient, while at the same time curtailing the sexual-political disorder inherent in his 'unnatural' veneration of the female beloved. Erotic melancholy functions as the cure for

Platonic love, rendering lovesickness the necessary precursor to marital health.

Davenant's masque *The Temple of Love* was written for Henrietta Maria when the fashion for Platonic love was at its height (one year after Howell treats the cult as 'news'). It was performed at Whitehall on Shrove Tuesday, with the queen and fourteen of her ladies taking part.[82] The queen was clearly pleased with the masque, and she performed it three more times within the week. *The Temple of Love* depicts the triumph of chastity over sensuality, achieved through the example of Queen Indamora of Narsinga (played by Henrietta Maria). At the opening of the masque, the queen is informed by Divine Poesy that the time has come for the Temple of Chaste Love to be reinstated in Britain. However, the magicians who control the world of sensual pleasures oppose the queen's attempts at reformation and call upon nature to combat this new, sterile philosophy. Through an antimasque they present the elements of nature—earth, fire, air, and water—in excessive and corrupted forms. The magicians fail and the masque ends with an image of the royal marriage as an ideal pattern of chaste affection.

The title suggests a celebration of Platonic love; however, the valorization of chaste affection within the masque is qualified by an admission that the physical world cannot be entirely effaced (something presumably evident to Davenant himself, whose nose was severely disfigured from a bout of syphilis). In the first half of the masque, the vulgar magicians playfully exaggerate the implications of Neoplatonism, intimating that if the courtiers fully pursue their interest in the spiritual realm, then the very finery for which the court is reputed will be rendered obsolete. According to the magicians, Persian quilts, embroidered couches, beds and clothing are mere 'Bodily implements' and should be relinquished, as they are of no use to a refined soul.[83] In addition, while the female followers of Platonic fashion may be exalted by their doctrine, they are simultaneously described as carrying 'frozen Winter in their blood'. Those who seek to woo Platonic women must attempt to court their minds and, rather than seek any physical consummation, practice 'generation not | Of bodies but of souls' (sig. B2ʳ).

Whilst faithfully reflecting the popularity of Neoplatonic doctrine among the women of the court, the masque nonetheless questions the

---

[82] Edmond, *Rare*, 56–7.   [83] Jones and Davenant, *Temple of Love*, sig. B2ᵛ.

desirability of a wholly intellectual interaction between the sexes. In a number of asides, the magicians joke with the women in the audience, insinuating that Platonic love, although delightful in theory, is unlikely to satisfy their every need. The Persian Page describes how the philosophy has transformed his master:

> One heretofore that wisely could confute
> A lady at her window with his Lute.
> There devoutly in a cold morning stand
> Two howres, praysing the snow of her white hand;
> So long, 'till's words were frozen 'tween his lips,
> And's Lute-strings learnt their quav'ring from his hips.
> And when he could not rule her to's intent,
> Like *Tarquin* he would proffer ravishment.
> But now, no fear of Rapes, untill he find
> A maidenhead belonging to the mind.
> The rest are all so modest too, and pure,
> So virginly, so coy, and so demure,
> That they retreat at kissing, and but name
> *Hymen*, or Love, they blush for very shame!
>
> (sig. B2ᵛ)

Here the traditional wooing of the lover is replaced by a display of coy and squeamish chastity; the only indication of his desire evident in his blush. Although the male Platonic lover thus fulfils a fundamental tenet of Neoplatonic doctrine (achieving wholeness through the integration of qualities traditionally associated with women, such as shame and modesty), the effect is to make him effete; while women who adhere to Neoplatonic doctrine become frigid, men are emasculated.

The magicians insist upon the impossibility of transcending the body, and they call upon nature to battle this new and strange doctrine of Neoplatonism, invoking the spirits of earth, air, fire and water to infect the bodies of mankind. Nature is represented by the four elements of the physical universe, appearing in the guise of the four bodily humours. The fiery spirits enter 'all in flames, and their visards of a Cholericke Complexion', the airy spirits enter in feathers 'with sanguine vizards', the watery spirits enter with fish scales and the earthy spirits wear branches without leaves (sig. B3ᵛ). The effect of the antimasque is to contrast the materiality of the physical universe, 'the faction of | the flesh', with the abstraction of Neoplatonic philosophy, a 'hum'rous virtue' favoured by a 'queasie age'. The antimasque, whilst depicting the physical world as riotous and immoral, nonetheless serves as a symbolic expression of the body given free reign. Its function is to remind the audience of the existence of physical and sinful appetites, thereby idealizing Platonic love by providing it with a lascivious and immoral foil. However, the magicians emphasize that this eruption of sensuous physicality is a product of nature itself; as they remark 'Nature, our weaknesse must be thought our crime' (sig. B3ʳ).

The construction of Davenant's masque, contrasting the language of Neoplatonic courtship with an antimasque of sinful appetites, appears to suggest that the physical and spiritual realms are irreconcilable. However, the final tableau of *The Temple of Love* seeks to resolve this conflict, integrating a discourse of Platonic love into a wider vision of nature as orderly, regenerative, and fertile. The song of Reason and Will serves to reconcile desire and virtue: 'Come melt thy soule in mine, that when unite, | We may become one virtuous appetite' (sig. C4ᵛ). Amianteros, or 'Chast Love,' descends to earth, celebrating her return with images of fecundity:

> Softly as fruitfull showres I fall,
> And th'undiscern'd increase I bring,
> Is of more precious worth than all
> A plenteous Summer payes a Spring.
>
> (sig. Dᵛ)

By likening herself to 'fruitfull showres', Amianteros indicates that the chaste love she represents is compatible with the fecundity of nature. Her song, with its images of fertility and natural increase, serves as a counterpoint to the sterile philosophy of Indamora and her followers, who 'carry frozen Winter in their blood'. Rather than seeking to efface the physical world, Amianteros celebrates the arrival of Spring, which reawakens the earth to *Fructifie each barren heart, | And give eternall growth to Love*' (sig. Dᵛ). Through Amianteros' song, Davenant thus offers his audience a redefinition of the Neoplatonic conception of 'virtue'. The political importance of this distinction is made manifest in the closing lines of the masque, which address the royal family directly:

To CHARLES, the mightiest and the best,
And to the Darling of his breast,
     (Who rule b'example as by power)
May youthfull blessings still increase,
And in their Off-spring never cease,
     Til Time's too old to last an hower.

(sig. D^v)

This tribute to the continuing fecundity of the royal marriage reworks the earlier song of Amianteros, with its celebration of natural abundance. The emphasis on Charles's children reminds the audience of the physical responsibilities of Henrietta Maria as wife and royal mother. Davenant does not seek to challenge the identity of the queen as a paradigm of chastity and virtue; rather, by insisting upon the possibility of 'virtuous appetite', the masque suggests that the abstract language of Neoplatonism is reconcilable with the material demands of the physical, political world.

Davenant's *The Platonick Lovers*, performed at court and at the Blackfriars Theatre in the season of 1635–6, further examines the tension between the spiritual abstraction of Platonic love and the material reality of human sexuality. Despite the fact that Theander and Eurithea, the lovers of the title, are idealized in the play, *The Platonick Lovers* also appears to criticize non-corporeal affection as an impractical and unnatural code for human behaviour; as Wendell Broom suggests, Davenant takes Platonic love seriously, 'but also satirically undercuts the assumptions and values on which it rests'.[84] Theander's idealistic view of love is shown to spring from ignorance, and his idealization of his mistress is lampooned in the behaviour of Gridonell, whose inexperience of women causes him to fall in love with an impoverished, old woman. Significantly, chaste and sterile Platonic affection is shown to demand a physical cure. The doctor Buonateste heats the blood of Theander and Eurithea, thereby engendering in them the symptoms of erotic melancholy. This prompts the two lovers to join in marriage, repudiating their former philosophy and reaffirming the traditional gender hierarchy and the 'natural' function of human desire.

The play opens with the arrival of Theander and Phylomont, who represent their friendship in Neoplatonic language as the sharing of

---

[84] Broom, 'Introduction', in Davenant, *Platonick Lovers*, ed. Broom, 19.

souls. The two friends are also linked through their love of one another's sisters. However, as each friend hurries to greet his beloved, differences between the two couples are revealed: whereas Eurithea runs to embrace Theander, Ariola's response to Phylomont is cold and stand-offish. Fredeline attributes this disparity to contrasting philosophies of love; Theander and Eurithea

> are Lovers of a pure
> Coelestiall kind, such as some stile Platonicall:
> (A new Court Epethite scarce understood)
> But all they wooe, Sir is the Spirit, Face,
> And heart, therefore their conversation is
> More safe to Fame.[85]

Ariola and Phylomont, on the other hand 'still affect | For naturall ends'

> such a way as Libertines call Lust,
> But peacefull Politicks, and cold Divines
> Name Matrimony Sir; therefore, although
> Their wise Intent be good and lawfull, yet
> Since it infers much Game and Pleasure i'th event,
> In subtle bashfulnesse, shee would not seeme
> To entertaine with too much forwardnesse,
> What shee (perhaps) doth willingly expect.

> (sig. B4^v)

Unlike Theander and Eurithea, who have a greater freedom to express their love physically, Phylomont and Ariola act awkwardly because of their anticipation of the 'Game and Pleasure' that awaits them in the marriage bed.

Although Platonic love is mocked by Fredeline as 'A new Court Epethite scarce understood,' the relationship of Theander and Eurithea is idealized. Their detachment from sexual desire gives them a greater freedom to express physical affection, and their scenes together are romantic and unrestrained. Unlike Phylomont, who is discouraged from entering Ariola's room before their marriage, Theander goes into Eurithea's room in the middle of the night to kiss and admire her. The Neoplatonic emphasis on spiritual love and mutual esteem also promotes a greater level of intimacy and equality between the lovers:

[85] Davenant, *Platonick Lovers*, sigs. B4^r–B4^v.

Eurithea is Theander's 'Virgin friend' in whom he confides and whom
he trusts. It is only when Theander's sexual desires emerge that he starts
to keep secrets from Eurithea, and asks that she keep her face covered.
Sexual desire is depicted as the force that establishes the gender hierarchy, and requires that women be modest. Events within the play make
it necessary for Theander and Eurithea to recognize their sexual nature.
However, rather than celebrating this awakening, the play represents it
as a fall from innocence.

The emergence of Theander's sexual desire resonates within the wider
theological context of the fall of man. He describes lovesickness as both
morally and physically damaging: his flaming heart, boiling liver and
'scorched veines' warm him 'to a guilt' which will 'burne [him] after
death'. The physiological language of the medical tradition is conflated
with a confessional language of sin and damnation, so that the fire
in his blood is identified with the flames 'kindled and bred in Hell'.
In addition, his sexual excitement results in a self-conscious desire to
conceal himself. He beckons Eurithea to hide with him in the garden,
but she recognizes the strangeness of his request and asks him why they
should hide, when they 'know | Not guiltinesse to cause a bashfull feare'
(sig. F3ʳ). Significantly, Theander's shame prompts him to cover, not
his own body, but the face of his beloved. He tells her, 'Hide, hide thy
beauty e're | Thou speak'st; put on thy vaile: nay, closer yet' (sig. Gʳ).
His actions substantiate the claim attributed to Bembo in Castiglione's
The Courtier that the beauty of women is not inherently sinful, but
is made to seem so by the intemperate response of men to its display.
Rather than exercise self-control, Theander displaces the responsibility
for sexual desire onto the body of his lover.

Although Theander constructs his newfound sexuality as an immoral
sickness, the play also criticizes Neoplatonism as a sterile and emasculating affection, which leads Theander to regard all forms of sexuality
as a 'secret sicknesse'. Theander's abhorrence of human sexuality leads
to a mistaken belief that marriage is a form of lust. When asked by
Phylomont for permission to marry Ariola, Theander reacts with hor-
ror, protesting that 'Your soules are wedded Sir, | I'm sure you would
not marrie bodies too' (sig. E1ᵛ). Just as his own experience of desire
prompts him to cover Eurithea's face, so Theander's awareness of his
sister's sexual desires causes him to lose respect for her and he tries to

have her locked up. Theander's disgust, however, may betray his naivety. Fredeline suggests that Theander's Platonism is simply an elaborate cover for his sexual ignorance, which will ultimately leave him without an heir; 'ignorant | O th'use of marriage', the only babies Theander will be making are those produced by gazing into Eurithea's eyes (sig. C1ᵛ).

The suggestion that Theander's adherence to non-corporeal affection stems from ignorance rather than spiritual elevation is reinforced by the subplot, which burlesques Theander's adulation of his mistress in the behaviour of Gridonell. Gridonell has been sent away by his father Sciolto to grow up without books and has never seen a woman. The first woman he lays eyes on is Amadine, the old and impoverished sister of Castraganio. Uncertain as to what she is, Gridonell gazes at her in fascination, exclaiming:

> This is a rare sight
> One of the Angels sure, and a great Gallant among 'em,
> Had it but blew wings on the shoulders, it
> Could not be of lesse degree then an Angell.
>
> (sig. C3ᵛ)

Gridonell's clownish attempt to praise Amadine as 'One of the Angels' offers a parody of the Platonic lover's idealization of the mistress, poking fun at the philosophy's insistence upon the quasi-divine status of women. Sciolto dismisses his son as 'one of *Plato's* Lovers' and assumes that he will fail to beget an heir (sig. [C4ʳ]). Through the figure of Gridonell, Davenant suggests that the philosophy of Neoplatonism encourages foolishness and self-delusion. Theander eventually realizes as much, confessing that his earlier preference for spiritual abstraction over physical desire was not in fact 'a virtue', but rather 'a dull mistake' (sig. G3ᵛ).

The figure who is responsible for awakening Theander and Gridonell to their sexual impulses is Buonateste, a 'generous Artist', who represents an ideal of sexual morality (sig. A3ᵛ). Maintaining that Plato's writings have been misinterpreted by women keen to invent their own theory of love and attribute it to the philosopher, he beseeches Fredeline 'not to wrong | My good old friend *Plato*, with this court calumnie', claiming that the women

> father on him a Fantastick Love
> Hee never knew, poore Gentleman, upon
> My knowledge sir, about two thousand yeares
> Agoe, in the high street yonder
> At *Athens*, just by the corner as you passe
> To *Diana's* Conduit (a Haberdashers house)
> It was (I thinke) hee kept a wench.
>
>   (sigs. D4ʳ–D4ᵛ)

Buonateste undermines the credibility of non-corporeal love by emphasizing Plato's sexual identity: he places the philosopher within a material, historical context, imagining him walking down the high street on the way to meet his mistress. Regarding Platonic love as a naïve and artificial doctrine devised by women, the doctor takes it upon himself to cure those devoted to virginity. When Ariola decides to convert to Platonism, her frustrated fiancé knows to ask Buonateste for assistance. '*Plato* shall lose one fond disciple sir' he assures Phylomont, 'Or I'le goe burne my bookes, and sindge my beard | Off in the flame' (sig. K1ᵛ).

Although Buonateste rejects Neoplatonic philosophies that depict love as a spiritual abstraction, neither does he construct love as a wholly sexual appetite. Instead, he repeatedly asserts that there is a difference between non-corporeal affection and erotic desire, maintaining that love cannot be induced artificially. It is rather Fredeline who articulates a cynical materialist view of love. He rejects Buonateste's assertion that Eurithea's affection cannot be compelled, maintaining that once she 'comes to relish Man' her entire psychological and ethical character will be transformed:

> then like a Spring
> Too long imprison'd in her Ice, shee'l spread
> Into a lib'rall streame, that ev'ry thirsty Lover may
> Carouse, untill his heat be quench'd.
>
>   (sig. G2ᵛ)

Like the women in *The Temple of Love* who 'carry frozen Winter in their blood', Eurithea's adherence to Platonism is depicted as endowing her with an inhuman iciness. Nevertheless, Fredeline's cynical attitude to women and his belief that love is merely the product of a sexual impulse is ultimately shown to be as reductive as Theander's Platonism; just as

Buonateste administers a cure for Theander's extreme chastity, so too does he give Fredeline a medicine to temper his 'lust'.

Buonateste is represented as embodying a harmonious balance between a philosophy that depicts love as a bodily instinct and one that represents it as an intangible abstraction. He recognizes the spiritual and physical components of love and gives each a separate aetiology: fascination, the theory outlined by Ficino in Book Speech Seven of his *Commentary on Plato's Symposium on Love*, is located as the origin of abstract affection, whereas 'the blood, and not the Eyes' is the corporeal basis of erotic desire (sig. D3ᵛ). Buonateste's cure thus reconciles spiritual and sexual appetites; his medicine works in agreement with the body's innate system, inciting a 'nat'rall appetite' for sex in the Platonic lovers by 'heat[ing] their bloods into desire' (sig. C2ʳ). Described in the play as a descendent of Diogenes, he is also depicted as the servant of nature: 'Wise Nature is my Mistrisse', he asserts, 'I shall | Demeane my selfe most stoutly in her cause' (sig. Lᵛ).

Theander's cure precipitates a change in the way in which he treats Eurithea. Fredeline suggests that Theander's sexual awakening provokes his recognition of the actual purpose of women:

> the Ice is melted that hath kept his vaines
> So frozen and condenc'd; hee must find out,
> That Nature made a woman for some use
> More consequent, than to converse with, and admire
> Besides, this our belov'd and knotty Sophister
> Hath fill'd me with such Potent arguments
> Divine and Morall, to perswade the Rites
> Of Marriage, wise, and seemly too, as hee
> Shall needs consent in's reason and his will,
> That hee was once begotten, and must now beget.
>
> (sig. G1ᵛ)

Desire is depicted as revealing and engendering 'natural' gender relations, prompting Theander to recognize that beyond being companions with whom to converse, or objects to admire, women have 'more consequent' uses. A woman's sexual identity is constructed as her chief function; it is the reason that 'Nature made a woman'. Fredeline's statement that Theander 'shall needs consent in's reason and will | That hee was once begotten, and must now beget' echoes the conclusion of *The*

Temple of Love in which Reason and Will sing together during the royal apotheosis, and both works end with a new form of love that promises fecundity and renewal. However, whereas in the masque Reason and Will are joined in a celebration of a new form of Platonism, here they act to prompt Theander to renounce Platonic love.

Theander's cure is thus represented as a move from an artificial, sterile philosophy to a natural, procreative one. Once again, this shift corresponds to the pattern found in *The Temple of Love*. Buonateste and the magicians, the chief agents who effect this change, are portrayed as devotees of nature, and where Buonateste engenders the symptoms of lovesickness in Theander to effect his cure, the magicians treat the body of mankind by infecting it with the four humours. Paradoxically, although both of these cures are represented as an illness and associated with sin, the destructive aspects of this cure—depicted in the antimasque of the former work and in Theander's illness in the latter— allow for a harmonious balance to be restored. As in *The Temple of Love*, in which nature unites with Platonic love resulting in a love which is both chaste and fertile, Buonateste is portrayed as uniting the lover's spiritual and corporeal desires.

When Phylomont is finally given permission to marry Ariola, he looks forward to taking control of their relationship. Ariola, who is no longer cold, but is free with her kisses, is told that her period of amorous governance is almost finished. Phylomont, accepting her affectionate embrace, tells her:

> This bounty had been excellent, when you
> Had privilege to give, or to deny; but now
> Your charter's out of date, and mine
> Begins to rule: the Priest attends below
> To celebrate our Nuptiall rites, which is
> The happy houre that doth advance
> The husband's government; come, to the Chappell, Love.
>
> (sig. H3^r)

Marriage, along with being a 'sweet | And sudden cure' for lovesickness, is depicted as restoring a man to his traditional place in the gender hierarchy, ushering in the 'husband's government'. Ariola, however, tells Phylomont that she has recently converted to Platonism and is therefore no longer interested in marrying him. Phylomont, weary and frustrated, threatens to find sexual satisfaction elsewhere if she will not agree to marry him. Invoking the name of Hercules, Phylomont threatens to 'seeke some downe right virgin out, that knowes | Natures plaine lawes, though not the Art of love' (sig. H3^r).

Platonic love is depicted as empowering women in that it extends the period of courtship, perpetuating the limited phase in which a woman has the 'privilege to give, or to deny' her lover favours. The philosophy's emphasis on chastity prevents men from consummating their relationships, leaving them in a frustrating role of sexual passivity. Phylomont, for example, complains that the position he is expected to take up in Platonic love is ridiculously effete, claiming that he is unfit for 'sighing thus (*Ariola*) Vnder a Poplar Tree, or whining by | A River side', and Gridonell is described by his father as being transformed 'from a tame | Soldier to a towne Bull' when he awakens to his sexual appetites (K1^r). Sexual intercourse is seen to affirm masculinity and ensure a man's possession of his beloved. Phylomont tells Theander that he should

> Possesse your Ladies Bed your selfe, y'are the
> Best sentinell to hinder th'onslaught of
> The Enemie, whining and puling Love is fit
> For Evenuches and for old revolted Nunnes.
>
> (sigs. L1^r–L1^v)

Phylomont regards Platonic love as an emasculating philosophy fit only for 'Evenuches'. Whereas Platonic love is represented earlier in the play as engendering peace, equality, and harmony between lovers, marriage is described through metaphors of war and domination. The epilogue emphasizes that Platonic love is effeminate, and it is women who promote this 'Ladies Paradox' despite that fact that it 'recreate[s] the mind and not the blood'. The traditional structure which associates men with rational thought and women with bodily instincts is reversed, so that the sensual and corporeal aspects of love are equated with men, whereas women prefer mental and spiritual forms of affection. Neoplatonism, in Davenant's play, ultimately suggests that it is women who are the chaste and cerebral gender.

Neoplatonism and medical ideas regarding love brought with them other philosophical and cultural assumptions, advocating a different relation between the body and soul; between spiritual affection and sexuality; and a different goal in the amorous process, whether spiritual enlightenment, or procreative marriage. The doctrine of Platonic love offers an alternative construction of love to that found in natural philosophy, formulating it as ideal, chaste, and spiritual, rather than disorderly and pathological. Emphasizing chastity over consummation, courtship over marriage, and desire over fulfilment, Platonic love inverts much of the medical advice for what Renaissance doctors hold to be healthy in romantic love. The most obvious contradiction between the two philosophies lies in their conflicting attitude towards sexuality. Whereas in Platonic love, abstinence and contemplation of the beloved might lead to spiritual transcendence, medical discourses posit sexual frustration and obsession as the main causes of lovesickness. Both traditions also suggested a different relation between the lover and beloved, each of which presupposes a different gender power hierarchy. Although initially constructed as a homoerotic discourse, Platonic love is also increasingly associated with women in the early modern period. In Neoplatonic gatherings, women 'quickly learned to use the reigning language to their own advantage'.[86] And in practical and esoteric ways Platonic love was beneficial to women: it justified a prolonged period of courtship, granted the female beloved an elevated spiritual significance, and endorsed flirtation as morally educative. With its emphasis on friendship, equality, and reciprocity, Neoplatonism offered women a new way of envisaging love, in which one was encouraged to find, not a lord and master, but a second self.

---

[86] Jones, *Currency*, 10.

5

'Griefs Will Have their Vent':
Physical and Psychological Remedies
for Lovesickness

Neither let any man call [love] the sweete passion or affection,
seeing of all other miseries, this is the greatest miserie, yea so great
as that all the tortures which have bin so exquisitely devised by
the wit of tyrants, wil never be able to exceed crueltie therof. The
Philosopher Thianeus knew well what to say to the K. of Babylon,
which praied him to invent some cruel torment for the punishing
of a gentleman whom he had found in bed with his paramour:
for (sayth he) let him live, and in time his love will punish him
sufficiently.

(M. Andreas Laurentius,
A Discourse of the Preservation of the Sight, 119)

This chapter investigates cures for lovesickness in early modern literature, detailing the divergent ways that writers depict medical treatments
in order to give them a charged dramatic meaning. In particular, I will
focus on four cures that are revealing for the ways in which gender
affects lovesickness: two physical treatments—phlebotomy (or bloodletting) and sexual intercourse—and two mental or psychological cures—
trickery (or performative healing) and humiliation. A final cure, which
involves the vilification of the beloved, will be treated separately in the
following chapter, due to the complexity of its history and significance.
These cures suggest the rich range of ways in which lovesickness is
conceptualized: bleeding and sexual intercourse assume the malady is
primarily physiological, trickery emphasizes the lover's mental fixation,
and humiliation illustrates how the degrading effects of love can act as
a cure.

In some instances, the therapies being examined function as medical cures in the loosest possible sense. On stage a doctor rarely administers a phlebotomy; rather, lovesick individuals are propelled by their passionate natures into incurring wounds that indirectly cure them. Bloodletting is thus represented as a lucky accident, dramatically engineered by the plot. Similarly, while humiliation acts to free the lover from his malady, it is never intentionally undergone as a cure. Nonetheless, the representations of these remedies convey different aspects of the cultural construction of lovesickness. Whereas bloodletting articulates the way in which disorderly sexuality is represented as being physically manifested in the body, sexual cures dramatize how desire precedes and is detached from the erotic object. Furthermore, trickery, which is aimed at dislodging the sufferer's mental fixation, suggests how the lover is enraptured not by the actual beloved, but by an internal vision; and cures achieved through the lover's humiliation dramatize the power struggles underlying courtship.

For men in particular, lovesickness is portrayed as a violent passion that can engender an emasculating loss of self-control and self-possession; because of this, remedies for erotic melancholy often function as social as well as psychosomatic cures, so that the sufferer's restoration to bodily health is also represented as a reconciliation with homosocial codes of honour. In bloodletting, for example, plays often align the purgative and punitive aspects of the remedy, in which the lover's wounding serves as both a cure for his excessive passion and a punishment for his ignoble behaviour. Alternatively, the lover's cure through humiliation is predicated upon the idea that love is effeminizing. An examination of cures for lovesickness thus illuminates wider cultural ideas about gender and sexuality, suggesting the fears and fantasies regarding erotic abandon, the sexual double standard concerning illicit sex, and what is at stake in curing the impassioned lover other than the lover's health.

PHYSICAL CURES: PURGING THE LOVER'S BODY

Polluted Blood

Bloodletting is frequently recommended as a cure for lovesickness, both because a sanguine disposition predisposed one to passionate emotion, and because blood was the material source of seed, or sperm, which was held by many to be the physiological source of erotic desire.[1] As medical texts suggest, phlebotomy expelled the lover's excess blood, rid the body of noxious humours, and reduced the amount of seed generated.[2] Despite the fact that the lover is stereotypically imagined as an emaciated figure, whose body is wasted away by passion, the discourse of phlebotomy suggests that the lover suffers from an excess of bodily fluids which require a cathartic discharge. Lovesick individuals may appear to waste away in a consumptive manner, but they also need to be purged of their excess passion, blood, and seed. John Ford's *The Broken Heart* draws upon this idea, in which Orgilus' death functions as both a punishment for his murder of Ithocles and a purging for his lovesickness. Orgilus is permitted to select the form of his demise, and asks, appropriately enough, 'to bleed to death'.[3] He tells Armostos that he will act as his own executioner: 'I am well skilled in letting blood. Bind fast | This arm, that so the pipes may from their conduits | Convey a full stream' (V.ii.100–3). Taking on the mantle of surgeon, Orgilus discharges his overfull veins, fulfilling his prediction that 'Griefs will have their vent' (IV.i.116). There is even a hint of pleasurable release as he slits his veins with his dagger, telling the spectators, 'Thus I show cunning | In opening of a vein too full, too lively' (V.ii.121–2). Orgilus' choice highlights the way in which his death also functions as a perverse cure, reinforcing the close conceptual link between death and sex, blood and seed.

Because blood is invested with symbolic and ethical meaning in early modern literature, phlebotomy is frequently depicted in moral as well as medical terms, in which the corrupt blood being released reveals an individual's degeneracy and purges the body politic of bad blood. The physical properties of an individual's blood are portrayed as being inexorably linked to his or her moral state. For women, in particular, adulterous sex is seen to pollute both the body and the bloodline. Unlike men, who were only thought to emit sperm during sex, women were believed both to emit and receive sperm; the male seed (thought to be composed of heated and refined blood) was said to turn back into blood

---

[1] See Ch 1.
[2] See Ferrand, *Erotomania*, 261; Hart, *Klinike*, 325; and Babb, 'Physiological Conception', 1021.
[3] Ford, *Broken Heart*, V.ii.99.

after being released into the woman's body, mingling with and tainting her own supply. Whereas in monogamous relationships a man's sperm was seen to strengthen a woman's body, providing it with beneficial nourishment, illicit sexual intercourse was regarded as physically harmful, regardless of whether or not the woman was a willing participant in the sexual act. Thomas Heywood suggests that illicit sexual intercourse taints the family bloodline, calling into question a woman's legitimacy and retrospectively corrupting her ancestors: 'for the mind, as the body, in the act of adulterie being both corrupted, makes the action infamous and dishonourable, dispersing the poyson of sinne ever amongst those from whom she derives her birth'.[4] Such a theory provided a physiological justification for the sexual double standard, suggesting it was women, rather than men, who carried the physical signs of sexual immorality. Adulterous women are not just sinful, but are also the receivers and bearers of men's sins; they are the 'common shoare, that still receives | All the townes filth'.[5]

Women who are raped in early modern literature are thus represented as being physically unclean, even if they are mentally pure. This is the distinction that Lucrece herself makes after she has been raped by Tarquin in Shakespeare's *The Rape of Lucrece*, consoling herself with the knowledge that 'Though my gross blood be stained with this abuse, | Immaculate and spotless is my mind'.[6] By stabbing herself in 'her harmless breast', Lucrece frees herself from her contaminated body (described as a 'poisoned closet' and 'polluted prison') and reveals how her rape has tainted her blood:

> bubbling from her breast it doth divide
> In two slow rivers, that the crimson blood
> Circles her body in on every side,
> Who like a late-sacked island vastly stood,
> Bare and unpeopled in this fearful flood.
> Some of her blood still pure and red remained,
> And some looked black, and that false Tarquin stained.
>
> (ll. 1726, 1659, 1737–43)

---

[4] Heywood, *Gunaikeion*, 164, quoted by Fletcher, *Gender, Sex and Subordination*, 110.
[5] Dekker, *Honest Whore I*, I.i.   [6] Shakespeare, *Rape of Lucrece*, ll. 1655–6.

Lucrece's suicide disrupts and exposes her blood's putrefaction at the point of its transformation; the blood that flows from her body divides into two distinct streams: one red and pure, and the other dark and polluted by Tarquin's assault.

A similar depiction of the physical consequences of rape is found in Davenant's *The Cruel Brother* (1630), in which Foreste decides that he must kill his sister, Corsa, after he discovers that the Duke has raped her. For Foreste, it is of little consequence that Corsa's defilement is the result of physical force rather than by her consent; either way he believes that she has been contaminated. Foreste urges his sister to submit to her own death willingly, pressing her to think of her husband, whom he sees as the main victim of the Duke's actions: 'Could you indure to see your Lord, defil'd, | Polluted as you are?' he asks accusingly, 'Can you | Survive a wrong so eminent: a wrong | Committed a'gainst your Husband, and my Patron?'[7] His obsessive concern with his sister's blood shifts the focus away from the violence of rape to the 'staine' of female impurity, and eventually Corsa consents to having her brother 'slit her Wrist-vaynes', giving 'Liberty, to her polluted Blood' (sigs. [I4ʳ], I3ᵛ). If control of women often manifests itself through the regulation of their bodily apertures, such as their mouth and vagina, then Foreste reclaims his sister's body in her husband's name by opening his sister's veins and draining her body of blood.[8] Foreste's instructions to his sister suggest that he envisages her murder as a perverse form of bloodletting:

FORESTE: Come, stretch downe your Arme: and permit this Scarfe
   To fastne it to th'Chaire. Then vaile your Eies.
   We must not trust a Woman's vallour so—
CORSA: Oh, oh, oh.
FORESTE: The torture's past. Thy wrist vaynes are cut, Heere
   In this Bason bleed.

(sig. I1ʳ)

For Foreste, Corsa's death functions as a cure for her physical degradation, purifying her body and her husband's lineage. Foreste locates his sister's corrupt blood as the site of her defilement, and laments how

---

[7] [Davenant], *Cruel Brother*, sig. I1ʳ.
[8] Stallybrass, 'Patriarchal Territories', 129.

her rape has tainted it all; 'O could I separate | The blood defil'd from what is pure', he bemoans, 'I would | Shed that; then restraine the current'. Even Corsa's husband, who recognizes that his wife is merely a victim of the Duke's violent passions, nonetheless shares Foreste's sense of her physical pollution. Rebuking Foreste for his cruelty, he imagines a reconciliation with his dead wife, in which her raped body would be cleansed by 'her owne Teares', which 'Might soone have wash'd away her Bodys staine. | And she againe seeme cleane' (sig. [I4^r]).

Another instance in which the language of phlebotomy is employed to articulate revulsion at a woman's supposed physical corruption is found in Middleton and Rowley's *The Changeling* (1622). Like Lucrece and Corsa, Beatrice-Joanna is (at least at first) an unwilling participant in her sexual liaison with De Flores, who blackmails her into having sex with him. However, despite initially finding De Flores repulsive, Beatrice-Joanna seemingly undergoes a psychological transformation as a result of her sexual indiscretion and comes to love him. Sex with De Flores also changes Beatrice-Joanna's body, as is evident in the virginity test that her fiancé Alsemero administers to her.[9] Unlike the virginal Diaphanta, who yawns, sneezes, laughs, and becomes sleepy when given the potion from Jar M, Beatrice-Joanna remains unaffected by the substance. Although Beatrice-Joanna is able to pass Alsemero's virginity test through her clever mimicry of Diaphanta's behaviour (suggesting the ease with which women can fake everything from their orgasms to their innocence), her secret affair with De Flores is

---

[9] The idea that one could test a woman's virginity is not just a theatrical invention. Frances Howard, the woman on whom Beatrice-Joanna is often thought to be based, also underwent a virginity test in 1613 to attain an annulment from Robert Devereux, the third Earl of Essex. Howard was married to Essex at the age of 13, but eventually became involved with Robert Carr, the King's favourite, and sought a divorce from Essex, claiming that the marriage had not been consummated. Howard and her family 'In order to refute Essex's claim that Frances was physically incapable of the sexual act, while simultaneously establishing that she was a virgin . . . proposed that Frances submit herself to a gynaecological examination by a panel of midwives and married ladies'. The panel 'testified that they found her as straight as a child of nine or ten years of age' and was both 'fit for canal copulation and still a virgin'. Nonetheless, her detractors claimed that she sent a substitute in her place wearing a veil, a rumour alluded to in the play when Beatrice-Joanna sends Diaphanta to take her place on her wedding night. Somerset, *Unnatural Murder*, 146–7. For a relation of this case to *The Changeling*, see Heinemann, *Puritanism and Theatre*, 178–9; Malcolmson, 'As Tame as the Ladies', 142–58; and Simmons, 'Diabolical Realism', 290–306.

finally revealed just before she dies.[10] After being stabbed by De Flores, Beatrice-Joanna describes her own impending death as a necessary phlebotomy which will purify the family line. Just as Beatrice-Joanna's virginity can be empirically tested by Alsemero, so too does she imagine that her sexual corruption is physically manifested. She tells her father:

> Oh come not near me, sir, I shall defile you:
> I am that of your blood was taken from you
> For your better health; look no more upon't,
> But cast it to the ground regardlessly,
> Let the common sewer take it from distinction.[11]

Beatrice-Joanna warns her father to stay away, imagining her blood is that part of her father's that has become corrupt, and therefore must be let. As Deborah Burks argues, her cast-aside body 'is a literalization of the kind of cutting-off prescribed by the law to separate a family from the daughter whose body has betrayed them. In life as on stage, honour could only be salvaged through a ritual purging of the defiled part: the woman.'[12] Beatrice-Joanna here accepts the necessity of her death for her family's continued health, anticipating and mimicking the patriarchal voices that condemn her.

Although women are held to be particularly susceptible to the damaging physiological effects of illicit sex, men's indiscretions were also depicted as physically corrosive. In Beaumont and Fletcher's *The Maid's Tragedy*, for example, when Evadne kills her lover, the King, she describes her action as a remedial purging for his corrupted body. The King awakens to find Evadne tying him to the bed; believing that his lover is engaged in some new erotic game, he is eager to know what her latest 'pretty new device' is.[13] Evadne's offer of therapy is not, however, the kind of sexual healing the King has in mind:

---

[10] See Garber, 'The Insincerity of Women', 19–38. Garber sees Diaphanta's reactions as suggesting orgasm, but they also resemble the symptoms of hysteria, reinforcing the sense that whilst virginity is prized in Renaissance England, it is also imagined as a state prone to illness.

[11] Middleton and Rowley, *Changeling*, V.iii.149–53.

[12] Burks, 'Women's Complicity', 181.

[13] Beaumont and Fletcher, *Maid's Tragedy*, V.i.47.

EVADNE: Stay, sir, stay:
  You are too hot, and I have brought you physic
  To temper your high veins.
KING: Prithee, to bed then; let me take it warm;
  Here thou shalt know the state of my body better.
EVADNE: I know you have a surfeited foul body,
  And you must bleed.
KING: Bleed!
EVADNE: Ay, you shall bleed, lie still, and if the devil
  Your lust will give you leave, repent.

                                  (V.i.52–61)

In the dialogue between Evadne and the King, the connotation of 'physic' oscillates between bloodletting and sexual intercourse: both lovers wish to 'temper' the King's 'high veins', but whereas the King prefers to take his remedy 'warm', Evadne has determined that the King 'must bleed'. Like other revengers, Evadne imagines the King's murder as a necessary phlebotomy which will purge the body politic of corrupt blood. Her actions also resemble a kind of rape; as Alison Findlay suggests, 'The violent delight she experiences in avenging herself is a specifically male form of pleasure: eroticized despoliation.'[14]

The 'cures' discussed thus far are purgative rather than remedial, and their outcome is invariably death. However, there are other instances in which phlebotomy not only rids society of the 'bad blood' that threatens to corrupt its ethical foundation, but also heals the lovesick individual. In plays such as *The Nice Valour* and *A Very Woman,* bloodletting brings about an immediate physical cure, releasing men from their passionate obsessions and returning them to their right minds. Interestingly, in both plays it is not a doctor who carries out the phlebotomy; rather the bloodletting is the result of an act of violence. Such plots grant the lover's cure an element of moral instruction: under the spell of love, the man acts in a dishonourable way, inciting another individual to inflict the very injury that returns him to mental and physical health.

This is the case in Fletcher and Middleton's *The Nice Valour* (*c*.1615), in which the Passionate Lord is cured only after he is wounded and loses blood. As his name suggests, the Passionate Lord 'runs through all the

---

[14] Findlay, *Feminist Perspective*, 74. See also Alfar's discussion of Evandne in 'Masochism in *The Maid's Tragedy*'.

Passions of mankind', suffering in turn from violent love, melancholic despair, and wrathful fury. Although several methods are attempted to cure him, including sexual intercourse, it is only after being stabbed by the Soldier that the Passionate Lord recovers. The Duke informs the Soldier, 'where hope fail'd, nay Art it selfe resign'd, | Thou'st wrought that cure, which skil could never find'.[15] According to the First Gentleman, when the Passionate Lord revives after his brush with death he has undergone

> the most admired change
> That living flesh e're had; he's not the man my Lord;
> Death cannot be more free from passions, sir,
> Then he is at this instant: hee's so meek now,
> He makes those seem passionate, were never thought of:
> And for he fears his moods have oft disturb'd you sir,
> Hee's only hasty now for his forgivenesse.
>
> (V.iii.154–60)

The Passionate Lord's stabbing is the equivalent of a severe bloodletting: the wound releases his surplus blood and the malignant humours contained therein, and the Lord awakens drained of his violent emotions. Similarly, in *A Very Woman* (*c*.1616) Don Martino is cured only after being stabbed by Don John, his rival in love. Like the Passionate Lord in *The Nice Valour*, Don Martino is blinded by his extreme emotions and he ignominiously taunts his rival, who treats him with courteous respect. His wound provides the necessary purge that drains away his passionate love for Almira, allowing him to recognize that he has behaved dishonourably towards Don John. Still weakened from his wounds, Don Martino asserts his newfound scorn of love, suggesting that his overindulgence in matters of the heart has cured him of its effects; talk 'no more of love', he tells the Doctor, 'It was my surfeit, and I loath it now, | As men in Feavers meat they fell sick on'.[16] Like *A Very Woman*, *The Nice Valour* represents excessive love as a threat not only to the rational control of the male protagonist, but also to men's bonds with one another; Don Martino is both cured and chastised,

---

[15] [Fletcher and Middleton], *The Nice Valour*, in Beaumont and Fletcher, *Dramatic Works*, vol. vii, V.iii.192–3.

[16] [Fletcher and Massinger], *A Very Woman*, in Beaumont and Fletcher, *Dramatic Works*, vol. vii, IV.ii.50–1.

his disorderly love is expelled, and loving relations between men are restored. His revival thus goes hand in hand with his acceptance of the proper modes of courtly behaviour, rendering the act of bloodletting both his psychosomatic and social cure.

Although it is only the final two examples in which an act of violence cures an individual of his lovesickness, on closer inspection there is really very little difference between instances of bloodletting that kills and those that cure. In both cases the language of phlebotomy is employed to explain and justify an act of violence, in which the corruption in the blood is depicted as being moral as well as physical. There is, however, a notable distinction in the way that these representations differ in terms of gender. For women who have been raped or who are promiscuous, bloodletting is a means of cleansing the family bloodline and of re-establishing ownership of the violated female body. Medical ideas about blood thus provide a rational for the sexual double standard, justifying acts of violence against women, so that murder and suicide are depicted as cleansing therapeutic acts. For men bloodletting is similarly punitive as well as healing, although in these instances it is not the family bloodline, but rather expectations about men's proper behaviour which are at stake. Whereas for women bloodletting is often used to purge the female body of the stain of illicit sex, in men it is the passionate emotions which must be purged.

Sexual Cures

By the early modern period, sexual intercourse had long been considered one of the most effective remedies for lovesickness. As Burton writes, 'The last refuge and surest remedy, to be put in practise in the utmost place, when no other meanes will take effect, is to let them goe together, and enjoy one another.'[17] According to early modern writers, sex expelled the lover's excess blood and seed, which accumulated in the body and putrefied, releasing harmful vapours that could cause melancholy. As seed was considered by many to be the physiological source of desire, sex (like bloodletting) directly diminished the lover's lust; Platter writes how erotic desire 'is raised by seed that itcheth the Genital vessels

---

[17] Burton, *Anatomy*, iii.242.

which desireth to get forth'.[18] And Vaughan offers a purely corporeal explanation of the beneficial effects of sexual intercourse:

for surely, by this carnall copulation, the vaporous fumes of the seede are taken away from the Patient, which doe infect his braine, and lead him into melancholy. By how much the more and longer they continue in the body, so much the more thoughts doe they engender, which at last will turne to folly or madnesse.[19]

However, while therapeutic intercourse was popular as a remedy in the early Middle Ages (at least in so far as it appears in a number of medical texts), some writers clearly felt unease at advocating extramarital intercourse, recommending marriage as a cure instead.

Although sex with the beloved is the most beneficial physical cure, from a purely physiological point of view the identity of the sexual partner is irrelevant, as any sexual encounter will ultimately release the lover's surplus blood and seed.[20] Nonetheless, the lovesick individual only wants to have sex with the object of desire, so doctors often have to resort to tricks and disguises to get their patients to engage in therapeutic intercourse. An example of this is found in William Vaughan's *Directions for Health*, which tells the story of a 'Lawyer of Tholouza' whose obsession with a Venetian woman drives him to madness:

The Gentlewoman with bitter threatning repulsed him. All which could not cause him to disist from his idle enterprise, so unbrideled was his affection, so violent his motion. But at the last perceiving his purpose frustrate and hopelesse, hee fell into a franticke humour, and one morning among the rest, in the *Church of Saint Marke*, casting himselfe through the Guard, endevoured to murther the Duke; but this amorous foole, as *God* would have it, was resisted, & led into prison. The matter was examined very straightly, & at the last it was found that Love had made him mad. The wise *Senate* upon grave deliberation dismissed him, committing his cure to that famous Physician *Fracastorius*, who at that time dwelt in *Venice*. This learned man undertaking his charge and cure, disguised a Courtezan like the Gallants mistrisse, to lye with him a whole night, and to yeeld him his amorous contentment, untill hee was weary. Then hee caused him to be well covered with clothes, til he fell into a sweat. His phantasie and lust being thus partly pleasured, he proceeded to other

---

[18] Platter and Culpeper, *Histories*, 155.   [19] Vaughan, *Directions*, 237.
[20] Platter, Culpeper, *Histories*, 155.

meanes, to purge him of his melancholike humors, so that at length he restored him to his former state.[21]

Fracastorius, recognizing the cause of the young man's lunacy, employs therapeutic intercourse as the first stage of his cure: coitus purges the man's body, and his belief that he has been with his beloved satisfies his mental obsession.

The therapeutic effect of sexual intercourse is dramatized in a number of plays. In Shakespeare's *The Two Noble Kinsmen*, for example, the doctor suggests that the Wooer should have sex with the Jailer's Daughter in order to cure her madness, while in Fletcher's *The Mad Lover*, Calis is expected to ask for 'a Man to cure her' of her lovesickness.[22] More typically the beneficiaries of such cures are men, a fact that counters the idea that men's lovesickness rarely had a genital origin in the early modern period.[23] In *The Nice Valour*, the Passionate Lord's former lover, who is pregnant and disguised as Cupid, believes that sex will function as a purge which will 'draw all his wilde passions, | To one point only, and that's love, the maine point' (III.i.12–13). And in Brome's *The Court Beggar* (*c*.1632), Ferdinand feigns lovesickness in order to gain entry to Lady Strangelove's house, where he attempts to rape her; as Mr Citwit informs the rest of the suitors, 'The Physician thought to have cur'd his patient...between my Ladies | legs'.[24] Ferdinand confesses to Frederick:

> And for my shew of madnesse; 'twas put on
> For my revenge on this impetuous Lady
> To coole these flames (as much of anger as
> Desire) which her disdaine, and tempting malice
> Had rais'd within mee.
>
> (sig. [R5ᵛ])

Beneath the lovesick victim lies the violent rapist, whose lovesick agonies mask a desire for vengeance. Despite his claim that the flames of passion and anger are indistinguishable, Ferdinand's desire to have sex with Lady Strangelove clearly springs from a desire to overpower and hurt

---

[21] Vaughan, *Directions*, 236–7.

[22] Fletcher, *Mad Lover*, in Beaumont and Fletcher, *Dramatic Works*, vol. v, III.vi.27.

[23] Rousseau suggests that male lovesickness only rarely has a genital origin in the Renaissance ('A Strange Pathology', 113–14).

[24] Brome, *Court Beggar*, sig. Q8ʳ.

her, rather than from any loving impulse. As in phlebotomy, the lover's cure is here conceptualized as a form of punishment, but this time it is directed at the disdainful woman.

As discussed in Chapter 1, the belief that sexual intercourse with someone pretending to be the beloved could cure lovesickness provides a rationale for the 'bed trick' in early modern drama, in which some other, more willing, sexual partner is substituted for the lover's unattainable object of desire.[25] Such substitutions generally take place under the cover of night, leaving the lover unaware of the swapping, and are facilitated by the lover's mental fixation. Lovers are easily tricked into believing that someone in disguise is their beloved: transfixed by an inner vision, the sufferer displaces all other sensory impressions, projecting the beloved's image onto others. In *The Two Noble Kinsmen*, for example, the rustic Wooer is presented to the Jailer's Daughter 'in the habit of Palamon', the prince with whom she is infatuated. And in *The Mad Lover*, Polidor suggests a similar cure for his brother, Memnon (the mad lover of the title), who is infatuated with the Princess Calis. As in Vaughan's story of the 'Lawyer of Tholouza', Polidor proposes that 'an handsome whore' be brought to his brother 'Rarely drest up' and taught to speak like the Princess, so that Memnon will believe it is his beloved and have sex with her (III.ii.144, 145).

In both medical and literary texts, the intensity of desire is thus related to the failure to attain physical satisfaction. As Suckling pithily observes, 'Men most enjoy, when least they doe'.[26] By contrast, sexual satiety can obliterate desire altogether, as in the case of Ursini in Harding's *Sicily and Naples*, who brags of Felicia: 'I loved her once, | Til I enjoyed her'.[27] Because of this, a number of women hesitate before consummating their relationships, lest their suitor's feelings of passionate love transform into hate or indifference. In Brewer's *The Love-Sick King* (1617), for example, Cartesmunda is doubtful as to whether King Canutus' interest in her will continue once they have had sex, despite his hyperbolic claims that he will die if she does not give in to his advances; she shrewdly observes, 'Men that lust for women once, no more indure 'em, | In health they loathe the physick that did cure 'em'.[28]

---

[25] See Desens, *Bed-Trick in English Renaissance Drama*; Doniger, *Bedtrick: Tales of Sex*; Briggs, 'Shakespeare's Bed-Tricks'.
[26] Suckling, 'Upon A. M', in *Non-Dramatic Works*, 27.
[27] Harding, *Sicily and Naples*, 70.   [28] Brewer, *Love-Sick King*, sig. [C4ᵛ].

And in Marston's *The Dutch Courtesan*, Malheurex recognizes that sex with Francischina will not only to extinguish his passion, but also to fill him with remorse and self-disgust:

> For appetite and sensual end, whose very having,
> Loseth all appetite and gives satiety,
> That corporal end remorse and inward blushings,
> Forcing us loathe the stream of our owne heat.[29]

Other individuals seem less disturbed by such moral qualms, suggesting that to purge oneself of passion one must satisfy it, eradicating desire by yielding to it; love, as Suckling observes, is 'easier cured with Surfets than abstinence'.[30] The Duke in *The Nice Valour* takes this approach, instructing the court to overindulge the Passionate Lord's humours so that he will sicken of them:

> let every passion
> Be fed ev'n to a surfet, which in time
> May breed a loathing: let him have enough
> Of every object, that his sence is rapt with;
> And being once glutted, then the taste of folly
> Will come into disrellish.
>
> (I.i.67–72)

Like Orsino in Shakespeare's *Twelfth Night*, who desires an 'excess' of music, 'the food of love' so that 'surfeiting, | The appetite may sicken and so die', so too does the Duke in *The Nice Valour* conceptualize love as an appetite which can be overfed to the point of nausea and distaste (I.i.1–3). Thus far I have focused on physiological cures of the diseased lover. However, sexual intercourse clearly remedies both the lover's body and mind—whilst the physical act freed the body from excess seed, sex with someone believed to be the beloved satisfied the lover's mental craving. In the next two sections I will turn to the mental components of lovesickness, exploring the lover's internalized image of the beloved and the techniques used either to satisfy or destroy this mental fixation.

---

[29] Marston, *Dutch Courtesan*, II.ii.212–15.
[30] Sucking, 'Letter 52' ['A disswasion from Love'] (*c*.1640), in *Non-Dramatic Works*, 159.

PSYCHOLOGICAL CURES

Dislodging the Lover's Mental Fixation

Lovers suffer from a particular type of psychological affliction, known as a mental fixation, in which the image of the beloved completely takes over the lover's memory and imagination.[31] This is particularly the case for individuals prone to melancholy, whose brains are believed to be dry and hard, enabling sense impressions to become deeply engraved.[32] Burton describes how the figure of the beloved is carved into the lover's mind beyond the threshold of consciousness, so that all thoughts are dominated by the image of the beloved: the 'impression of her beauty is still fixed in his minde . . . as he that is bitten with a mad dogge, thinkes all he sees dogges, dogges in his meat, dogges in his dish, dogges in his drinke, his mistris is in his eyes, eares, heart, in all his senses'.[33] The lover dotes obsessively, not on the true physical form of the beloved object, but on the phantasm: the perceived, imaginary image that is impressed upon the mind. Sexual intercourse is curative not only because it satisfies a physical desire, but also because it answers a mental craving.

Some cures for lovesickness seek to satisfy the lover's mental fixation, either by manipulating the patient's delusion or by replacing the image of the beloved with a different, less harmful phantasm. Several stories in the early modern period illustrate the first instance, in which the doctor colludes with the patient's aberrant imagination to effect a therapy. In this context, lovesickness resembles any other mental delusion, in which the hallucinations of fixated patients are dispelled through the cunning of the physician; here, the doctor colludes with the patient's aberrant imagination, satisfying his or her mental fixation before coaxing the patient back to health through more conventional methods. One story, for example, describes a woman who was convinced that she was possessed by an evil spirit; the woman was cured when the priest made a small cut in her arm and released a bat he had hidden in a bag, reassuring her that the spirit had been driven out.[34] Another describes how a

---

[31] See also Burton, *Anatomy*, i.152; Laurentius, *Preservation of the Sight*, 97; and Wack, *Lovesickness*, 56.

[32] Burton, *Anatomy*, i.152; Laurentius, *Preservation of the Sight*, 97.

[33] Burton, *Anatomy*, iii.156.   [34] Thomas, *Religion*, 249–50.

doctor cured a woman who believed that she had swallowed a serpent by causing the woman to vomit into a basin where he had secretly placed snakes.[35] In another instance, a man refused to leave his study when he became convinced that his nose was dangerously large; his cure was effected by a doctor who pretended to cut off his nose, showing a large slab of meat he had kept hidden in his hand as proof. Another patient was cured in this fashion:

There have been seene very melancholike persons, which did thinke themselves dead, and would not eate any thing: the Phisitions have used this sleight to make them eate. They caused some one or other servant to lie neere unto the sicke partie, and having taught him to counterfeite himselfe dead, yet not to forsake his meate, but to eate and swallow it, when it was put into his mouth: and thus by this craftie devise, they perswaded the melancholike man, that the dead did eate as well as those which are alive.[36]

The doctor, failing to convince the sick individual of the error of his judgement, manipulates his patient's delusion in a beneficial manner, tricking the individual into eating and thereby removing him from immediate physical danger.

The effectiveness of medical trickery was corroborated by the early modern belief in the powerful influence of the imagination, which was held to be overactive in lovers and those with psychological illnesses.[37] Noting that 'some ascribe all vices to a false and corrupt imagination', Burton gives several examples of how an individual's irrational imaginings can cause real physical harm; he maintains that people can catch diseases simply by fearing them, and that a strong sympathetic identification with a condemned man at his execution can lead to one's own death. Similarly, Burton affirms the popular notion that an unborn child's features can be shaped by a woman's imagination; he writes: 'if a woman . . . at the time of her conception, thinke of another man present, or absent, the childe will be like him.' Alternatively, the role-playing and trickery used to heal individuals are sometimes seen as cures in and of themselves. William Vaughan in his *Directions for Health*, for example,

---

[35] Jorden, *Briefe Discourse*, 25.

[36] Laurentius, *Preservation of the Sight*, 101, 102. See also Burton, *Anatomy*, i.401.

[37] Burton writes, 'In *Melancholy* men this faculty is most Powerfull and strong, and often hurts, producing many monstrous and prodigious things' (*Anatomy*, i.152). See also Laurentius, *Preservation of the Sight*, 97; Kinsman, 'Introduction', in *Darker Vision*, 8.

suggests that art has a therapeutic quality, cleansing and fortifying the imagination:

> The Physitian therefore that will cure these spirituall sicknesses, must invent and devise some spirituall pageant, to fortifie and help the imaginative facultie, which is corrupted and depraved; yea, hee must endevour to deceive, and imprint another conceit, whether it be wise or foolish, in the Patients braine, thereby to put out all former phantasies.[38]

Images and pictures could either distract the sufferer from his or her delusion, or remove the image altogether. Just as one can *drive out one love with another, as they doe a pegge, or pinne with a pinne*', so too can one drive out the image of the beloved with a new, more beneficial phantasm.[39] From the perspective of the early modern physician, the absurd credulity of the lovesick patient was both the cause of the affliction and the means to achieve a lasting cure; as Burton writes, 'As by wicked incredulity many men are hurt...wee finde in our experience, by the same meanes many are relieved.'[40]

In lovesickness, the most straightforward way of satisfying the lover's psychological craving is via therapeutic intercourse with either the beloved or someone believed to be the beloved; for while sexual intercourse in and of itself frees the body from excessive blood and corrupt seed, only sex with the object of desire is capable of satisfying the lover's phantasm. There are even instances in which the lover's mental fixation is satisfied by a purely imaginary encounter with the beloved; here, the lover's disorderly imagination is also responsible for producing the mental images that satisfy it. Laurentius describes a case of a young man whose lovesickness is occasioned by a courtesan who refused to have sex with him unless she received an 'excessive summe of silver'.[41] Fortunately for him, the young man has an erotic dream, which provides the mental images (and one assumes the physical release) which cure him of his malady:

> It happened that this miserable love-slave dreamed on a night, that hee held his mistresse in his armes, and that she was altogether at his commaund: whereupon when he awaked, he wel perceived that this inward fire which whilome fed greedily upon him, and thereby about to consume him, was become cold & utterly quenched, so that he sought not any more after the Curtisane.

[38] Vaughan, *Directions*, 230–1.   [39] Burton, *Anatomy*, i.251–2.
[40] Ibid. i.254.   [41] Laurentius, *Preservation of the Sight*, 122.

The conclusion that Laurentius draws from this story is 'to shew that this rage and furie of erotike love, may be staied by the injoying of the thing beloved'.[42] Significantly, however, it is not the Courtesan's actual body that the young man enjoys, but rather her phantasmic mental image. Alternatively, one might dislodge the lovesick patient's mental fixation by introducing a new erotic object. Burton, typically figuring the lovesick victim as male, recommends that the individual should 'have two mistresses at once, or goe from one to another: as he that goes from a good fire in cold weather, is loth to depart from it, though in the next roome there be a better, which will refresh him as much; there's as much difference of *hæc* as *hic ignis*'.[43] Here, the permanence of the erotic need (imagined by Burton as the desire to warm oneself) is contrasted with the transitory and replaceable nature of the beloved (who is likened to one of many possible sources of heat).

Early modern plays often foreground the powerful impact of performance and theatrical illusion, which are capable of curing individuals' mental illnesses and satisfying its audiences' unconscious desires; in a time when theatrical illusion is often disparaged as illicit and immoral, such plays provide a counter-model for the theatre as cathartic therapy. In Brome's *The Antipodes*, for example, Perigrine is cured of his obsession with travel after a doctor persuades the other characters in the play to stage a fictional trip to the Antipodes.[44] Like Laurentius' young man whose inflamed passion for a beautiful woman is quenched by a dream in which he has sex with her, Perigrine is also cured by an imaginary attainment of his heart's desire. Other plays depict doctors engaging in the kinds of trickery and role-playing that are described in early modern medical texts. Harding's *Sicily and Naples*, for example, contains an episode which appears to be taken directly from the story in Laurentius, in which a physician resorts to a 'craftie devise' to cure a man who believes himself to be dead. In the play, Calantha stops eating and sleeping when her father is killed by the man she loves, and as a consequence suffers a complete breakdown and believes herself to be dead. As in the Laurentius story, Bentivogli (the doctor of the play) cures Calantha by indulging her in her 'false supposition', and by

---

[42] Ibid.   [43] Burton, *Anatomy*, iii.215–16.

[44] An alternative example can be found in Webster's *The Duchess of Malfi*, in which Ferdinand attempts to drive his sister to despair by organizing a masque of madness. See Sutherland, *Masques*, 76–8.

manipulating her delusion so that she eats and sleeps: he organizes a fictional funeral for Calantha after which characters dressed as ghosts sit down at a banquet. The cure works: Calantha is persuaded to eat, and her desire for death is gratified fictitiously. Mental fixations thus vanish by being indulged; as Bentivogli observes, 'The nature of her disease…yields not unto cure, till it be | wrought up to the height'.[45]

Bentivogli's cure, which treats both Calantha's weakened physiological state and her mental delusion, typifies a number of theatrical cures, which focus on both the lover's somatic illness and troubled mind. As discussed previously, in Fletcher and Massinger's *A Very Woman* (*c*.1616) Don Martino is cured only after being stabbed by Don John. However, while this wound functions like a necessary bloodletting, purging Martino's violent passion, it does not minister to his mind, which is haunted by his guilt over his bad behaviour; as the Doctor observes, the 'strong imagination of [his] wrongs' has 'rent his minde into so many pieces', subjecting him to 'various imaginations'.[46] Consequently, the Doctor attempts to cure Don Martino through a series of performances, transforming Don Martino's room into a kind of ministage, complete with costumes and trapdoors. Like a skilled actor, the doctor emerges first as a friar, then as a soldier, then as a philosopher, and finally in his original shape to heal his patient, while Martino's family watch on like audience members (V.ii.165). The doctor's success is thus predicated upon his excellence as a performer. Don Martino tells the Doctor:

> Doctor, thou hast perfected a Bodies cure
> T'amaze the world; and almost cur'd a Mind
> Neer phrensie. With delight I now perceive
> You for my recreation have invented
> The several Objects, which my Melancholy
> Sometimes did think you conjur'd, otherwhiles
> Imagin'd 'em Chimera's. You have been
> My Friar, Soldier, my Philosopher,
> My Poet, Architect, my Physitian;
> Labor'd for me more then your slaves for you

---

[45] Harding, *Sicily and Naples*, 71.
[46] [Fletcher and Massinger], *A Very Woman*, in Beaumount and Fletcher, *Dramatic Works*, vol. vii, IV.ii.3, 5, 6.

> In their assistance: In your moral Song
> Of my good Genius, and my bad, you have won me
> A chearful heart, and banish'd discontent;
> There being nothing wanting to my wishes,
> But once more, were it possible, to behold
> *Don John Anthonio.*
>
> (IV.ii.170–85)

As in Vaughan, the Doctor here invents a 'spirituall pageant, to fortifie and help the imaginative facultie, which is corrupted and depraved': he plays upon Don Martino like 'a musical Instrument', bringing the discordant aspects of his melancholic mind into a harmonious balance, while simultaneously instructing him in the proper code of conduct for a soldier and courtier (IV.ii.22). The Doctor thus provides moral and social instruction as well as a psychological cure. By the end of the doctor's performance, Don Martino's cure is complete: he seeks forgiveness from Don John and rejects love altogether, pronouncing himself freed from the emasculating and dishonourable effects of excessive passion. Martino's plans for matrimony give way to his homosocial bonds with other men. It is not Almira he now cries for from his sickbed, but Don John.

Ford's *The Lover's Melancholy* dramatizes a more complex use of performance as a means of dislodging a lovesick individual's mental fixation. Corax, the court physician, is called upon to cure the melancholy afflicting Prince Palador, and soon discovers that the Prince is lovesick for Eroclea, who, prior to the action of the play, has fled the court after Palador's father had attempted to seduce her. Unbeknownst to Palador, however, Eroclea has returned to court disguised as a young man, Parthenophill. From one perspective, it seems that all Corax has to do to cure the Prince's melancholy is unite Palador with Eroclea. However, Aretus, tutor to the Prince, emphasizes that the treatment of the Prince must be gradual as 'Passions of violent nature by degrees | Are easiliest reclaimed'.[47]

Corax instructs Palador in a range of practical measures that will help ease his melancholy, such as his diet and choice of pastimes, but the

---

[47] Ford, *Lover's Melancholy*, ed. Hill, II.i.25–6; all quotations taken from this edition. See Hopkins, who argues that the play investigates the slow ways in which emotional changes occur ('Staging Passion').

turning point in Palador's cure comes when Corax stages a 'Masque of Melancholy'. In many respects, the highly visual nature of the masque, with its emphasis on harmonious forms and intricate architecture, seems like the ideal type of 'spirituall pageant' both to 'fortifie . . . the imaginative facultie' and create new phantasms.[48] Like emblems, which employ a visual language thought to supersede normal speech, masques were thought to contain complex stage pictures that the mind could grasp without the medium of language. Because of this, it is a genre highly suitable to Palador, who as well as being highly responsive to images ('what most he takes delight in | Are handsome pictures'), is locked in a private world of contemplation where the pictorial world of phantasms reign (I.i.76–7). Most especially, Palador dotes on his internalized image of Eroclea, which, like the miniature of her that secretly hangs around his neck, exists independently of her in an idealized and unchanging form. Corax's masque presents various types of melancholy, such as lycanthropy, hydrophobia, intellectual melancholy, and pride, but he deliberately excludes love melancholy. At the end of the masque Corax leaves the characters in the play gazing at an empty stage. When Palador asks the meaning of the blank space, Corax responds:

> One kind of melancholy
> Is only left untouched; 'twas not in art
> To personate the shadow of that fancy.
> 'Tis named Love Melancholy.
>
> (III.iii.94–7)

For a tense moment, it seems that Corax is going to expose the secret source of the prince's melancholy, and indeed Corax gestures towards the disguised Eroclea, placing the 'real' characters within the masque but to a rather different end; he instructs Palador:

> Admit this stranger here—young man, stand forth—
> Entangled by the beauty of this lady,
> The great Thamasta, cherished in his heart
> The weight of hopes and fears, it were impossible
> To limn his passions in such lively colours
> As his own proper sufferance could express.
>
> (III.iii.98–103)

---

[48] Vaughan, *Directions*, 230–1.

Corax focuses on 'Parthenophill's' supposed lovesickness in order to draw Palador's attention to his disguised mistress; Palador recognizes something oddly familiar about the beautiful youth and feels himself strangely moved by his/her presence. Although critics disagree as to whether Corax is aware of Parthenophill's real identity, it seems likely that he does and that this is a deliberate strategy on his part: through the masque, Corax offers the Prince distracting images to fortify his mind, whilst simultaneously presenting him with an image of his lost love, preparing him for her reappearance.[49] Corax also uses the masque to reproach Palador indirectly for giving in to lovesick grief; he warns: 'Love is the tyrant of the heart; it darkens | Reason, confounds discretion; deaf to counsel, | It runs a headlong course to desperate madness' (III.iii.105–7).

The masque thus prepares Palador for the return of Eroclea and in this way follows the general pattern for the play, 'which is not of concealed facts suddenly disclosed but a process of healing in which known facts are slowly disclosed'.[50] Indeed, when Eroclea eventually removes her disguise, Palador shows some resistance to accepting the reality of her reappearance. Accusing her of being a 'Cunning imposter' and 'seducing counterfeit', Palador both worries that Eroclea is not who she claims to be, and also that she is the imperfect copy of his cherished internal image (IV.iii.80, 107). He is only convinced of her authenticity once she reveals her miniature of him, which, like her lover, she wears secretly on a chain around her neck; as in Neoplatonic philosophy, the lover recognizes the beloved through the image of the self buried within.

However, if Palador's recognition of Eroclea seems designed to enact a central principle of Neoplatonism (that the beloved contains a cherished image of the self), the play ultimately reverses the philosophy's hierarchical relationship between the ideal and real, suggesting that abstract ideals must ultimately give way to the living, material world. For Palador's cure not only enables him to relinquish a private world of contemplation for the public world of political sovereignty, but also to exchange his private internal image of Eroclea for the real flesh and blood woman. This is made explicit in Act V when Palador sends Melander, Eroclea's father, his daughter's miniature. Palador asks Melander:

[49] For Corax's knowledge of Parthenophill's real identity see Hill, 'Introduction', in Ford, *Lover's Melancholy*, 16.
[50] Ibid.

> Where's the picture
> I sent thee? Keep it, 'tis a counterfeit;
> And in exchange of 'that I seize on this,
> The real substance.
>
> (V.ii.222–5)

Palador exchanges his 'picture' of Eroclea for 'the real substance', aban-
doning the miniature of Eroclea for the woman herself. Palador's cure
thus offers an optimistic view of love, in which the solitary pleasures
of introspective melancholy are exchanged for the companionate joys
of marriage. As in *The Lover's Melancholy*, the final cure I will be
discussing also focuses on the mental fixation of the lover; here too
the lover is cured when the idealized image of the beloved gives way
to an understanding of the woman's 'real substance'. However, in these
instances, intimacy with the beloved brings not the companionate joys
of marriage, but rather a repudiation of love itself.

Curing Love through Humiliation

The humiliating consequences of immoderate love are sometimes the
means through which men free themselves of the bonds of their affection. By submitting to the whims of a cruel mistress, male sufferers grow
to loathe love. Just as love of the divine will make you spiritual, 'this
effeminate love of woman doth so womanize a man that, if you yield
to it, it will make you . . . a launder, and distaff-spinner'.[51] Such 'cures'
show how erotic desire effeminizes men and reverses the conventional
gender hierarchy: just as the lover is subjugated by his 'feminine' passions, so too is he dominated by his female mistress; lovesick men are
thus

commonly slaves, captives, voluntary servants, [for] a lover is the slave of his
beloved . . . Is he a free man over whom a woman domineers, to whom she
prescribes Laws, commands, forbids what she will herself? that dares deny
nothing she demands; she asks, he gives; she calls, he comes; she threatens,
he fears.[52]

Whereas individuals overcome by lust are power-hungry and seek to
control others, melancholic lovers exhibit a desire for submission and

---

[51] Sidney, *Old Arcadia*, 20.   [52] Burton, *Anatomy*, iii.149.

self-abasement. Early modern writers keen to dramatize the dangers of immoderate passion cite the myth of Circe and her ability to transform men into animals as the key symbol for love's ability to dehumanize; Geoffrey Whitney's *A Choice of Emblems* (1586), for example, interprets this myth as suggesting that 'those foolishe sorte, whome wicked love dothe thrall, | Like brutishe beastes do passe theire time, and have no sence at all'. Nor do lovesick individuals lament their fallen state, but rather wish to stay captivated by their passion and 'still brutishe to remaine'.[53] In Book II of *The Faerie Queene* Spenser draws on this myth; Acrasia lures knights into the Bowre of Bliss where men wallow in 'lewd loves, and wastfull luxuree' and are physically transformed: just as they are turned from brave warriors to idle paramours, so too they turn 'into figures hideous, | According to their mindes like monstrous'.[54] And in Milton's *Comus*, or *A Mask presented at Ludlow Castle* (1634), Comus, like Acrasia, offers the 'pleasing poison' of sensual enjoyment, transforming the face of those that drink into 'the inglorious likeness of a beast . . . unmoulding reasons mitage | Charactered in the face'.[55]

The depiction of love as an emasculating force is represented in John Ford's *The Queen* (*c*.1625–30), in which Velasco, besotted by the widow Selassa, is portrayed as being controlled by his feminine passions as well as by his female mistress.[56] In a bid to win her love, Velasco pledges to do anything Selassa demands, but her request is a symbolic castration that only serves to dramatize the humiliating effects of being doubly controlled by passion and by a woman:

> I command,
> For two years space, you shall not wear a sword,
> A dagger, or stelletto; shall not fight
> On any quarrel be it neer so just.[57]

Velasco immediately recognizes the meaning of her request: 'Happy was I, that living liv'd alone', he laments, '*Velasco* was a man then, now is none'. His newfound meekness is a source of wonder for everyone, and

---

[53] Whitney, *Emblems*, 82. [54] Spenser, *Faerie Queene*, 296, 297.
[55] Milton, *Mask* [Comus], ed. Carey, 527–8. See also Whitney, *Emblemes*, 82.
[56] For a reading of this play in relation to Essex's 1601 uprising see Dawson, 'Trials of History'.
[57] [Ford], *Queene*, sig. C4ᵛ.

Mopas suspects he knows the cause of his newfound passivity; he asserts 'I'll lay my life, his lady sweet heart hath given him the Gleek, and he in return hath gelded himself, and so both lost his courage and his wits together' (sigs. C4ᵛ, D2ʳ). Mopas's analysis literalizes the emasculating process of passionate love, suggesting the way in which excessive passion can be seen to turn men into 'a strumpet's fool', or even into women.[58] Selassa's tyrannous treatment of Velasco indicates the debilitating and humiliating effects of being at a woman's mercy. 'Was ever man so much a slave as I?' he asks (sig. D1ᵛ).

However, Salassa's behaviour eventually backfires. When the Queen needs a champion to defend her, Salassa pledges her life that she can command Velasco to fight. Velasco, however, remains true to his vow and Salassa is threatened with execution. Velasco, unable to fight for the Queen, is publicly humiliated and regrets that he has ever allowed himself to be so subjected to his desires. Too late he finds 'How passions at their best are but sly traytors | To ruin honour' (sig. E2ᵛ). Salassa, on the other hand, regrets her behaviour and falls in love with her disgraced lover. The plot is thus structured in such a way as to reveal to Salassa her dependency upon the very male strength she has impaired, compelling her to recognize the way in which her honour is safeguarded by Velasco's strength. Although he is finally reunited with Salassa at the end of the play, by this time it is Salassa who is lovesick and subjected both to her affections and her lover: the process that 'cures' Velasco simultaneously enacts a restoration of 'proper' gender relations.

Ford's *Love's Sacrifice* also dramatizes the way in which humiliation can act as a cure. Fiormonda, also a widow, scorns her lover's affection and is instrumental in his banishment. In order to return to court, Roseilli disguises himself as a fool and eventually is presented to Fiormonda. His physical transformation literalizes the anxiety that men can become clowns and servants when enslaved by their affections, so that his disguise is ironically made to figure what he has actually become (Fiormonda's fool). However, while acting in this role, Roseilli witnesses his beloved's malicious plotting and passionate desire for Fernando, which cures him of his lovesickness. Throwing off the role of fool (in both senses), Roseilli reveals to Fiormonda his knowledge of her scorn and machinations; he tells her:

[58] Shakespeare, *Antony and Cleopatra*, I.i.13.

> Wonder not, madam, here behold the man
> Whom your disdain hath metamorphosèd:
> Thus long have I been clouded in this shape,
> Led on by Love.[59]

Fiormonda is humbled by his revelations, declaring 'Thy truth, | Like a transparent mirror, represents | My reason with my errors' (V.iii.9–11). She asks Roseilli for forgiveness, offering both herself and the dukedom to him, and promising that if her 'heart can entertain | Another thought of love, it shall be thine' (V.iii.13–14). Roseilli's love has turned to disgust, however, and although he welcomes the marriage, he refuses to have sex with Fiormonda; he declares, 'henceforth I here dismiss | The mutual comforts of our marriage bed. | Learn to new-live, my vows unmoved shall stand' (V.iii.156–8). Significantly, Roseilli's renunciation of sexuality occurs as he assumes political power, in which matrimony is made subordinate to his bonds with other men. Whereas the play aligns lovesickness with servitude, the rejection of passion is empowering for the male lover, granting him both the capacity to rule himself and others.

Ford's *The Queen* and *Love's Sacrifice* show how submitting oneself to the beloved can enact a cure, as it reveals the negative characteristics of the beloved and leaves the lover with a distaste for both love and the object of desire. The plays thus explore the gender power inversion that accompanies courtship, dramatizing the anxiety of the male lover, whose affection makes him subject to his mistress. The woman's attempts to humiliate her lover rebound so that she is ultimately the one humiliated by her actions. However, the discomfort felt by such women is radically different: whereas the men are portrayed as mastering their desires, female characters respond to their own humiliation by submitting themselves to their lovers. Thus, while mortification breeds repugnance in men, it engenders love in women, implying that women secretly wish to be abased, and even find it erotic.

However, there is at least one example of a woman who is cured of her love via humiliation. In Shirley's *A Lady of Pleasure* (1635) Lady Aretina Bornwell is infatuated by Alexander Kickshaw, but does not wish to compromise either her reputation or her marriage. In order to protect her identity, she engages Decoy, a bawd, to arrange a secret

---

[59] Ford, *Love's Sacrifice*, V.iii.1–4.

midnight tryst with Alexander. Blindfolded, Alexander is taken to the bawd's house where Decoy, disguised as an old woman, propositions him. Alexander, unaware that it is actually Aretina who is waiting for him in the bedroom, nevertheless agrees to have sex with Decoy, believing her to be a devil and that 'succubi must not be crossed'.[60] The following day, Alexander gets drunk and divulges his strange midnight encounter to Aretina, unwittingly describing his night to the very woman with whom he spent it. Showing her the gold he was given for his 'services', he explains to Aretina how his financial position has been remedied:

ALEXANDER: What think you first of an old witch, a strange ill-favoured hag, that for my company last night has wrought this cure upon my fortune? I do sweat to think upon her name.
ARETINA: How sir, a witch?
KICKSHAW: I would not fright your ladyship too much at first, but witches are akin to spirits. The truth is—nay, if you look pale already, I ha' done.
ARETINA: Sir, I beseech you.
KICKSHAW: If you have but courage, then, to know the truth, I'll tell you: in one word; my chief friend is the devil.

(V.ii.145–55)

Aretina's charade seems to have worked a little too well: Alexander actually believes that he has slept with 'a she-devil', and Aretina is forced to hear horrified descriptions of her affair. Alexander describes his lover as 'a most insatiate, abominable devil with a tail thus long', and Aretina is overcome with guilt (V.ii.157–8). ''Tis a false glass; sure,' she bemoans, 'I am more deformed . . . My soul is miserable' (V.ii.178–9). Humiliated and full of remorse, Aretina is cured of her lovesickness. However, unlike the previous examples, it is not disgust with the beloved but *self-disgust* which acts as her cure.

There is clearly more at stake in the cure of lovesickness than simply returning the individual to bodily health. For the male sufferer in particular, love threatens not only his body and ethical constitution, but also his gender identity. Indeed, a man's cure frequently corresponds to his return to political and martial power, in which union with the beloved is eschewed in favour of bonds with other men. The corrective

[60] Shirley, *Lady of Pleasure,* IV.i.83.

'cures' thus serve to re-establish the traditional gender hierarchy, in which anxieties about the power of love are reconfigured in such a way that male romantic authority and self-mastery are restored. There are of course exceptions to this. Ford's *The Lover's Melancholy*, for one, ends not with a rejection of love or women, but rather with passion's tempering and transformation into mutual affection; but in most cases, the man's return to rational self-control is also a return to a world in which men dominate their mistresses as well as their passions. There are also instances in which women are cured of lovesickness. However, despite shifts in the construction of female erotic melancholy, sexual intercourse is still predominantly seen as the most beneficial cure for women, and in a number of texts the boundaries of the female body signify the authority and purity of her husband and family. In the next chapter I will focus on a final cure for lovesickness, which reveals, more than any other, the complicated mental and emotional stratagems that the male lover can employ to overcome his desire. In the menstrual cure for lovesickness, the lover deliberately reimagines his beloved's body as filthy and disgusting, unleashing on her a vituperate misogyny which is ultimately the product of (and screen for) his vulnerability and frustration.

6

Menstruation, Misogyny, and the Cure for Love

medio de fonte leporum
surgit amari aliquid quod in ipsis floribus angat.

(Lucretius, *De rerum natura*, IV.1133–4)

from the middle of the spring of delights arises something bitter
to choke him amidst the very flowers.

(trans. Brown, *Lucretius on Love and Sex*, 155)

In Jonathan Swift's 'The Lady's Dressing Room' Strephon steals into his mistress Celia's chamber, only to find that it is utterly unlike the paradise he has been imagining. Filled with cosmetics and dirty clothing, the squalid room reveals the artistry that goes into creating Celia's beauty and the ordinary bodily functions her glamorous image conceals. In a lengthy '*inventory*' he examines her spit, sweat-stained smock, grimy towels, and dirty combs before concluding his visit by searching a cabinet, from which emanates a putrid smell.[1] Utterly crushed and disillusioned by what he finds there, Strephon leaves the dressing room in disgust:

> Thus finishing his grand survey,
> The swain disgusted slunk away,
> Repeating in his amorous fits,
> 'Oh! Celia, Celia, Celia shits!'
>
> (ll. 115–18)

Strephon, who has clearly been conditioned by pastoral and Petrarchan conventions to view women as celestial, non-corporeal creatures, is horrified to discover that his mistress is an ordinary mortal with a fully

[1] Swift, 'The Lady's Dressing Room', in *Complete Poems*, ed. Rogers, 10.

functioning body; he 'looks behind the scene' and discovers that his idealistic notions about Celia are the products of mere pretence and literary cliché. By foregrounding Celia's physicality—her sweat, spit, and shit—Swift criticizes the idealistic fictions generated about women. According to the poem, romantic philosophical conceptions of love that elevate the female beloved can only be maintained through distance and unfamiliarity.

Although Swift's 'excremental vision' is often ascribed either to a perverse personal fixation or frustrated sexual desire, he is in fact following a long tradition that draws attention to a woman's bodily functions in order to challenge unrealistic ideas about women and romantic love.[2] The Roman poet and Epicurean philosopher Lucretius (early to mid-first century BCE) offers a very similar account in *De rerum natura* (*On the Way Things Are*), a book that Swift knew well and read with great care.[3] Swift's interest in Lucretius, evident in a number of references and quotations, makes the *De rerum natura* a likely source for the 'The Lady's Dressing Room' and for Swift's scatological poems about women in general.[4] Lucretius' attack on love in Book IV mocks the men whose worshipful behaviour towards women blinds them to their ordinary humanness. Describing a stock romantic scenario from Latin love poetry—the lover outside his mistress's door[5]—Lucretius suggests that the lover's rarefied image of his beloved would be destroyed if only he could actually enter her room:

> sed tamen esto iam quantovis oris honore,
> cui Veneris membris vis omnibus exoriatur:
>
> .   .   .   .   .   .
>
> nempe eadem facit, et scimus facere, omnia turpi
> et miseram taetris se suffit odoribus ipsa,
> quam famulae longe fugitant furtimque cachinant.
>
> .   .   .   .   .   .
>
> quem si, iam admissum, venientem offenderit aura
> una modo, causas abeundi quaerat honestas

---

[2] For a discussion of the ways in which Swift's scatology fits into a wider satirical tradition see Lee, *Swift and Scatological Satire*.

[3] On Swift's copy of Lucretius see Davis, 'Introduction', in *Prose Works*, ed. Davis, vol. v, p. xxxi.

[4] For Lucretius as a possible source for 'The Lady's Dressing Room' see Fleischmann, *Lucretius and English Literature*, 246–7.

[5] Brown, *Love and Sex*, 297.

et meditata diu cadat alte sumpta querella,
stultitiaque ibi se damnet, tribuisse quod illi
plus videat quam mortali concedere par est.
nec Veneres nostras hoc fallit; quo magis ipsae
omnia summo opere hos vitae postscaenia celant
quos retinere volunt adstrictosque esse in amore

(IV.1171–2, 1174–7, 1180–7)

But let her be as fine of face as she can be and let the power of Venus arise from all her limbs, still . . . she does just the same in everything, and we know it, as the ugly, and reeks, herself, poor wretched thing, of foul odors, and her housemaids flee far from her and giggle in secret . . . Yet if he were finally let in, and if just one whiff of that smell should meet him as he came in, he would think up a good excuse to go away, and his deep-drawn lament, long planned, would fall silent, and on the spot he would condemn his own stupidity, because he sees that he has attributed more to her than it is correct to grant to any mortal. Nor are our Venuses in the dark about this. That's why they are all the more at pains to conceal the backstage side of their lives from those whom they want to keep held fast in love.[6]

No matter how beautiful the beloved is, she nevertheless has a body that behaves in the same manner as any other woman's. Here too, bodily functions serve to counteract the inappropriate overestimation of the beloved, elevated by a lover who has 'attributed more to her than it is correct to grant to any mortal'. Lucretius thus criticizes 'the erotic distortion that overlays the realities of sex with sentimental poetic images',[7] advising men to relinquish their unrealistic expectations regarding women and 'yield to human life' ('humanis concedere rebus').[8] A similar conclusion is reached in 'The Lady's Dressing Room', in which Strephon is instructed to 'bless his ravished eyes to see | Such order from confusion sprung'.[9]

The quoted passage from *De rerum natura* has bewildered commentators through the ages who have offered a number of implausible interpretations as to the origin of the noxious smell.[10] Although in Swift's poem the odour clearly arises from excrement (and here, perhaps,

---

[6] Lucretius, *De rerum natura*, trans. Nussbaum, *Therapy of Desire*, 178.
[7] Brown, *Love and Sex*, 64.
[8] Lucretius, *De rerum natura*, IV.1191, trans. Nussbaum, *Therapy of Desire*, 178.
[9] Swift, 'Lady's Dressing Room', 142–3.
[10] See Nussbaum, *Therapy of Desire*, 179–81.

one can find evidence of Swift's 'scatological' mind), this is not the case in Lucretius. As Martha C. Nussbaum suggests, in this instance, 'a specifically female secret is being unmasked' (the beautiful woman 'does the same as the ugly'), necessitating the lover's exclusion from his mistress's room and causing her maids to 'flee far from her and giggle in secret'. Nussbaum argues convincingly that 'what is at issue is the smells associated with the menstrual period—surely more difficult to control in times before disposable paper products, and the subject, in all times, of intense negative concern and superstitious misogynistic loathing'.[11] Nussbaum's interpretation is further supported by the fact that Lucretius' rhetorical strategy for disrupting unrealistic ideas about sexual love draws upon a known cure for erotic melancholy, in which a man is shown the menstrual blood of his mistress in order to cure his romantic fixation. Swift's misinterpretation of the origin of the noxious smell in Lucretius marks the disappearance of the menstrual cure from literary texts. Menstrual blood, frequently used in early modern texts as a symbol of corruption and defilement, is instead subjected to a different kind of censure: that of silence.

Although the menstrual cure has a very long history, appearing in texts from the first century BCE to the seventeenth century, it has not generated a great deal of scholarly interest.[12] In this chapter I give an overview of this remedy, focusing in particular on its re-emergence in early modern English medical and literary texts, and suggesting how it throws important light on concepts of women and menstruation. In the menstrual cure for erotic melancholy, the lovesick man is shown the stained cloths of his mistress, so that rather than inciting desire, her body provokes revulsion. However, while the ostensible aim of the cure is to free the individual from his obsession, there is more at stake in remedying the lovesick man than merely returning him to psychological and physical health. Overwhelming erotic passion had the potential to disrupt male gender identity (men are seen to be effeminized by passionate emotions) and to upset conventional gender power structures. In several instances the corrective cure serves to re-establish

---

[11] See ibid. 180.
[12] Some exceptions to this are: Wack, who refers to the menstrual cure as one type of 'aversive therapy' (*Lovesickness*, 70); Neely, who discusses it as the most graphic form of the 'misogyny cure' (*Distracted Subjects*, 102); Schiesari (*Gendering of Melancholia*, 100); and Coulianu, *Eros*, 20.

the traditional gender hierarchy, resolving anxieties about the power of love and restoring male sexual authority and self-mastery. Where Lucretius seems intent to disrupt both the lover's idealization and his equally self-deceptive misogyny, the cure for lovesickness deliberately harnesses sexual disgust as a crucial aspect of the lover's therapy. In the menstrual therapy, misogyny is not the object of satire, but a means for a man to achieve mental health.

The patriarchal conception of the menstruating woman stands in stark contrast to the language of Petrarchan and Neoplatonic philosophy, which elevates the beloved object and effaces her real corporeal presence. By foregrounding the physicality of the beloved—her bodily odours and excretions—early modern writers could suggest that the Neoplatonic view of women as a source of purity or means of spiritual transcendence is absurd. The misogynistic discourse that associates menstruation with physical and moral corruption both denigrates women and mocks the men who subscribe to elevated philosophical conceptions of desire. The radical reversal in the way the lover conceptualizes his mistress reflects what critics such as Mary Beth Rose have termed the 'polarization' in the medieval and Renaissance construction of the female sex, in which women are alternatively configured as desirable or disgusting, saintly or whorish.[13] These seemingly opposed constructions of female sexuality go hand in hand; traditions that conceptualize women as objects worthy of either veneration or revulsion keep women from their more obvious role as man's partner and fellow human. Narratives associating menstruation with male revulsion project this polarity onto the female body itself, creating the division that Lear sees between women's celestial upper bodies and their devilish lower regions: 'But to the girdle do the gods inherit, beneath is all the fiend's.'[14]

The lover's misogynistic reaction to the female body reveals a deep-seated anxiety about the disruptive force of erotic desire and suggests a close affiliation between sexual attraction and repulsion. This corresponds to a Freudian model of desire that presupposes the inescapable intimacy between desire and disgust, pleasure and pain. For Freud, there is 'something in the nature of the sexual function itself which denies us full satisfaction', so that the constituent elements of erotic

---

[13] Rose, *Expense of Spirit*, 47.   [14] Shakespeare, *King Lear*, IV.vi.122–3.

excitement are concomitant with impulses that lead to its destruction.[15] Leo Bersani, in his analysis of Freud and aesthetics, notes how Freud repeatedly 'speaks of a sexuality which is its own antagonist', finding that 'destructiveness is constitutive of sexuality' which is itself 'indissociable from masochism'.[16] Through its explicit sexual descriptions designed to attract and repel, the menstrual therapy for erotic melancholy enacts a similar destructiveness, as if the very descriptions of erotic excitation result in the extinction of desire and denigration of the erotic object. Within this framework, the menstrual cure articulates the contradictory and self-destructive nature of desire and projects these internal contradictions onto the female body; here, it is not the lover but his mistress who is divided. Such a strategy both mitigates the contradictions of male emotion and renders them justifiable: conflicting responses are not the product of internal inconsistencies but are rather the inevitable result of being confronted by two seemingly different bodies. Male sexual insecurity is thus projected onto the female body, so that the lover's misogyny functions as a means of compensating for his sense of vulnerability and powerlessness.[17]

Although the roots of the menstrual cure go back at least to Lucretius and Ovid,[18] medical texts often suggest that the remedy derives from a story about Hypatia of Alexandria (d. 415 CE), a pagan Neoplatonic philosopher and mathematician. According to various sources, Hypatia cured a man who was besotted with her by producing a menstrual rag, which she then threw at her admirer. Eunapius of Sardes (347–414 CE) recounts the story in his *De vitis philosophorum et sophistarum* (fifth century CE) and it is also found in the lexicon *Suda* (tenth century CE), both of which were translated in the Renaissance.[19] In addition to this, it features in almost all of the chapters on love written by the

---

[15] Freud, *Civilization and Its Discontents*, in *Complete Psychological Works*, ed. Strachey, xxi.105.

[16] Bersani, *The Freudian Body*, 17, 18, 61.

[17] Clack regards this type of projection as typifying a wider cultural phenomenon, in which 'the fear of the mutability and animality of the body is projected onto women, who in turn are identified with those aspects of humanity which relate to physicality' (*Sex and Death*, 74).

[18] Wack argues that the cure eventually functioned as 'a lightning rod for clerical misogyny' (*Lovesickness*, 70). See also Demaitre, *Bernard de Gordon*, 26–7.

[19] Eunapius of Sardes, *De vitis philosophorum*, trans. Junius (1568); *Suidae historica*, trans. Wolfius (1581).

Arab physicians, including Avicenna.[20] Bernard de Gordon includes this cure in his *De conservatione vitae humanae* (1574), after which it appears in several Renaissance texts, including Theodor Zwinger's *Theatrum humanae vitae* (1586) and Robert Burton's *Anatomy of Melancholy*.

The menstrual cure is part of a wider tradition that suggests that an effective way of remedying the lovesick sufferer is to sully the lover's conception of the beloved. As Jacques Ferrand advises, 'By probable sounding arguments it must be proved that what he finds attractive is, in the judgement of those who see better, actually ugly and deformed.'[21] The quickest means of transforming the lover's idea of his beloved is to engender physical disgust. Any physical malady, providing it is gruesome or shocking, is thought sufficient to awaken the lover out of his amorous reverie. One story describes a scholar who was infatuated with a chaste young woman until she 'flung open her bosome, and offer'd a most filthy, stinking, ulcer'd Cancer of her Breast to his view' to break the spell of love.[22] Apparently this did the trick. Vaughan's version of this story uniquely depicts the emotional conversion as having charitable effects. The young woman shows her admirer her diseased breast, 'At which hideous sight his courage sodainely quailed, and cooled in such sort, that his lustful love was coverted into a charitable love to study for some extraordinary Physicke to helpe her'.[23] Physical revulsion could also be engendered through use of the imagination, in which the lover would visualize his mistress as either sick or old. Alternatively, the lover could mentally anatomize his beloved, stripping her of her skin in order to recognize what lies beneath. Paraphrasing St John Chrysostom, Burton writes: 'Take her skinne from her face, and thou shalt see all loathsomenesse under it, that beauty is a superficiall skinne … within she is full of filthy fleame, stinking, putride, excrementall stuffe.'[24]

Burton's discussion of the menstrual remedy appears in the third section of his *Anatomy of Melancholy*, which treats pathological forms of desire. According to Burton, in order to cure erotic melancholy it is essential to remove the ideal image of the beloved that is deeply engraved in the lover's mind, dominating his imagination. To this end, a doctor

---

[20] Ferrand, *Treatise*, 529 n. 8.   [21] Ferrand, *Erotomania*, 314.
[22] Harvey, *Morbus Anglicus*, 54.   [23] Vaughan, *Directions*, 235.
[24] Burton, *Anatomy*, iii.226.

or friend should malign the erotic object. Old women are seen as being particularly skilled in denigrating the beloved, as they are better than the doctor at revealing another woman's faults. Burton writes:

Paretur aliqua vetula turpissima aspectu, cum turpi & vili habitu: & portet subtus gremium pannum menstrualem, & dicat quòd amica sua sit ebriosa, & quòd mingat in lecto, & quòd est epilepita & impudica, & quòd in corpore suo sunt excrescentiæ enormes, cum fœtore anhelitus, & aliæ enormitates, quibus vetulæ sunt edoctæ: si nolit his persuaderi, subitò extrahat pannum menstrualem, coram facie portando, exclamando, talis est amica tua, & si ex his non demiserit, non est homo, sed diabolus incarnatus.

Let some old woman of the vilest appearance, in dirty and disgusting clothes, be prepared: and let her carry a [menstrual] towel under her apron, and let her say that her friend is drunken, and that she pisses her bed, and that she is epileptic and unchaste; and that on her body there are enormous growths, that her breath stinks, and other monstrous things, in which old women are knowledgeable: if he will not be persuaded by these arguments, let her suddenly produce that [menstrual] towel, and brandish it before his face, crying 'This is what your loved one is like!', and if he doesn't give up at this, he is not a man but a devil incarnate.[25]

The lover's cure is effected through an imaginative transformation of the female body: not only is the mistress unchaste, but her breath is said to stink, her body is covered in growths and she wets her bed. The display of menstrual blood is, in fact, only the final method adopted when other strategies fail to dislodge the lover's romantic image of his mistress. More than just a disturbing bodily discharge, the woman is equated with the menstrual fluid she produces; as the old woman proclaims, 'This is what your loved one is like!' Unlike the idealizing tradition of courtly love, which elevates the mistress and temporarily grants her the upper hand, such misogyny returns the woman to a subordinate place in the gender power hierarchy; no longer idealized and elevated, the mistress is associated with a tradition that regards all women as inherently dangerous and unclean.

In Gideon Harvey's version of the remedy it is the mistress who performs the cure. Harvey describes how one young woman

---

[25] Burton, *Anatomy*, iii.214–15 (trans. vi. 139). I have used 'menstrual' in place of the translator's 'sanitary'.

discovered to herself an ingenious cure, to remedy the poor Schollar of his menaced insanity (madness) in order whereunto, knowing him to be master of a great deal of reason, she muster'd a great bundle of her menstrual rags together (as the wise man calls them) and spread them all open before him; saying, you men that so admire at the Elegant shape, and Notorious Complexion of Womens upper parts, behold now, O Scholar! the constitution of their lower, the object of all your Lascivious Loves; what a filthy, nasty, detestable sight is here?[26]

Just as Lear describes women as centaurs, the mistress divides women into their elegant 'upper parts' and their filthy lower regions. Menstrual blood, historically associated with both fertility and defilement, becomes the strange, hidden truth of the feminine, which when exposed reveals to the man his illusions about the female sex.[27] Often a key sign of a woman's otherness, here menstrual blood is also the mark of her monstrousness. For Sandra Gilbert and Susan Gubar, such images are part of a wider paradigm whereby women are repeatedly figured throughout history as either angels or monsters, paradigms of virtue or embodiments of vice; as Sherry Ortner puts it, 'women can appear from certain points of view to stand both under and over (but really outside of) the sphere of culture's hegemony'.[28] In Harvey's rendition, the revelation of menstrual blood transforms the angelic beloved into something foreign and disturbing, giving added meaning to Gilbert and Gubar's claim that for women 'the monster may not only be concealed behind the angel, she may actually turn out to reside within (or in the lower half of) the angel'.[29]

When one looks at medical, biblical and literary texts, it becomes clear that the male lover's horrified reaction to the display of menstrual blood is not only due to visceral disgust, but also to the moral misgivings such blood engenders about the beloved. Associated with prostitution,

[26] Harvey, *Morbus Anglicus*, 55.
[27] For symbolic and sociological interpretations of menstruation see Delaney, Lupton, and Toth, *The Curse*.
[28] Ortner, 'Female to Male', quoted by Gilbert and Gubar, *Madwoman in the Attic*, 19.
[29] Gilbert and Gubar, *Madwoman in the Attic*, 29. Gilbert and Gubar argue that 'the female freak is and has been a powerfully coercive and monitory image', illustrating 'Simone de Beauvoir's thesis that woman has been made to represent all of man's ambivalent feelings about his own inability to control his own physical existence, his own birth, and death' (p. 34).

poison, corruption, and sexual depravity, menstrual blood is more than just a bodily fluid in the early modern period, it is the symbol for anything immoral or defiled. Within this context, menstrual blood could be interpreted as both the sign of, and the symbol for, a woman's deceitful character; as well as serving as 'a reminder of the axiom that women had inferior bodies', menstruation could also be employed to suggest the beloved's inconstancy, unpredictability, or promiscuous sexuality.[30] Francis Lenton, for example, in his character sketch of 'An Old Bawd' describes a prostitute as 'menstrous' to convey her moral and physical filth, both of which are associated with her bad smell; he writes, 'An old bawd is a menstrous beast, engendred of diverse most filthy excrements, by the stench of whose breath the Ayre is so infected, that her presence is an inevitable contagion.'[31]

Although there is evidence to suggest that more positive and humane approaches to menstruation existed in the early modern period, physiological accounts of women's monthly bleeding served on the whole to reinforce traditional notions about female inferiority, justifying women's subordinate position in society.[32] The two dominant medical theories available in the Renaissance to explain menstruation both regard women's bodies as less functional and wholesome than their male counterparts. The Hippocratic model maintains that menstruation purifies a woman's blood through a process likened to fermentation, bringing impurities to the surface to be washed away. Men do not undergo this process because they have warmer bodies and a more active disposition, features that allow them to release impurities through sweat. Alternatively, medical writers who follow a Galenic model argue that menstruation is a means of removing an excess of blood. This excess accumulates every month because women are physiologically incapable of transforming all of the food they eat into life-giving blood.[33] During pregnancy or while breast-feeding, the excess blood is used to nourish the child in the womb or is converted into breast milk; at all other times it is released through menstruation. The fact that men do not menstruate is regarded as a sign of their

---

[30] Crawford, 'Attitudes to Menstruation', 73.   [31] Lenton, *Characters*, sig. C3.
[32] For more positive approaches to menstruation see Maclean, *Notion*, 40; Wood, 'Sin, Salvation', 710–27. For the way in which menstruation supported notions of female inferiority see Crawford, 'Attitudes to Menstruation', 47–73.
[33] Crawford, 'Attitudes to Menstruation', 50–3.

physiological superiority.[34] Although the two medical theories were incompatible, they were frequently combined when treating menstrual disorders.

Although blood is often praised as a life-giving substance in the Renaissance, the blood produced from menstruation is generally regarded as waste material and referred to as excrement. Mary Douglas describes the blood produced from menstruation as a classic example of 'matter out of place', a substance judged to be a pollutant because it has escaped its natural boundaries (in this case the body).[35] Dangerously impure, menstrual blood is held to emit venomous fumes and have a noxious smell.[36] There are also a variety of superstitions surrounding menstruating women, 'which ironically gave them a good deal of power over their immediate environment'.[37] According to Pliny (second century CE), the mere presence of a menstruating woman will cause wine to sour, mirrors to discolour, grass to die, and knives to blunt. Despite a general decline in magical beliefs, these ideas remained current in the seventeenth century. Rather bizarrely, the powerful properties infused in menstrual blood also made it an ideal substance for a number of cures and potions. Foremost of these was its use in manufacturing love-potions. Whereas the sight of menstrual blood could cure lovesickness, its ingestion was believed to provoke intense feelings of erotic desire.[38] The primary illness related to menstruation in the early modern period was green sickness, thought to afflict young women who had passed puberty but were still virgins.[39] Although phlebotomy was often suggested, sexual intercourse was thought to be the most effective cure as it would loosen the vaginal passage, and release corrupted seed that might be trapped in the womb (See Chapter 2).[40] Within this context, a woman who menstruated was regarded as more 'open' than her closed, green-sick counterpart, so that 'menstruation

---

[34] For the role menstrual blood was believed to play in conception and pregnancy see Needham, *Embryology*, 149–50; Blackham, Woodward and Richards, 'Popular Theories', 56–88; and Tuana, 'The Weaker Seed', 147–71.

[35] Douglas, *Purity and Danger*. Douglas later modified her argument somewhat in 'Self-Evidence' (276–318). For a summary of Douglas's influence on studies of menstruation see Buckley and Gottlieb, 'A Critical Appraisal', 26.

[36] Crawford, 'Attitudes to Menstruation', 51.

[37] Katz, 'Shylock's Gender', 444.

[38] Crawford, 'Attitudes to Menstruation', 59–60.

[39] King, 'Green Sickness', 386. See Ch. 2.   [40] King, *Disease of Virgins*, 79–82.

comes to resemble other varieties of female incontinence—sexual, urinary, linguistic—that served as powerful signs of woman's inability to control the workings of her own body'.[41] Crucially, the discourse regarding green sickness assumes a correlation between a woman's loss of virginity and her achievement of a healthy menstrual flow. This correlation may help to explain why menstruation is frequently regarded as a sign of promiscuity in early modern literary texts, in which the mature, well-functioning female body is simultaneously interpreted as being marked by signs of sexual availability: menstruation functions in the Renaissance as another sign of the open and leaky female body, conceptualized as being both promiscuous and, to use Bakhtin's term, 'grotesque'.

The Bible, which had an enormous impact on how menstruation was perceived in the seventeenth century, represented menstrual blood as unclean by definition. Leviticus, the text from which most sexual taboos in the Judaeo-Christian tradition derive, depicts the menstruating women as both polluted and polluting: she is herself unclean and capable of infecting others (20:18; 15:24). Because of this, sexual intercourse with a menstruating woman was prohibited and punishable by death. In addition, the intimate association between menstruation and contamination allowed the image of the menstruating woman and the menstrual cloth to function as symbols for anything profane or defiled. In the King James Bible the sinful city of Jerusalem is described as 'a menstruous woman' in Lamentations 1:77, and the coverings used to conceal 'graven images of silver' are to be cast away 'as a menstruous cloth' in Isaiah 30:22.[42]

Renaissance writers adopted this discourse, employing images of menstruation to suggest profound corruption. Whilst some writers use menstruation to suggest physical squalor,[43] more frequently they use it to evoke spiritual degradation and sin. The devil in Barnabe Barnes's *The Devil's Charter* (1607), for example, compares Pope Alexander VI's soul to 'a menstruous cloth, | Polluted with unpardonable sins', and the speaker in Richard Brathwait's *The Golden Fleece* (1611) contrasts Christ's 'precious bloud' to his own spiritual corruption, which

---

[41] Paster, 'Spirit of Men', 287. See also Paster, *Embarrassed*, 23–63.
[42] Both quoted by Crawford, 'Attitudes to Menstruation', 57–8.
[43] See, for example, Gerbier d'Ouvilly, *False Favourite Disgrac'd*, 91.

is compared to a 'menstrous cloth'.[44] Several poems paraphrase the lamentations of Jeremiah, comparing Jerusalem with a menstruating woman.[45] As Barnes demonstrates in his depiction of the Pope, Catholicism is often slandered in terms that affiliate it with menstruation. Jonson parodies this kind of abuse in *The Alchemist*, in which the puritan Tribulation maintains his own religion's ability to 'stand up for the beauteous discipline, | Against the menstruous cloth, and rag of Rome'.[46] As F. H. Mares has noted, critics of Catholicism regarded Rome as the 'Scarlet Woman' of Revelation, 'drunken with the blood of the saints and with the blood of the martyrs'. Tribulation's depiction of Rome as a cloth stained with menstrual discharge therefore represents 'an apt—if revolting—metonymy'.[47] Superstitions regarding menstrual blood are also referred to in literature of the period; the idea that menstrual blood has the potential to harm its environment allows menstruation to be employed to convey anything that has a noxious effect, from 'menstruous blasts' of wind to the 'menstruous poison' of a corrupt individual's breath.[48]

As many of the metaphors make clear, menstruation marks the moment at which a woman is transformed from a beloved object to one of scorn. George Sandys in his 'A Paraphrase upon the Lamentations of Jeremiah', for example, laments 'Jerusalem, O thou of late belov'd; | Now like a Menstrous Woman art remov'd'.[49] At times, the close affiliation between a menstruating woman and corruption grants an added association of sexual promiscuity, as if the substance being referred to is hymeneal as well as menstrual blood. Matthew Stevenson, for example, in his poem 'To my lillie white Leda in Commendation of a pale face' (1645) praises the pale complexion of his lover, associating the colour red with menstruation, physical corruption, and sexual promiscuity.[50] Even more striking is the metaphoric use of the menstrual cloth in Abraham Cowley's *The Guardian* (1650). Truman is secretly visited by a woman whom he believes to be his beloved Lucia, but who is in fact

---

[44] Barnes, *Devil's Charter*, 108; Brathwaite, *Golden Fleece*, sig. D[1]ʳ. See also Stephens, *Cinthia's Revenge* (1613), sig. L3ᵛ [P4ᵛ].

[45] Quarles, 'The Lamentations of Jeremiah', in *Fons Lachrymarum*, 32; Sandys, 'A Paraphrase upon the Lamentations of Jeremiah', in *Divine Poems*, 2.

[46] Jonson, *The Alchemist*, ed. Mares, III.i.30–3.   [47] Ibid. 95 n. 33.

[48] Moffett, *Silkewormes* (1599), 67; Barnes, *Devil's Charter*, 13.

[49] Sandys, 'Jeremiah', 2.

[50] Stevenson, 'To My Lillie White Leda', in *Occasions Off-Spring*, 18 [30].

the disguised Aurelia. Refusing to speak, the disguised Aurelia presents Truman with a letter in which she offers herself to him sexually. Stunned and horrified that his beloved is not the 'angel' he thought her to be, he sets her letter on fire, declaring:

> May all remembrance of thee perish with thee,
> Unhappie paper, made of guilty linen.
> The menstruous reliquis of some lustful woman:
> Thy very ashes here will not be innocent,
> But flie about, and hurt some chaste mens eyes,
> As they do mine.[51]

Truman's comparisons implicitly construct the menstruating woman as sexually corrupt and available: not only does he conflate 'Lucia's' letter with 'guilty linen' stained by menstrual blood, but he also envisages this cloth to be the product of 'some lustful woman'. In both instances, menstruation is depicted as being closely affiliated with a woman's immorality and sexual promiscuity: a woman's outspoken sexual desire is as disgusting as a bloody cloth, and both are seen to extinguish the male lover's desire. Menstruation, in fact, figures as part of a wider paradigmatic shift in the way in which Truman imagines his mistress and women in general, who are now regarded as 'poisonous Spiders' driven by lust (sig. C3ᵛ).

Katherine Duncan-Jones regards menstrual revulsion as an important feature in Shakespeare's sonnets, contributing to the sense of misogynistic disgust in the 'dark lady' poems and emphasizing the youth's superiority as an object of desire. In Sonnet 18, for example, the youth's beauty is praised as being more steadfast and 'temperate' than that of a female beloved, at least in part because he does not menstruate: his loveliness will not 'fade' because it is not subject to 'nature's changing course' (menstrual bleeding was known as 'monthly courses' in the early modern period).[52] The difference between the youth's steady progression to maturity and the physical and emotional fluctuations of the dark lady is further evident in the numerical arrangements of Shakespeare's sonnets. Whereas the opening poems addressed to the youth which persuade him to marry and procreate add up to seventeen (18 being the age at which young men were believed to be ready for consummated marriage), the

---

[51] Cowley, *The Guardian*, sig. [C3ʳ].
[52] Duncan-Jones, 'Introduction', in Shakespeare, *Shakespeare's Sonnets*, 48–9.

'dark lady' sequence contains in total twenty-eight poems, a figure that is likely to allude to the lunar month and to the female menstrual cycle. As Duncan-Jones writes, 'in enclosing the great central, Sidneian, sequence of 108 sonnets between the two shorter units of 17 and 28 sonnets, Shakespeare may have designed a contrast between the steadfast growth to physical perfection of the young man and the emotional and moral turbulence of the "dark lady" cycle, with its images of sex-crazed lunacy'.[53] Menstruation here comes to be the sign of female inconstancy, providing a physiological basis for women's false nature and fickle heart.

The menstrual cure for lovesickness may lie behind the literary trope whereby a woman's genitals are revealed to be disgusting when exposed. Paolo Cherchi argues that Bernard de Gordon's account of the aversion therapy is a source for Dante's depiction of the 'femmina balba' [stammering woman] in *Purgatory* Canto 19.[54] There are similar occurrences in Ariosto's *Orlando Furioso* and Spenser's *Faerie Queene*, although the primary source for both these incidents is scripture;[55] Revelation 17:16 and 18:16 tell of a time when the great whore will be 'desolate and naked' and Isaiah 3:17 maintains of the daughters of Zion, that 'the Lord shal discover their secret partes...in stead of swete savour, there shal be stinke'.[56] Aversion therapy is also evident in the 'misogynist letter dissuading a friend from marriage', an epistolary genre popularized by Nicholas Breton in 1602 in *A Poste with a Packet of Madde Letters*, and later developed and expanded by Suckling, whose letters were collected and printed after his death.[57] These letters, as well as rehearsing a number of physiological cures for erotic melancholy, malign women in order to free men from lovesickness and dissuade them from marriage.[58] Suckling's 'Letter 52', for example, suggests that the lover qualify his passion by visiting his mistress 'when she is in sicknes' or by 'draw[ing]

---

[53] Ibid. 99.   [54] Cherchi, 'Per la femmina "balba," ', 228–32.

[55] Ariosto, *Orlando Furioso*, V.ii.72–4; Spenser, *Faerie Queene*, I.iix.46–8.

[56] See the notes for Stanza 46 in Spenser's *Faerie Queene*, 117. More frequently, men in literature are depicted as being cured of their lovesickness through a more general reappraisal of the female sex. In Turner's *Constant Lusina* (1599), for example, King Egistus cures his son Paurinio of his desire for an impoverished maid by maligning women as 'the very refuse of Natures excrements' (sigs. B3ᵛ, C2).

[57] Clayton, editor's note to Letter 51(a), in Suckling, *Non-Dramatic Works,* 331. Although such correspondence is probably just a rhetorical exercise, it is important in that it employs contemporary misogynist discourses as a means of curing lovesickness.

[58] Robertson, *Art of Letter Writing*, 26, 68–9.

her to discourse of things she understands not'.[59] As in Ferrand's *Erotomania*, Suckling suggests that whatever sort of woman is chosen, there
is always some way of finding her faulty: either she is too chaste or
too wanton, too tall or too short, too young or too old. Women, it
seems, are hardly ever in season: they are 'like Melons: too green, or too
ripe.'[60]

The use of the menstrual cure is related to a recurring motif that
Sandra Clark refers to as the 'nice wanton', evident in a number of
plays written solely by Fletcher, including *The Faithful Shepherdess*
(*c*.1608–9), *Monsieur Thomas* (*c*.1610–13), *The Loyal Subject* (1618),
and *The Humorous Lieutenant* (*c*.1619–25). It is also a feature of *The
Coxcomb* (*c*.1612), a play written in collaboration with Beaumont, and
also of one written with Rowley, entitled *The Maid in the Mill* (1623).
In this device, a lascivious man is cured of his desires when the woman
he is pursuing pretends to be attracted to him and willing to accept
his advances. With one exception, the men are unanimously outraged
and repelled by this unexpected display of sexual desire, and withdraw
their attention immediately, seemingly reformed.[61] The 'nice wanton'
device clearly has affinities with the menstrual cure, in which sexual
disgust is deliberately engendered in order to free a lustful man of
his obsession. What is so remarkable about Beaumont and Fletcher's
contribution to this tradition is that here it is not the sight of a diseased
breast or a menstrual cloth which repulses the lover, but merely the
woman's open expression of sexual desire which engenders the man's
disgust.

Whilst the depiction of the 'nice wanton' may, in Sandra Clark's
words, 'function to resolve the sexual anxieties of men' (titillating the
men in the audience with the appearance of intemperance whilst affirming a woman's ability to remain chaste), these scenes also signal the
extent to which polarized constructions of female sexuality reinforce
and justify the lover's contradictory responses.[62] The lover's oscillation
between sexual desire and repulsion is caused, not by his own emotional

---

[59] Suckling, 'Letter 52' ['A disswasion from Love'], in *Non-Dramatic Works*, 158.
[60] Suckling, 'Letter 53' [Perhaps to Charles Suckling of Bracondale], in *Non-Dramatic
Works*, 160.
[61] The exception is Fletcher's *A Wife for a Month* (*c*.1624).
[62] Clark, *Sexual Themes*, 154. See also Cotton, who suggests that the plays provide a
'soothing, wish-fulfilling reassurance to audiences indoctrinated with a horror of wifely
unchastity and the dishonor it brought to the husband' (*Fletcher's Chastity Plays*, 68).

ambivalence, but rather by his mistress, who alternates between appearing chaste and lascivious. Within such contexts, chastity is constructed
not as the ability to temper and restrain one's sexual impulses but
rather as the complete absence of such impulses. Nevertheless, there
is a tension within these plays between the male protagonists' rigid
constructions of female sexuality and the protean roles adopted by the
heroines. The fact that the beloved is usually found to be innocent and
uncorrupted reinforces the male lover's belief in absolute and polarized
conceptions of female sexuality. However, the plays also reveal a chaste
woman's ability to play both the innocent virgin and the predatory
wanton, adopting and manipulating paradoxical constructs of female
sexual behaviour to her own ends; the dramaturgical structure, with its
emphasis on tricks, disguises and pretence, introduces a more fluid and
interchangeable definition of female sexual identity.

The menstrual cure throws new light on a key scene in John Fletcher's
The Mad Lover (*c*.1616), which is related to the 'nice wanton' device.[63]
The Mad Lover, which focuses upon soldiers in times of peace, is
structured around the clash between male and female codes of honour,
in which military values are contrasted with those of the court. The
play opens with Memnon returning victorious from battle. A man's
man, whose soul is 'conceiv'd a Souldier', Memnon can feel nothing but
contempt for the activities of 'lazie' peace (I.i.14, 52). However, despite
Memnon's rejection of the 'oylie language' of the court, his strength as a
military leader is subverted by his desire for Princess Calis, whose beauty
transfixes him in silent awe (I.i.62). Determined to win her hand, he
offers the princess possession of his heart; 'I would you had it in your
hand sweet Ladie', he tells her, 'To see the truth it beares ye' (I.ii.90–1).
For Memnon, however, this is no idle, metaphoric promise, but a vow
given in complete seriousness: he intends to have his heart cut from his
body and sent to his mistress in a 'goblet of pure gold' (I.ii.101). Such an
offer literalizes the conceit whereby lovers exchange hearts, burlesquing
the Petrarchan conventions of love, while simultaneously hinting at the

---

[63] *The Mad Lover* has always been considered as Fletcher's composition exclusively,
despite the fact that the entry in the Register's record attributes the plays generally to
Beaumont and Fletcher. The prologue declares it to be the work of a single author, and
Sir Aston Cokayne ascribes the play to him in a poem praising the deceased playwright.
See John Fletcher, *The Mad Lover*, ed. Turner in Beaumont and Fletcher, *Dramatic Works*,
ed. Bowers, v.3.

darker, pathological side of desire. Memnon's lack of familiarity with the codes of courtship leads him to offer his mistress not promises of amorous devotion, but pledges of masochistic self-sacrifice.

Memnon's lovesickness is regarded by his fellow soldiers as emasculating, transforming the war hero into an object of pity and ridicule. His passion undermines the male codes of honour in the play and jeopardizes the country's safety. Polidor feels 'shame and scorn' at his brother's undignified metamorphosis, lamenting the way in which a man previously hailed for his good governance of others is no longer able to regulate himself (III.ii.97). Eventually Polidor decides that sexual intercourse will cure his brother's insanity, discharging his brother's excessive heat and returning him to reason. Sending for a 'handsome whore', he tells the assembled soldiers that she must be taught to look and speak like Princess Calis; if all goes to plan, Memnon will believe the women is his beloved and have sex with her (III.ii.144) (see Chapter 5). Initially all seems to be going well: the men are amazed at how cleverly the woman has disguised her unseemly background and Memnon seems convinced that she is indeed his beloved. However, despite the woman's superficial resemblance to the princess, she cannot disguise her horrible smell. '[B]y heaven she stinkes', Memnon declares, likening her odour to 'rotten Cabbage' and 'a poyson'd Ratt behind a hanging' (IV.v.43–5). Overcome with disgust every time he approaches her, Memnon questions whether the woman before him is an impostor and threatens to bring in the Numidian lion to test her royal identity:

> For if she be a Princesse, as she may be
> And yet stink too, and strongly, I shall find her;
> Fetch the *Numidian* Lyon I brought over,
> If she be sprung from royall blood,—the Lyon
> He'l doe ye reverence, els
>
> .   .   .   .
> He'l teare her all to pieces.
>
> (IV.v.52–9)

The woman, however, is not prepared to stand the trial; terrified of being torn from limb to limb, she confesses herself to be only a 'poore retaining whore', and Memnon bursts into laughter (IV.v.61). The encounter marks a turning point in the play: from this point forward, Memnon begins to regain his wits and his face appears 'not so clouded as it was' (IV.v.66).

Memnon's reaction to the impoverished whore dramatizes the way in which sexual disgust can act as a cure, freeing the lover from his passionate affliction. While the woman's odour is ostensibly the product of her poverty and circumstance, repeated reference to the woman's blood suggests that it is an important aspect of Memnon's revulsion. Different potential meanings of blood are drawn together, including menstrual blood, hymeneal blood, and the purified blood of semen (in the Renaissance semen was believed to be composed of refined, concocted blood). The woman's blood is an indicator not only of her social class, but also of her physical identity as a woman. Questions of the woman's social rank merge with those of her sexual status: she is unable to act the part of the noble lady and is physically unclean.

The first reference to the woman's blood occurs when the disguised prostitute is first brought before the company of men for their approval, and the Captain announces she has 'smockt away her blood' (IV.v.18). The use of 'smockt' here is unusual. The *OED*'s earliest citations of 'smock' as a verb are 'to render effeminate' (1614) and 'to consort with women' (1719), neither of which make sense in the given context. The most plausible and straightforward reading of the line is offered by the editors of the Cambridge edition, who propose that 'smockt' refers to the whore's transformation in appearance. Clearly impressed with the woman's disguise, the men admire how the whore has concealed both her humble birth and her profession, appearing instead like a 'good round Virgin' (IV.v.8). However, the substance to which the Captain refers may be physical rather than metaphoric, in which case 'smockt' would mean 'wiped away'. The editor of the Cambridge edition recognizes this possibility, suggesting that the blood referred to might be that lost 'through sexual intercourse'.[64] In this instance the line could refer either to hymeneal blood (so that the woman is in effect erasing the physical signs that disclose her loss of virginity) or 'seed' (composed of refined blood), which women were thought to emit during sexual intercourse. It could also refer to semen (see above).

The substance in question may also be menstrual blood. Fletcher's frequent use of the aversion cure is reminiscent of that described in medical texts, some of which include the use of menstrual blood in

<hr/>

[64] Turner, ed., John Fletcher, *The Mad Lover*, in Beaumont and Fletcher, *Dramatic Works,* ed. Bowers, v.110 n. 18.

the treatment of lovesickness. In addition, it is the woman's odour that leads Memnon to question the woman's identity, and menstruation is repeatedly associated with a noxious smell.[65] An odd piece of stage business may well strengthen this interpretation. Upon first encountering the disguised courtesan, Memnon offers to kiss the woman's 'royall hand' (IV.v.31); but when her hands are revealed, the male onlookers are disgusted. Noting the state of her gloves the Captaine remarks, 'The Lees of baudie prewnes [prunes]: mourning gloves? | All spoyl'd by heaven' (IV.v.35–6). The woman has failed to remove her gloves while eating, ruining the fashionable accessory that should be the sign of her supposed status; prunes in particular are associated with prostitutes in the Renaissance, as the staple dish offered in bawdy-houses was stewed prunes. It is, however, possible to interpret the red and purple marks in another manner: as stains from menstrual blood hastily cleaned up before her appearance on stage. This would both make sense of the Captain's claim that the woman has 'smockt away her blood' and explain the intense reaction of the soldiers, who instantly repudiate her as a 'dam'd foule one' and 'clawing scabby whore' (IV.v.34, 37). Either way, the soiled gloves that the disguised prostitute reluctantly offers for Memnon's kiss trigger his emotional volte-face. Torn between hopeless idealization and visceral disgust, he threatens to bring on the Numidian lion as a means of determining the purity of the woman's 'royall blood'.

Although Memnon locates blood as the substance that will determine the true identity of the woman before him, the play's burlesque treatment of him suggests that all idealizing fantasies about women are faulty. The mythical lion may be able to distinguish the wholesome noble woman from the foul-smelling whore, but the misogynist tradition on which the menstruation cure draws maintains no such distinction. In the cure for lovesickness outlined above, all women—regardless of their rank, clothing, smell, and chastity—are capable of producing revulsion in the male lover. Menstruation, which associates women with pollution and corruption, extinguishes the lover's passion and undermines idealistic notions of women and physical intimacy. Sexual frustration re-emerges as vituperative disgust, as the lover's elevated image of his mistress is transformed to one of scorn. Within this context, misogyny

---

[65] Crawford, 'Attitudes to Menstruation', 51.

is a product of vulnerability rather than power, expressing the lover's subjugation to his commanding mistress, as well as his passivity and sexual frustration.

The menstrual cure for lovesickness promotes a construction of women as duplicitous (women are not what they seem) and corrupt, in which the female sexual organs are imagined to be both physically repellent and ethically corrosive; in the words of Lear, 'there's hell, there's darkness, there is the sulphurous pit, burning, scalding, stench, consumption'.[66] Because of this men are advised, as in Shakespeare's Sonnet 129, 'To shun the heaven that leads men to this hell', avoiding an intimate knowledge of the female body as it might occasion the destruction of amorous passions and idealistic dreams of love, rather than their fulfilment (the 'hell' of the lover's disillusionment thus engendered by the 'hell' of the beloved's disturbing genitalia).[67] Men are thus defeated by their very erotic success, so that feelings of intense desire ultimately give way to those of hatred and disgust; as Burton suggests, 'burning lust is but a flash, a gunpowder passion, and hatred oft followes in the highest degree, dislike and contempt'.[68] The lover's conflicting emotions of love and hate, longing and loathing, suggest the destructive and ambivalent aspect of erotic affection, and the ways in which sexual desire, as well as being a bittersweet pleasure, can be a source of anger and resentment to the disempowered and sexually frustrated male. As the menstrual cure makes clear, elevated philosophical conceptions of love are intimately related to discourses that denigrate women as monstrous and disgusting, and both of these viewpoints obstruct a more realistic assessment of the beloved, which includes bodily functions such as menstruation. In the fraught context of erotic passion, the female beloved can be damned, as well as exalted, by exaggerated praise.

[66] Shakespeare, *King Lear*, IV.vi.123–5.
[67] Shakespeare, 'Sonnet 129', in *Sonnets*, 14.   [68] Burton, *Anatomy*, iii.222.

Bibliography

PRIMARY SOURCES

Manuscripts

The Ashmole Manuscripts are fully described in William H. Black, comp., *A Descriptive, Analytical and Critical Catalogue of the Manuscripts Bequeathed...by Elias Asmole* (Oxford, 1845).

Richard Napier's case notes
  Bodleian, Ashmole MS 182.
  Bodleian, Ashmole MS 196.
  Bodleian, Ashmole MS 198.
  Bodleian, Ashmole MS 406.
  Bodleian, Ashmole MS 414.

Plays and Masques

Anonymous, *The Faire Maide of the Exchange* (1607), ed. Arthur Brown (Oxford, 1962).
—— *The Wit of a Woman* (London, 1604).
Barnes, Barnabe, *The Devil's Charter: A Tragedy Containing the Life and Death of Pope Alexander the Sixth* (1607), ed. Nick de Somogyi (London, 1999).
Barry, Larding, *Ram-Alley* (London, 1610).
Beaumont, Francis, and John Fletcher, *The Dramatic Works in the Beaumont and Fletcher Canon,* gen. ed. Fredson Bowers, 10 vols. (Cambridge, 1966–96).
—— *The Maid's Tragedy*, ed. T. W. Craik, Revels Plays (Manchester, 1988, repr. 1999).
—— *The Maid's Tragedy*, ed. Howard B. Norland, Regents Renaissance Drama Series (Lincoln, NE, 1968).
Brewer, Anthony, *The Love-Sick King*, ed. A. E. H. Swaen (Louvain, 1907).
Brome, Richard, *The Antipodes*, ed. David Scott Kastan and Richard Proudfoot, Globe Quartos (London, 2000).
—— *The City Wit, or, The Woman Wears Breeches* (London, 1653).
—— *The Court Beggar* (London, 1653).
—— *The Northern Lasse* (London, [1632]).
—— *The Queen and Concubine*, in Richard Brome, *Five New Playes* (London, 1659).

—— *The Sparagus Garden* (London, 1640).

Cartwright, William, *Comedies, Tragi-Comedies, with Other Poems* (London, 1651).

Cavendish, Jane, and Elizabeth Brackley, 'The Concealed Fancies', in S. P. Cerasano and Marion Wynne-Davies (eds.), *Renaissance Drama by Women: Texts and Documents* (London, 1996).

C[hamberlain], R[obert], *The Swaggering Damsell* (London, 1640).

Chapman, George, *A Humerous Dayes Myrth* (London, 1597).

—— *Monsieur D'Olive* (London, 1606).

—— *The Widow's Tears*, ed. Akihiro Yamada (London, 1975).

Cokayn [Cokain], Aston, *The Obstinante Lady* (London, 1657).

—— *Trappolin Creduto Principe, Or, Trappolin Suppos'd a Prince* (London, 1658).

Cowley, Abraham, *The Guardian* (London, 1650).

[Davenant, William], *The Cruel Brother* (London, 1630).

—— *The Platonick Lovers* (London, 1636).

—— *The Platonick Lovers: An Old-Spelling Critical Edition of William Davenant's The Platonick Lovers*, ed. Wendell W. Broom, Jr. (New York, 1987).

—— *The Wits* (London, 1636).

Dekker, Thomas, *The Honest Whore, Parts One and Two*, ed. Nick de Somogyi, Globe Quartos (London, 1998).

—— and John Webster, *North-ward Hoe* (London, 1607).

Fletcher, John, *The Captaine* (London, 1647).

—— *The Elder Brother* (London, 1637).

Ford, John, *The Broken Heart*, ed. Brian Morris, New Mermaids (London, 1966).

—— *The Broken Heart*, ed. T. J. B. Spencer, Revels Plays (Manchester, 1980).

—— *The Ladies Triall* (London, 1639).

—— *The Lover's Melancholy*, ed. R. F. Hill, Revels Plays (Manchester, 1985).

—— *Love's Sacrifice*, ed. A. T. Moore, Revels Plays (Manchester and New York, 2002).

—— *The Queene, or the Excellency of her Sex* (London, 1653).

—— *'Tis Pity She's a Whore*, ed. Martin Wiggins, New Mermaids (London and New York, 2003, repr. 2006).

—— and Tho[mas] Dekker, *The Sun's-Darling: A Moral Masque* (London, 1656).

Gerbier d'Ouvilly, George, *The False Favourite Disgrac'd* (London, 1657).

Glapthorne, Henry, *The Hollander* (London, 1640).

—— *The Ladies Priviledge* (London, 1640).

Goffe, Thomas, *The Tragedy of Orestes* (London, 1632).

Harding, S[amuel], *Sicily and Naples, or, the Fatall Union*, ed. Joan Warthling Roberts (New York and London, 1986).

Hausted, Peter, *The Rivall Friends* (London, 1632).

Heywood, Thomas, *The Dramatic Works of Thomas Heywood Now First Collected with Illustrative Notes and a Memoir of the Author in Six Volumes* (London, 1874).

—— *Loves Maistresse: Or, The Queens Masque* (London, 1636).

—— *The Wise-Woman of Hogsdon* (London, 1638).

—— *A Woman Killed with Kindness*, ed. Brian W. M. Scobie, New Mermaids (London, 1985).

Jones, Indigo, and William Davenant, *The Temple of Love* (London, 1634).

Jonson, Ben, *The Alchemist*, ed. F. H. Mares, Revels Plays (Manchester, 1967, repr. 1997).

—— *Complete Plays of Ben Jonson*, ed. G. A. Wilkes, 4. vols. (Oxford, 1981–2), based on vols. iii–iv of the edition by C. H. Herford and P. and E. Simpson (Oxford, 1925–52).

—— *Ben Jonson: Selected Masques*, ed. Stephen Orgel, the Yale Ben Jonson (New Haven and London, 1970), vol. iv.

—— *The Case is Alterd* (London, 1609).

—— 'Chloridia, Rites to Chloris and Her Nymphs', in *Ben Jonson: The Complete Masques*, ed. Stephen Orgel, the Yale Ben Jonson (New Haven and London, 1969), 462–72.

—— *Every Man Out of his Humour* (London, 1599).

—— *The New Inn* (1631), ed. Michael Hattaway, Revels Plays (Manchester, 1984).

—— *The Staple of Newes*, ed. Anthony Parr, Revels Plays (Manchester, 1999).

—— and Inigo Jones, *Loves Triumph Through Callipolis* (London, 1630).

Knevet, Ralph, *Rhodon and Iris* (London, 1631).

Kyd, Thomas, *The Spanish Tragedy*, ed. Andrew S. Cairncross (Lincoln, NE, 1967).

Lyly, John, *Midas*, ed. Anne Begor Lancashire (Lincoln, 1969).

—— *Sappho and Phao*, ed. David Bevington, in G. K. Hunter and David Bevington (eds.), *John Lyly: Campaspe, Sappho and Phao* (Manchester, 1991).

[Mabbe, James], *The Spanish Bawd, Represented in Celestina: Or, The Tragicke-Comedy of Calisto & Melibea* (London, 1631).

Manuche, Cosmo, *The Loyal Lovers* (London, 1652).

Marlowe, Christopher, *Dido Queene of Carthage and The Massacre at Paris*, ed. H. J. Oliver, Revels Plays (London, 1968).

Marmion, Shackerley, *A Fine Companion* (London, 1632).

—— *Hollands Leaquer* (London, 1631).

Marston, John, *The Dutch Courtesan*, ed. David Crane, New Mermaids (London, 1997).

—— *The Insatiate Countesse* (London, 1613).

—— *The Malcontent*, ed. George K. Hunter, Revels Plays (London, 1999).

—— *The Tragedy of Sophonisba*, in Peter Corbin and Douglas Sedge (eds.), *Three Jacobean Witchcraft Plays*, Revels Plays (Manchester, 1986).

Massinger, Philip, *The Plays and Poems of Philip Massinger*, ed. Philip Edwards and Colin A. Gibson, 5 vols. (Oxford, 1976).

—— *The Picture* (London, 1629).

May, Thomas, *The Heire* (London, 1633).

—— *The Old Couple* (London, 1658).

[Mayne, Jasper], *The Citye Match* (Oxford, 1639).

Middleton, Thomas, *Women Beware Women*, ed. William C. Carroll (London and New York, 1994).

Middleton, Thomas, and William Rowley, *The Changeling*, ed. Michael Neill, New Mermaids (London and New York, 2006)

—— *The Changeling*, ed. N. W. Bawcutt, Revels Plays (London, 1961).

Milton, John, *A Mask Presented at Ludlow Castle* [Comus], in *John Milton: Complete Shorter Poems*, ed. John Carey (London, 1997).

Nabbes, Thomas, *The Bride* (London, 1638).

—— *Microcosmus, A Morall Maske* (London, 1637).

—— *The Springs Glorie* (London, 1638).

[Peaps, William], *Love in it's Extasie: Or the Large Prerogative* (London, 1649).

S.S., *The Honest Lawyer* (London, 1616).

Shakespeare, William, *William Shakespeare: The Complete Works*, ed. Stanley Wells and Gary Taylor (Oxford, 1988, repr. 1990).

Shirley, James, *The Arcadia* (London, 1640).

—— *The Ball* (London, 1632).

—— *The Bird in a Cage* (London, 1633).

—— *Changes: Or, Love in a Maze* (London, 1632).

—— *The Constant Maid* (London, 1640).

—— *A Critical Edition of James Shirley's St. Patrick for Ireland*, ed. John P. Turner, Jr. (New York, 1979).

—— *The Gamester* (London, 1633).

—— *The Gratefull Servant* (London, 1629).

—— *The Humorous Courtier* (London, 1640).

—— *The Lady of Pleasure* (1635), ed. Ronald Huebert, Revels Plays (Manchester, 1986).

—— *Love's Crueltie* (London, 1640).

—— *The Young Admirall* (London, 1633).

Stephens, John, *Cinthia's Revenge: Or Maenanders Extasie* (London, 1613).

Strode, William, *The Floating Island* (London, 1655).

Suckling, John, *Aglaura* (London, 1638).

Townshend, Aurelian, *The Poems and Masques of Aurelian Townshend*, ed. Cedric Brown (Reading, 1983).

Turner, Richard, *Constant Lusina: The Amorous Passions of Paurinio a Surfeiting Lover* (London, 1599).

Webster, John, *The Devil's Law-Case*, in John Webster, *The Complete Works of John Webster*, ed. F. L. Lucas (London, 1927).

—— *The White Devil*, ed. John Russell Brown, Revels Plays (Manchester, 1996).

—— *The Works of John Webster: An Old-Spelling Critical Edition*, ed. David Gunby, David Carnegie, Antony Hamond, Doreen DelVecchio, 3 vols. (Cambridge, 1995–2007).

Other Primary Texts

Adams, Thomas, *Diseases of the Soule: A Discourse Divine, Morall, and Physicall* (London, 1616).

Alciati, Andrea, *Emblemata cum commentariis* (Padua, 1621; repr. New York, 1976).

—— *Emblemata* (1550), trans. Betty I. Knott (Chippenham, 1996).

[Anonymous], *A Rational Account of the Natural Weaknesses of Women, and of the Secret Distempers Peculiarly Incident to Them* (London, 1716).

Aristotle, *Problems*, trans. W. S. Hett, 23 vols. (London and Cambridge, MA, 1957), vol. xvi.

Arnald of Villanova, *Tractatus de amore heroico*, in *Opera Omnia* (Basileae, 1585).

Aubrey, John, *Aubrey's Brief Lives*, ed. Oliver Lawson Dick (Harmondsworth, 1972).

Bacon, Francis, *The Essayes or Counsels, Civill and Morall*, ed. Michael Kiernan (Oxford, 1985).

—— 'Narcissus, or Philautia (Self-Love)', in *The Wisdom of the Ancients, The Works of Francis Bacon*, ed. James Spedding, Robert Leslie Ellis, and Douglas Denon Heath, 15 vols. (Boston, 1860–64), xiii. 89–90.

Bacon, Francis, *The Works of Francis Bacon*, ed. James Spedding, Robert Leslie Ellis, and Douglas Denon Heath, 15 vols. (Cambridge, 1992).

Barrough, Philip, *The Method of Physicke, Containing the Causes, Signs, and Cures of Inward Diseases in Man's Bodie from the Head to the Foote* (London, 1633).

B[astard], T[homas], *Chrestoleros. Seven Bookes of Epigrames* (London, 1598).

B[enlowes], E[dward], *Theophilia, or Loves Sacrifice* (London, 1652).

Boaistuau, Pierre, *Theatrum Mundi*, trans. John Alday (London, 1581).

Bradwell, Stephen, *Mary Glovers Late Woeful Case, Together with her Joyfull Deliverance* (London, 1603), repr. in Michael MacDonald (ed.), *Witchcraft and Hysteria in Elizabethan London* (London and New York, 1991).

Brant, Sebastian, *The Shyp of Folys of the Worlde*, trans. Alexander Barclay (London, 1509).

[Brathwait, Richard], *The Golden Fleece* (London, 1611).

—— *The Honest Ghost, or a Voice from the Vault* (London, 1658).

—— *Panaretees Triumph: or Hymens Heavenly Hymne* (London, 1641).

Breton, Nicholas, *The Arbor of Amorous Devices*, ed. Hyder Edward Rollins (Cambridge, MA, 1936).

—— *Two Pamphlets of Nicholas Breton: Grimellos Fortunes (1604) An Olde Mans Lesson (1605)*, ed. E. G. Morice (Bristol, 1936).

—— *Melancholike Humours*, ed. G. B. Harrison (London, 1929).

Bright, Timothie, *A Treatise of Melancholie. Containing the Causes Thereof & Reasons of the Strange Effects it Worketh in our Minds and Bodies: With the Phisicke Cure, and Spirituall Consolation for Such as have thereto Adioyned an Afflicted Conscience* (London, 1586).

Bruno, Giordano, *The Heroic Frenzies*, ed. and trans. Paul Eugene Memmo, Jr. (Chapel Hill, NC, 1964).

Burton, Robert, *The Anatomy of Melancholy*, eds. Nicolas K. Kiessling, Thomas C. Faulkner, and Rhonda L. Blair, 3 vols. (Oxford, 1989–94).

Campion, Thomas, *The Works of Thomas Campion: Complete Songs, Masques, and Treatises with a Selection of Latin Verse*, ed. with intro. by Walter R. Davis (London, 1969).

Carew, Thomas, *The Poems of Thomas. Carew*, ed. Rhodes Dunlap (Oxford, 1957).

Carter, Angela, 'John Ford's *'Tis Pity She's a Whore*', in Angela Carter, *American Ghosts and Old World Wonders* (London, 1994), 20–44.

Castiglione, Count Baldassare, *The Book of the Courtier*, ed. and trans. Virginia Cox (London, 1994).

Cavendish, Margaret, *A True Relation of my Birth, Breeding and Life*, from *Nature's Pictures Drawn by Fancy's Pencil to the Life* (1656), in Elspeth Graham, Hilary Hinds, Elaine Hobby, and Helen Wilcox (eds.), *Her Own Life: Autobiographical Writings by Seventeenth-Century Englishwomen* (London, 1989) 87–100.

Cavendish, William, *The Phanseys of William Cavendish, Marquis of Newcastle, Addressed to Margaret Lucas, and her Letters in Reply*, ed. Douglas Grant (London, 1956).

C[leveland], J[ohn], *The Character of A London-Diurnall: With Severall Select Poems* (London, 1647 [1646]).

C[leveland], J[ohn], *Poems with Additions Never before Printed* ([London], 1653).

Clifford, Lady Anne, *The Diaries of Lady Anne Clifford*, ed. D. J. H. Clifford (Stroud, 1990).

Coëffeteau, F. N., *A Table of Humane Passions,* trans. Edw[ard] Grimeston (London, 1621).

Cokain, Aston, *Small Poems of Divers Sorts* (London, 1658).

Collop, John, *Poesis Rediviva: Or Poesie Reviv'd* (London, 1656 [1655]).

Cowley, Abraham, *The Collected Works of Abraham Cowley*, 2 vols. (Newark, NJ, London, and Toronto, 1993).

Culpeper, Nicholas, *A Directory for Midwives* (London, 1675).

Donne, John, *John Donne*, ed. John Carey, The Oxford Authors (Oxford, 1990).

—— *The Complete English Poems*, ed. C. A. Patricles (London, 1994).

Drayton, Michael, *Poly-Olbion. or, a* Chorographicall *Description of* Tracts, Rivers, Mountaines, Forests, *and other Parts of this Renowned* Isle *of* Great Britaine (London, 1613).

Du Bartas, Guillaume de Saluste, *Du Bartas: His Divine Weekes, and Workes with all the Other Workes,* trans. Joshuah Sylvester (London, 1621).

Elizabeth I, *The Letters of Queen Elizabeth I*, ed. G. B. Harrison (London, 1935).

E[lys], E[dmund], *Dia Poemata: Poetick Feet Standing upon Holy Ground: Or, Verses on Certain Texts of Scripture* (London, 1655).

Erasmus, Desiderius, *The Praise of Folly*, ed. and trans. Hoyt H. Hudson (Princeton, 1941, repr. 1970).

Evelyn, John, *The Diary of John Evelyn*, ed. E. S. de Beer (Oxford, 1959, repr. 2000).

Ferrand, Jacques, *A Treatise on Lovesickness*, ed. and trans. Donald Beecher and Massimo Ciavolella (Syracuse, NY, 1990).

—— *Erotomania, or a Treatise Discoursing of the Essence, Causes, Symptomes, Prognosticks, and Cure of Love, or Erotique Melancholy*, trans. Edmund Chilmead (Oxford, 1640).

Ficino, Marsilio, *Marsilio Ficino and the Phaedran Charioteer*, intro. and trans. Michael J. B. Allen, Publications of the Center for Medieval and Renaissance Studies 14 (Berkeley and London, 1981).

—— *Marsilio Ficino's Commentary on Plato's Symposium on Love*, ed. and trans. Sears Jayne (Dallas, 1985).

F[lesher], M[iles], *Cupids Messenger: Or, a Trusty Friend Stored with Sundry Sorts of Letters* (London, 1629).

Ford, John, *A Line of Life*, in *The Nondramatic Works of John Ford*, ed. L. E. Stock et al., The Renaissance English Text Society 15, Seventh Series (Binghamton, NY, 1991), 299–327.

—— *The Works of John Ford*, ed. William Gifford and Alexander Dyce, 3 vols. (London, 1895).

Fregosos, Giovan Battista, *L'anteros ou contramour de Messire Baptiste Fulgoses*, trans. Thomas Sibilet (Paris, 1581).

Galen, Claudius, *Galeni exhortatio ad bonas arteis, praesertim medicinam, de optimo docendi genere*, trans. Erasmus (Basle, 1526).

Gawdy, Philip, *Letters of Philip Gawdy*, ed. I. H. Jeayes (London, 1906).

Greene, Robert, *Mamillia*: *A Mirrour or Looking Glasse for the Ladies of England*, in Robert Greene, *The Life and Complete Works of Robert Greene in Prose and Verse*, ed. Alexander B. Grosart, 15 vols. (New York, 1881–6).

Guillemeau, Jacques, *Child-Birth or The Happy Deliverie of Women* (London, 1612).

Hall, John, *Poems* (Cambridge, 1646).

Hart, James, *Klinike, or The Diet of the Diseased* (London, 1633).

Harvey, Gideon, *Morbus Anglicus: Or, the Anatomy of Consumptions* (London, 1666).

Heath, Robert, *Clarastella: Together with Poems Occasional, Elegies, Epigrams, Satyrs* (London, 1650).

Henslowe, Philip, *Henslowe's Diary*, ed. R. A. Foakes and R. T. Rickert (Cambridge, 1961).

Herbert, Edward, *Occasional Verses (1665)*, facs. repr. (Menston, 1969).

Herbert, Mary Sidney, *The Collected Works of Mary Sidney Herbert, Countess of Pembroke*, ed. Margaret P. Hannay, Noel J. Kinnamon, and Michael G. Brennan (Oxford, 1998).

Herrick, Robert, *The Poetical Works of Robert Herrick*, ed. L. C. Martin (Oxford, 1956).

Heywood, Thomas, *Gunaikeion: or Nine Books of Various History Concerning Women* (London, 1624).

H[ookes], N[icholas], *Amanda, a Sacrifice to an Unknown Goddesse, or A Free-will Offering of a Loving Heart to a Sweet-Heart* (London, 1653).

Howell, James, *Epistolae Ho-Elianae, The Familiar Letters of James Howell, Historiographer Royal to Charles II*, ed. J. Jacobs, 2 vols. (London, 1890).

Hutchinson, Lucy, *Memoirs of the Life of Colonel Hutchinson, with the Fragment of an Autobiography of Mrs. Hutchinson*, ed. James Sutherland (London, 1973).

James VI and I, *Political Writings*, ed. J. P. Sommerville (Cambridge, 1994).

Jones, John, *Adrasta: Or, the Woman's Spleene, and Lover's Conquest* (London, 1635).

Jorden, Edward, *A Briefe Discourse of a Disease called the Suffocation of the Mother. Written upon Occasion which hath Beene of Late Taken Thereby, to*

Suspect Possession of an Evill Spririt, or Some Such Like Supernaturall Power (London, 1603).

Lange, Johannes, *Medicinalium epistolarum miscellanea* (Basel, 1554), repr. in Helen King, *The Disease of Virgins: Green Sickness, Chlorosis and the Problems of Puberty* (London and New York, 2004) 142–3, trans. King, 46–8.

Laurentius, M. Andreas, *A Discourse of the Preservation of the Sight; of Melancholike Diseases; of Rheumes, and of Old Age,* trans. Richard Surphlet (London, 1599).

Lawes, Henry, *Ayres, and Dialogues, for One, Two, and Three Voyces. The Third Book* (London, 1658).

—— *The Treasury of Musick: Containing Ayres and Dialogues to Sing to the Theorbo-Lute or Basse-Viol in 3 Books* (London, 1669).

Lemnius, Levinus, *The Touchstone of Complexions*, trans. T[homas] N[ewton] (London, 1576).

Lenton, Frances, *Characters: Or, Wit and the World* (London, 1663).

Lovelace, Richard, *The Poems of Richard Lovelace*, ed. C. H. Wilkinson (Oxford, 1930, 1953).

M., Io., *Phillippes Venus, Wherin is Pleasantly Discoursed Sundrye Fine and Wittie Arguments in a Senode of Gods and Goddesses, Assembled for the Expelling of Wanton Venus, from among their Sacred Societie* (London, 1591).

Mercatus, Lodovicus, *De mulieribus affectionibus* (Venice, 1587).

—— *Operum tomus primus* (Frankfurt, 1620–9).

Moffett, Thomas, *The Silkewormes, and their Flies* (1599), intro. by Victor Houliston, facs. repr., Medieval and Renaissance Texts and Studies 56, 6th Series (Binghamton, NY, 1989).

Montaigne, Michel de, 'On Affectionate Relationships', *The Essays of Michel de Montaigne*, ed. and trans. M. A. Screech (London, 1987, 1991), 205–19.

Nashe, Thomas, *The Unfortunate Traveller. Or, the Life of Jacke Wilton* (London, 1594).

Needham, Joseph, *A History of Embryology*, 2nd edn. (Cambridge, 1959).

Osborne, Dorothy, *The Letters of Dorothy Osborne*, ed. Kingsley Hart (London, 1968).

Overbury, Thomas, *New and Choise Characters, of Severall Authors: Together with that Exquisite and Unmatcht Poeme, The Wife* (London, 1615).

Ovid, *The Art of Love, and Other Poems*, trans. J. H. Mozley (Cambridge, MA, 1979).

—— *His Remedie of Love* (London, 1600).

Oxenbridge, Daniel, *General Observations and Prescriptions in the Practice of Physick* (London, 1715).

Paré, Ambroise, *The Workes of the Famous Chirurgion Ambrose Parey, Translated out of the Latine and Compared with the French by Tho. Johnson* (London, 1649).

Pecke, Thomas, *Parnassi Puerperium: or, Some Well-Wishes to Ingenuity* (London, 1659).

Pierce, Robert, *Bath Memoirs: Or, Observations in Three and Fourty Years Practice, at the Bath, What Cures Have Been There Wrought* (Bristol, 1697).

Platter, Felix, Abdiah Cole, and Nich[olas] Culpeper, *A Golden Practice of Physick, in Five Books, and Three Tomes* (London, 1662).

—— and Nicholas Culpeper, *Histories and Observations upon Most Diseases Offending the Body and Mind* (London, 1664).

Plato, *Selected Dialogues of Plato: The Benjamin Jowett Translation*, trans. B. Jowett, revised with introduction by Hayden Pelliccia (New York, 2000).

Quarles, John, *Fons Lachrymarum* (London, 1648).

Raynalde, Thomas, *The Birth of Mankynde, Otherwise Named the Womans Booke* (London, 1565).

R[owlands], S[amuel], *The Melancholie Knight* (London, 1615).

Sadler, John, *The Sick Womans Private Looking-Glasse*, repr. in The English Experience (Amsterdam, 1977).

Sandys, George, *A Paraphrase upon the Divine Poems* (London, [1638]).

Scot, Th[omas], *Philomythie or Philomythologie. Wherein Outlandish Birds, Beasts, and Fishes, are Taught to Speake True English Plainely* (London, 1622).

Shakespeare, William, *Shakespeare's Sonnets*, ed. Katherine Duncan-Jones, The Arden Shakespeare (London, 1997).

Sidney, Philip, *The Poems of Sir Philip Sidney*, ed. William A. Ringler, Jr. (Oxford, 1962).

—— *Sir Philip Sidney, The Countess of Pembroke's Arcadia (The New Arcadia)*, ed. Victor Skretkowicz (Oxford, 1987).

—— *Sir Philip Sidney, The Countess of Pembroke's Arcadia (The Old Arcadia)*, ed. Jean Robertson (Oxford, 1973).

Spenser, Edmund, *The Faerie Queene*, ed. A. C. Hamilton (London and New York, 1977, repr. 1980).

—— *The Yale Edition of the Shorter Poems of Edmund Spenser*, ed. William Oram *et al.* (New Haven, 1989).

Stevenson, Matthew, *Occasions Off-Spring* (London, 1654).

Suckling, John, *The Works of Sir John Suckling: The Non-Dramatic Works,* ed. Thomas Clayton (Oxford, 1971).

Swift, Jonathan, *Jonathan Swift: The Complete Poems*, ed. Pat Rogers (New Haven, 1983).

—— *The Prose Works of Jonathan Swift*, ed. Herbert Davis, 14 vols. (Oxford, 1957–74).

Tofte, Robert, *The Poetry of Robert Tofte, 1597–1620*, ed. Jeffrey N. Nelson (New York, 1994).

Tomkis, Thomas, *Albumazar* (London, 1615).

Turner, Richard, *Constant Lusina: The Amorous Passions of Paurinio a Surfeiting Lover, with the Constancie of Lusina a Country Mayd* (London, 1599).

Vaughan, William, *Directions for Health, Both Naturall and Artificial* (London, 1617).

W[alkington], T[homas], *The Optick Glasse of Humors; Or, The Touchstone of a Golden Temperature, or the Philosophers Stone to Make a Golden Temper* (London, 1607).

Whitney, Geoffrey, *A Choice of Emblemes, and Other Devises, for the Moste Part Gathered out of Sundrie Writers, Englished and Moralized* (Leyden, 1586).

Whythorne, Thomas, *Autobiography of Thomas Whythorne*, ed. J. Osborn (Oxford, 1962).

W[right], Th[omas], *The Passions of the Minde in General*, ed. William Webster Newbold, The Renaissance Imagination 15 (New York and London, 1986).

W[roth], T[homas], *The Abortive of an Idle Houre: Or A Centurie of Epigrams* (London, 1620).

Wyatt, Thomas, *Collected Poems of Sir Thomas Wyatt,* ed. Kenneth Muir and Patricia Thomson (Liverpool, 1969).

SECONDARY SOURCES

Addyman, Marie E., 'The Character of Hysteria in Shakespeare's England', Doctoral Diss., University of York, 1988.

Adelman, Janet, *Suffocating Mothers: Fantasies of Maternal Origin in Shakespeare's Plays,* Hamlet *to* The Tempest (New York, 1992).

Alfar, Cristina Leon, 'Staging the Feminine Performance of Desire: Masochism in *The Maid's Tragedy*', *Papers on Language and Literature*, 31/3 (1995), 313–33.

Allen, Michael J. B., *The Platonism of Marsilio Ficino: A Study of his Phaedrus Commentary, its Sources and Genesis*, Publications of the Center for Medieval and Renaissance Studies, 21 (Berkeley, 1984).

Anderson, Donald K, Jr. (ed.), *'Concord in Discord': The Plays of John Ford 1586–1986*, AMS Studies in the Renaissance, 17 (New York, 1986).

—— *John Ford* (New York, [1972]).

—— 'The Heart and the Banquet: Imagery in Ford's *'Tis Pity* and *The Broken Heart*', *Studies in English Literature, 1500–1900*, 2/2 (1962), 209–17.

Armstrong, A. Hilary, *St Augustine and Christian Platonism* (Villanova, 1967).

Ashelford, Jane, *Dress in the Age of Elizabeth I* (London, 1988).

Babb, Lawrence, *The Elizabethan Malady: A Study of Melancholia in English Literature from 1580 to 1642* (East Lansing, MI, 1951).

—— 'The Physiological Conception of Love in the Elizabethan and Early Stuart Drama', *PMLA*, 56/4 (1941), 1020–35.

Baldwin, Anna, and Sarah Hutton (eds.), *Platonism and the English Imagination* (Cambridge, 1994).

Barton, Anne, *Ben Jonson, Dramatist* (Cambridge, 1984).

—— 'Oxymoron and the Structure of Ford's *The Broken Heart*', *Essays and Studies*, NS 33 (1980), 70–94.

Bates, Catherine, 'Astrophil and the Manic Wit of the Abject Male', *Studies in English Literature*, 41/1 (2001), 1–24.

—— *The Rhetoric of Courtship in Elizabethan Language and Literature* (Cambridge, 1992).

Beecher, Donald, 'The Lover's Body: The Somatogenesis of Love in Renaissance Medical Treatises', *Renaissance and Reformation*, NS 12/1 (1988), 1–11.

—— and Massimo Ciavolella, *Eros and Anteros: The Medical Traditions of Love in the Renaissance*, University of Toronto Italian Studies, 9 (Toronto, 1992).

—— and Massimo Ciavolella, 'Jacques Ferrand and the Tradition of Erotic Melancholy in Western Culture', in Jaques Ferrand, *A Treatise on Lovesickness* (Syracuse, NY, 1990), 1–202.

Beier, Lucinda McCray, *Sufferers and Healers: The Experience of Illness in Seventeenth-Century England* (London, 1987).

Bell, Rudolph, *Holy Anorexia* (Chicago, 1985).

Bergeron, David M., 'Brother–Sister Incest in Ford's 1633 Plays', in Donald K. Anderson (ed.), *'Concord in Discord': The Plays of John Ford 1586–1986*, AMS Studies in the Renaissance, 17 (New York, 1986), 195–219.

—— *Royal Family, Royal Lovers: King James of England and Scotland* (Columbia, MO, and London, 1991).

Berry, Philippa, *Of Chastity and Power: Elizabethan Literature and the Unmarried Queen* (London, 1989).

Bersani, Leo, *The Freudian Body: Psychoanalysis and Art* (New York, 1986).

Blackham, Janet, John Woodward and David Richards, 'Popular Theories of Generation: The Evolution of Aristotle's Works, the Study of an Anachronism', in John Woodward and David Richards (eds.), *Health Care and Popular Medicine in Nineteenth-Century England: Essays in the Social History of Medicine* (London, 1977), 56–88.

Boss, J. M. N., 'The Seventeenth-Century Transformation of the Hysterical Affection, and Sydenham's Baconian Medicine', *Psychological Medicine*, 9 (1979), 221–34.

Boulton, Jeremy, *Neighbourhood and Society: A London Suburb in the Seventeenth Century* (Cambridge, 1987).

Brain, Lord, 'The Concept of Hysteria in the Time of William Harvey', *Proceedings of the Royal Society of Medicine*, 56 (1963), 317–24.

Bray, Alan, *Homosexuality in Renaissance England* (London, 1982).

Bredbeck, Gregory W., *Sodomy and Interpretation: Marlowe to Milton* (Ithaca, NY, 1991).

Briggs, Julia, 'Shakespeare's Bed-Tricks', *Essays in Criticism*, 44/4 (October, 1994), 293–314.

Brown, Robert D., *Lucretius on Love and Sex: A Commentary on* De rerum natura *IV, 1030–1287 with Prolegomena, Text, and Translation*, Columbia Studies in the Classical Tradition, 15 (Leiden, 1987).

—— 'The Jailer's Daughter and the Politics of Madwomen's Language', *Shakespeare Quarterly*, 46/3 (1995), 277–300.

Buckley, Thomas, and Alma Gottlieb, 'A Critical Appraisal of Theories of Menstrual Symbolism', in Thomas Buckley and Alma Gottlieb (eds.), *Blood Magic: The Anthropology of Menstruation* (Berkeley, 1988), 3–50.

Bueler, Lois E., 'Role-Splitting and Reintegration: The Tested Woman Plot in Ford', *Studies in English Literature, 1500–1900*, 20/2 (1980), 325–44.

—— 'The Structural Uses of Incest in English Renaissance Drama', in Leonard Barkan (ed.), *Renaissance Drama*, NS 15 (1984), 115–45.

Burbridge, Roger T., 'The Moral Vision of Ford's The Broken Heart', *Studies in English Literature, 1500–1900*, 10.2. (1970), 397–407.

Burks, Deborah G., ' "I'll Want My Will Else": *The Changeling* and Women's Complicity with their Rapist', in Stevie Simkin (ed.), *Revenge Tragedy. New Casebooks* (Basingstoke, 2001), 163–207.

Butler, Martin, '*Love's Sacrifice*: Ford's Metatheatrical Tragedy', in Michael Neill (ed.), *John Ford: Critical Re-Visions* (Cambridge, 1988), 201–31.

—— *Theatre and Crisis 1632–1642* (Cambridge, 1984).

Bynum, Caroline Walker, *Holy Feast and Holy Fast* (Berkeley, 1987).

Camden, Carroll, 'On Ophelia's Madness', *Shakespeare Quarterly*, 15/2 (1964), 247–55.

Carson, Anne, *Eros The Bittersweet: An Essay* (Princeton, 1986).

Cassirer, Ernst, *The Platonic Renaissance in England* (New York, 1970).

Champion, Larry S., 'Ford's *'Tis Pity She's a Whore* and the Jacobean Tragic Perspective', *PMLA*, 90/1 (1975), 78–87.

Charney, Maurice, and Charney, Hanna, 'The Language of Madwomen in Shakespeare and His Fellow Dramatists', *Signs*, 3/2 (1977), 451–60.

Cherchi, Paolo, 'Per la femmina "balba" (*Purgatorio* 19)', *Quaderni d'italianistica*, 6 (1985), 228–32.

Cipolla, Carlo, *Public Health and the Medical Profession in the Renaissance* (Cambridge, 1976).

Clack, Beverley, *Sex and Death: A Reappraisal of Human Mortality* (Cambridge, 2002).

Clark, George, *A History of the Royal College of Physicians*, 2 vols. (Oxford, 1964, repr. 1966).

Clark, Sandra, *The Plays of Beaumont and Fletcher: Sexual Themes and Dramatic Representation* (New York, 1994).

Cotton, Nancy, *John Fletcher's Chastity Plays: Mirrors of Modesty* (Lewisburg, PA, 1973).

Coulianu, Ioan P., *Eros and Magic in the Renaissance*, trans. Margaret Cook (Chicago, 1987).

Crawford, Patricia, 'Attitudes to Menstruation in Seventeenth-Century England', *Past and Present*, 91 (1981), 47–73.

Culler, Jonathan, *On Deconstruction* (London, 1983).

Cyrino, Monica Silveira, *In Pandora's Jar: Lovesickness in Early Greek Poetry* (Lanham, MD, New York, London, 1991).

Davies, H. Neville, 'Beaumont and Fletcher's *Hamlet*', in Kenneth Muir, Jay L. Halio, and D. J. Palmer (eds.), *Shakespeare, Man of the Theater* (Newark, NJ, 1983), 173–81.

Dawson, Lesel, 'The Earl of Essex and the Trials of History: Gervase Markham's *The Dumbe Knight*', *Review of English Studies*, NS 53/211 (2002), 344–64.

—— 'Menstruation, Mysogyny and the Cure for Love', *Women's Studies*, 34/6 (2005), 461–84.

—— 'Misogyny, Psychology and Sedition: John Ford's *The Queen* and the Earl of Essex's 1601 Uprising', *Explorations in Renaissance Culture*, 33/1 (2007), 64–82.

—— ' "New Sects of Love": Neoplatonism and Constructions of Gender in Davenant's *The Temple of Love* and *The Platonick Lovers*', *Early Modern Literary Studies*, 8/1 (2002), 4.1–4.36.

Delaney, Janice, Mary Jane Lupton, and Emily Toth (eds.), *The Curse: A Cultural History of Menstruation* (New York, 1977).

Desens, Marliss C., *The Bed-Trick in English Renaissance Drama: Explorations in Gender, Sexuality, and Power* (Newark, NJ, 1994).

Diethelm, Oscar, *Medical Dissertations of Psychiatric Interest Printed Before 1750* (Basel, 1971).

Dixon, Laurinda S., *Perilous Chastity: Women and Illness in Pre-Enlightenment Art and Medicine* (Ithaca, NY, 1995).

Doniger, Wendy, *The Bedtrick: Tales of Sex and Masquerade* (Chicago, 2000).

Doran, Susan, *Monarchy and Matrimony: The Courtships of Elizabeth I* (London, 1996).

Douglas, Mary, *Purity and Danger: An Analysis of the Concepts of Pollution and Taboo* (London, 1969).

—— 'Self-Evidence', in Mary Douglas (ed.), *Implicit Meanings: Essays in Anthropology* (London, 1975), 276–318.

—— *Natural Symbols* (1970; New York, 1982).

Dubrow, Heather, *Echoes of Desire: English Petrarchism and its Counterdiscourses* (Ithaca, NY, and London, 1995).

Duffin, Jacalyn, *Lovers and Livers: Disease Concepts in History*, The 2002 Joanne Goodman Lectures (Toronto, Buffalo, and London, 2005).

Eagleton, Terry, *William Shakespeare*, Rereading Literature Series (Oxford and New York, 1967).

Edmond, Mary, *Rare Sir William Davenant* (Manchester, 1987).

Ellmann, Maud, *The Hunger Artists: Starving, Writing, and Imprisonment* (London, 1993).

Enterline, Lynn, *The Tears of Narcissus: Melancholia and Masculinity in Early Modern Writing* (Stanford, CA, 1995).

Ewing, S. Blaine, *Burtonian Melancholy in the Plays of John Ford* (Princeton, 1940).

Ezell, Margaret J. M., *The Patriarch's Wife* (Chapel Hill, NC, 1987).

—— ' "To Be Your Daughter in Your Pen": The Social Functions of Literature in the Writings of Lady Elizabeth Brackley and Lady Jane Cavendish', *Huntington Library Quarterly*, 51/4 (1988), 281–96.

Farr, Dorothy M., *John Ford and the Caroline Theatre* (London, 1979).

Findlay, Alison, *A Feminist Perspective on Renaissance Drama* (Oxford, 1999).

Finke, Laurie A., 'Painting Women: Images of Femininity in Jacobean Tragedy', *Theatre Journal*, 36/3 (1984), 357–70.

Fleischmann, Wolfgang Bernard, *Lucretius and English Literature* (Paris, 1964).

Fletcher, Anthony, *Gender, Sex and Subordination in England 1500–1800* (New Haven, 1995).

Folger, Robert, *Images in Mind: Lovesickness, Spanish Sentimental Fiction and Don Quixote* (Chapel Hill, NC, 2002).

Forker, Charles R., *Fancy's Images: Contexts, Settings, and Perspectives in Shakespeare and His Contemporaries* (Carbondale and Edwardsville, IL, 1990).

Freud, Sigmund, *The Standard Edition of the Complete Psychological Works of Sigmund Freud*, trans. James Strachey and Anna Freud, 24 vols. (London, 1953–73).

Frey, Charles H. (ed.), *Shakespeare, Fletcher and* The Two Noble Kinsmen (Columbia, MO, 1989).

Garber, Marjorie, 'The Insincerity of Women', in Valeria Finucci and Reqina Schwartz (eds.), *Desire in the Renaissance: Psychoanalysis and Literature*, (Princeton, 1994), 19–38.

Gatti, Hilary, 'Giordano Bruno and the Stuart Court Masque', *Renaissance Quarterly*, 48/4 (1995), 809–42.

Gilbert, Sandra M., and Susan Gubar, *The Madwoman in the Attic: The Woman Writer and the Nineteenth-Century Literary Imagination*, 2nd edn. (New Haven and London, 2000).

Gilman, Sander L., *Disease and Representation: Images of Illness from Madness to AIDS* (Ithaca, NY, 1988).

—— *Seeing the Insane* (New York, 1982).

—— Helen King, Roy Porter, G. S. Rousseau, and Elaine Showalter (eds.), *Hysteria Beyond Freud* (Berkeley, 1993).

Girard, René, *Deceit, Desire, and the Novel: Self and Other in Literary Structure* (1961), trans. Yvonne Freccero (Baltimore, 1966).

Giudici, Jose, 'De l'amour courtois à l'amour sacré: la condition de la femme dans l'oeuvre de B. Castiglione', in André Rochon (ed.), *Images de la femme dans la littérature italienne de la Renaissance* (Paris, 1980), 9–80.

Goldberg, Jonathan, *James I and the Politics of Literature* (Baltimore, 1983).

—— 'James I and the Theater of Conscience', *English Literary History* 46 (1979), 379–98.

—— *Sodometries: Renaissance Texts, Modern Sexualities* (Stanford, CA, 1992).

Graham, Elspeth, Hilary Hinds, Elaine Hobby, and Helen Wilcox (eds.), *Her Own Life: Autobiographical Writings by Seventeenth-Century Englishwomen* (London and New York, 1989, repr. 1998).

Greenblatt, Stephen, *Renaissance Self-Fashioning: From More to Shakespeare* (Chicago, 1980).

Gregerson, Linda, *The Reformation of the Subject: Spenser, Milton, and the English Protestant Epic* (Cambridge, 1995).

Groneman, Carol, *Nymphomania: A History* (New York, 2000).

Gutierrez, Nancy A., *'Shall She Famish Then?': Female Food Refusal in Early Modern England* (Aldershot and Burlington, VT, 2003).

Hackett, Helen, ' "A Book, and Solitariness": Melancholia, Gender and Literary Subjectivity in Mary Wroth's *Urania*', in Gordon McMullan (ed.), *Renaissance Configurations: Voices/Bodies/Spaces, 1580–1690* (Basingstoke and New York, 1988, 2001), 65–85.

—— *One Hundred Years of Homosexuality, and Other Essays on Greek Love* (New York, 1990).

Hamilton, Sharon, 'The Broken Heart: Language Suited to a Divided Mind', in Donald K. Anderson (ed.), *'Concord in Discord': The Plays of John Ford 1586–1986*, AMS Studies in the Renaissance, 17 (New York, 1986) 171–94.

Hamlin, Will, 'A Select Bibliographical Guide to *The Two Noble Kinsmen*', in Charles H. Frey (ed.), *Shakespeare, Fletcher and* The Two Noble Kinsmen (Columbia, MO, 1989), 186–216.

Hannay, Margaret P., *Philip's Phoenix: Mary Sidney, Countess of Pembroke* (New York and Oxford, 1990).

——Noel J. Kinnamon and Michael G. Brennan (eds.), *The Collected Works of Mary Sidney Herbert, Countess of Pembroke* (Oxford, 1998).

Hart, Vaughan, *Art and Magic in the Court of the Stuarts* (London, 1994).

Haskings, Susan, *Mary Magdalen: Myth and Metaphor* (London, 1993).

Hawkins, Harriet, 'Mortality, Morality, and Modernity in *The Broken Heart*: Some Dramatic and Critical Counter-Arguments', in Michael Neill (ed.), *John Ford: Critical Re-Visions* (Cambridge, 1988), 129–52.

Heilbrun, Carolyn, *Toward A Recognition of Androgyny* (New York, 1973).

Heinemann, Margot, *Puritanism and Theatre: Thomas Middleton and Opposition Drama under the Early Stuarts* (Cambridge, 1929).

Hill, R. F., 'Introduction', in John Ford, *The Lover's Melancholy* (Manchester, 1985), 1–42.

Hobby, Elaine, *Virtue of Necessity: English Women's Writing 1649–88* (London, 1988).

Hogan, A. P., '*'Tis Pity She's a Whore*: The Overall Design', *Studies in English Literature, 1500–1900*, 17/2 (1877), 303–16.

Holman, Peter, *Dowland: Lachrimae (1604)* (Cambridge, 1999).

Hopkins, Lisa, *John Ford's Political Theatre* (Manchester, 1994).

——'Judith Shakespeare's Reading: Teaching *The Concealed Fancies*', *Shakespeare Quarterly*, 47/4 (1996), 396–406.

——'Staging Passion in Ford's *The Lover's Melancholy*', *Studies in English Literature, 1500–1900*, 45/2 (2005), 443–59.

Huebert, Ronald, '"An Artificial Way to Grieve": The Forsaken Woman in Beaumont and Fletcher, Massinger and Ford', *English Literary History*, 44 (1977), 601–22.

——*John Ford, Baroque English Dramatist* (Montreal and London, 1977).

Hunter, Michael, *Science and Society in Restoration England* (Cambridge, 1981).

Hunter, Richard, and Ida Macalpine, *Three Hundred Years of Psychiatry: 1535–1860* (London, 1963).

Hutton, Sarah, 'Introduction to the Renaissance and Seventeenth Century', in Anna Baldwin and Sarah Hutton (eds.), *Platonism and the English Imagination* (Cambridge, 1994), 67–75.

Hyde, Thomas, *The Poetic Theology of Love: Cupid in Renaissance Literature* (Newark, NJ, 1986).

Jackson, Stevi, 'Women and Heterosexual Love: Complicity, Resistance and Change', in Lynne Pearce and Jackie Stacey (eds.), *Romance Revisited* (London, 1995), 49–62.

Jaeger, C. Stephen, *Ennobling Love: In Search of a Lost Sensibility* (Philadelphia, 1999).

Jardine, Lisa, *Still Harping on Daughters* (Brighton, 1983).

Jayne, Sears, 'Introduction to *Marsilio Ficino's Commentary on Plato's Symposium on Love*', in Ficino, *Ficino's Commentary on Plato's Symposium on Love*, ed. and trans. Sears Jayne (Dallas, 1985), 1–32.

Jones, Ann Rosalind, *The Currency of Eros: Women's Love Lyric in Europe, 1540–1620* (Bloomington and Indianpolis, 1990).

Jordan, Constance, *Renaissance Feminism: Literary Texts and Political Models* (Ithaca, NY, and London, 1990).

Katz, David S, 'Shylock's Gender: Jewish Male Menstruation in Early Modern England', *Review of English Studies*, NS 50/200 (1999), 440–62.

Kaufmann, R. J., 'Ford's Tragic Perspective', in R. J. Kaufmann (ed.), *Elizabethan Drama: Modern Essays in Criticism*, (New York, 1961), 356–72.

Kerrigan, John, *Motives of Woe: Shakespeare and the 'Female Complaint'* (Oxford, 1991).

—— *Revenge Tragedy: Aeschylus to Armageddon* (Oxford, 1996).

Kessel, Marie L., '*The Broken Heart*: An Allegorical Reading', *Medieval and Renaissance Drama in England*, 3 (1986), 217–30.

King, Helen, *The Disease of Virgins: Green Sickness, Chlorosis and the Problems of Puberty* (London and New York, 2004).

—— 'Green Sickness: Hippocrates, Galen and the Origins of the "Disease of Virgins"', *International Journal of the Classical Tradition*, 2/3 (1996), 372–87.

—— ' "Once Upon a Text": Hysteria from Hippocrates', in Gilman *et al.* (eds.), *Hysteria Beyond Freud* (Berkeley, 1993), 3–90.

King, Margaret L., *Women of the Renaissance* (Chicago, 1991).

Kingsley-Smith, Jane, 'Lovestruck: Cupid in England, 1557–1634', unpublished manuscript.

—— '*Gismond of Salerne*: An Elizabethan and Cupidean Tragedy', *Yearbook of English Studies* (forthcoming).

Kinsman, Robert (ed.), *The Darker Vision of the Renaissance* (Berkeley, 1974).

Klibansky, Raymond, Erwin Panofsky, and Fritzl Saxl, *Saturn and Melancholy. Studies in the History of Natural Philosophy, Religion, and Art* (London, 1964).

Klindienst, Patricia, 'The Voice of the Shuttle is Ours', *Stanford Literature Review*, 1 (1984), 25–53.

Kraye, Jill, 'The Transformation of Platonic Love in the Italian Renaissance', in Anna Baldwin and Sarah Hutton (eds.), *Platonism and the English Imagination* (Cambridge, 1994), 76–85.

Kristeva, Julia, *Black Sun: Depression and Melancholia* (New York, 1989).

—— *Desire in Language: A Semiotic Approach to Literature and Art* (New York, 1980).

Kuhl, E. P., 'Shakespeare's *Rape of Lucrece*', *Philological Quarterly*, 20 (1941), 352–60.

Lacan, Jacques, 'God and the Jouissance of The Woman', in Juliet Mitchell and Jacqueline Rose (eds.), *Feminine Sexuality: Jacques Lacan and the Ecole Freudienne* (London, 1982), 137–48.

Lamb, Mary Ellen, *Gender and Authorship in the Sidney Circle* (Madison, WI, 1990).

Laqueur, Thomas, *Making Sex: Body and Gender from the Greeks to Freud* (Cambridge, MA, and London, 1990).

Lee, Jae Num, *Swift and Scatological Satire* (Albuquerque, NM, [1971]).

Leech, Clifford, *John Ford* (London, 1964).

—— *Shakespeare's Tragedies and Other Studies in Seventeenth-Century Drama* (London, 1961).

Levin, Carole, ' "Lust Being Lord, There is No Trust in Kings": Passion, King John, and the Responsibilities of Kingship', in Carole Levin and Karen Robertson (eds.), *Sexuality and Politics in Renaissance Drama* (Lewiston, NY, 1991), 255–78.

Lewalski, Barbara K., 'Lucy, Countess of Bedford: Images of a Jacobean Courtier and Patroness', in Kevin Sharpe and Steven N. Zwicker (eds.), *Politics of Discourse: The Literature and History of Seventeenth-Century England* (Berkeley, 1987), 52–77.

Lewis, C. S., *The Allegory of Love* (New York, 1958, repr. 1967).

Lowes, John L., 'The Loveres Maladye of Hereos', *Modern Philology*, 11/4 (1914), 491–546.

Lyons, Bridget Gellert, 'The Iconography of Ophelia', *English Literary History*, 44/1 (1977), 60–74.

—— *The Voice of Melancholy: Studies in Literary Treatments of Melancholy in Renaissance England* (London, 1971).

Maaskant-Kleibrink, Marianne, 'Nymphomania', in Josine Blok and Peter Mason (eds.), *Sexual Asymmetry: Studies in Ancient Society* (Amsterdam, 1980), 275–96.

McCabe, Richard, *Incest, Drama and Nature's Law, 1550–1700* (Cambridge, 1993).

MacDonald, Michael, *Mystical Bedlam: Madness, Anxiety, and Healing in Seventeenth-Century England* (Cambridge, 1981).

—— (ed.), *Witchcraft and Hysteria in Elizabethan London: Edward Jorden and the Mary Glover Case* (London and New York, 1991).

—— 'Women and Madness in Tudor and Stuart England', *Social Research*, 53 (1986), 261–81.

McFarland, Ronald E., 'The Rhetoric of Medicine: Lord Herbert's and Thomas Carew's Poems of Green-Sickness', *Journal of the History of Medicine*, 30 (1975), 250–8.

MacFarlane, Alan, *The Family Life of Ralph Josselin, a Seventeenth-Century Clergyman: An Essay in Historical Anthropology* (Cambridge, 1970).

—— *Witchcraft in Tudor and Stuart England: A Regional and Comparative Study* (London, 1970).

McGovern, Barbara, *Anne Finch and Her Poetry* (London, 1992).

MacLean, Ian, *The Renaissance Notion of Woman: A Study in the Fortunes of Scholasticism and Medical Science in European Intellectual Life* (Cambridge, 1980).

McMullan, Gordon, *The Politics of Unease in the Plays of John Fletcher* (Amherst, MA, 1994).

—— (ed.), *Renaissance Configurations: Voices/Bodies/Spaces, 1580–1690* (Basingstoke and New York, 1988, repr. 2001).

—— 'A Rose for Emilia: Collaborative Relations in *The Two Noble Kinsmen*', in McMullan (ed.), *Renaissance Configurations* (Basingstoke and New York, 1988, repr. 2001), 129–47.

Malcolmson, Cristina, ' "As Tame as the Ladies": Politics and Gender in *The Changeling*', in Stevie Simkin (ed.), *Revenge Tragedy. New Casebook* (Basingtoke, 2001), 142–62.

—— 'Shakespeare's Comic Heroines, Elizabeth I, and the Political Uses of Androgyny', in Mary Beth Rose (ed.), *Women in the Middle Ages and the Renaissance: Literary and Historical Perspectives* (Syracuse, NY, 1986), 135–53.

Marotti, Arthur, ' "Love Is Not Love": Elizabethan Sonnet Sequences and the Social Order', *English Literary History*, 49 (1982), 396–428.

Marshall, Cynthia, *The Shattering of the Self: Violence, Subjectivity, and Early Modern Texts* (Baltimore and London, 2002).

Marshall, Rosalind K., *The Winter Queen: The Life of Elizabeth of Bohemia, 1596–1662* (Edinburgh, 1998).

Massé, Michelle A., *In the Name of Love: Women, Masochism, and the Gothic* (Ithaca, NY, and London, 1992).

Micale, Mark S., *Approaching Hysteria: Disease and Its Interpretations* (Princeton, 1995).

—— and Porter, Roy (eds.), *Discovering the History of Psychiatry* (New York and Oxford, 1994).

Miller, David Lee, *The Poem's Two Bodies: The Poetics of the 1590* Faerie Queene (Princeton, 1988).

Miller, Naomi J., *Changing the Subject: Mary Wroth and Figurations of Gender in Early Modern England* (Lexington, KY, 1996).

Montrose, Louis Adrian, '*A Midsummer Night's Dream* and the Shaping Fantasies of Elizabethan Culture: Gender, Power, Form', in Margaret W. Ferguson, Maureen Quilligan, and Nancy J. Vickers (eds.), *Rewriting*

the Renaissance: The Discourse of Sexual Difference in Early Modern Europe,
Women in Culture and Society Series (Chicago, 1986), 65–87.

Muir, Kenneth, 'Samuel Harsnett and King Lear', *Review of English Studies*, NS
2 (1951), 11–21.

Neely, Carol Thomas, *Distracted Subjects: Madness and Gender in Shakespeare
and Early Modern Culture* (Ithaca, NY, and London, 2004).

—— '"Documents in Madness": Reading Madness and Gender in
Shakespeare's Tragedies and Early Modern Culture', in Shirlay Nelson
Garner and Madelon Sprengnether (eds.), *Shakespearean Tragedy and Gender*
(Bloomington, IN, 1996), 75–104.

Neill, Michael, *Issues of Death: Mortality and Identity in English Renaissance
Tragedy* (Oxford, 1997).

—— (ed.), *John Ford: Critical Re-Visions* (Cambridge, 1988).

—— 'New Light on "The Truth" in *The Broken Heart*', *Notes and Queries*, NS
22 (1975), 249–50.

—— '"What Strange Riddle's This?": Deciphering *'Tis Pity She's a Whore*', in
Michael Neill (ed.), *John Ford: Critical Re-Visions* (Cambridge, 1988), 153–
74.

Nelson, John Charles, *The Renaissance Theory of Love: The Context of Giordano
Bruno's* Eroici Furori (New York, 1968).

Nohrnberg, James, *The Analogy of* The Faerie Queene (Princeton,
1976).

Nussbaum, Martha C., *The Therapy of Desire: Theory and Practice in Hellenistic
Ethics* (Princeton, 1994).

Oestreich-Hart, Donna J., ' "Therefore, Since I Cannot Prove a Lover" ', *Studies
in English Literature*, 40/2 (2000), 241–60.

O'Hara, Diana, *Courtship and Constraint: Rethinking the Making of Marriage in
Tudor England* (Manchester, 2000).

Orgel, Stephen, and Roy Strong, *Inigo Jones: The Theatre of the Stuart Courts*, 2
vols. (London, 1973).

Paster, Gail Kern, *The Body Embarrassed: Drama and the Disciplines of Shame in
Early Modern England* (Ithaca, NY, 1993).

—— ' "In the Spirit of Men there is no Blood": Blood as Trope of Gender in
Julius Caesar', *Shakespeare Quarterly*, 40 (1989), 284–98.

Patrides, C. A., *The Cambridge Platonists* (Cambridge, 1969).

Pearce, Lynne, and Jackie Stacey, 'The Heart of the Matter: Feminists Revisit
Romance', in Pearce and Stacey (eds.), *Romance Revisited* (London, 1995),
11–45.

—— (eds.), *Romance Revisited* (London, 1995).

Perry, T. Anthony, *Erotic Spirituality: The Integrative Tradition from Leone Ebreo
to John Donne* (University, AL, 1980).

Peterson, Kaara L., 'Fluid Economies: Portraying Shakespeare's Hysterics', *Mosaic*, 34/1 (2001), 35–59.

Pigeaud, Jackie, *La Maladie de l'âme: étude sur la relation de l'âme et du corps dans la tradition médico-philosophique antique*, Collection d'études anciennes (Paris, 1981).

Platt, Michael, '*The Rape of Lucrece* and the Republic for which it Stands', *Centennial Review*, 19/2 (1975), 59–79.

Porter, Roy, 'The Body and the Mind, the Doctor and the Patient: Negotiating Hysteria', in Sander M. Gilman, *et al.* (eds.), *Hysteria Beyond Freud* (Berkeley, 1993), 225–85.

—— *Disease, Medicine and Society in England, 1550–1860* (London, 1993).

—— *A Social History of Madness: Stories of the Insane* (London, 1987).

Poulton, Diana, *John Dowland* (Trowbridge, 1982).

Roberts, Jeanne Addison, 'Crises of Male Self-Definition in *The Two Noble Kinsmen*', in Charles H. Frey (ed.), *Shakespeare, Fletcher and* The Two Noble Kinsmen (Columbia, MO, 1989), 133–43.

Robertson, Jean, *The Art of Letter Writing* (London, 1942).

Rosaldo, Michelle Z., 'Towards an Anthropology of Self and Feeling', in R. A. Shweder and R. A. Levine (eds.), *Culture Theory* (Cambridge, 1984), 137–57.

Rose, Mary Beth, *The Expense of Spirit: Love and Sexuality in English Renaissance Drama* (Ithaca, NY, and London, 1988).

Rougemont, Denis de, *Love in the Western World*, trans. Montgomery Belgion (New York, 1956, rev. edn. 1983).

Rousseau, G. S., 'Depression's Forgotten Genealogy: Notes Towards a History of Depression', *History of Psychiatry*, 11 (2000), 71–106.

—— 'Nymphomania, Bienville, and the Rise of Erotic Sensibility', in Paul-Gabriel Bouce (ed.), *Sexuality in Eighteenth-Century Britain* (Manchester, 1982), 95–119.

—— ' "A Strange Pathology": Hysteria in the Early Modern World, 1500–1800', in Sander L. Gilman *et al.* (eds.), *Hysteria Beyond Freud* (Berkeley, 1993), 91–224.

Sawday, Jonathan, *The Body Emblazoned: Dissection and the Human Body in Renaissance Culture* (London, 1995).

Sawyer, Ronald C., 'Patients, Healers, and Disease in the Southeast Midlands, 1597–1634', Doctoral Dissertation, University of Madison, WI, 1986.

Schiesari, Juliana, *The Gendering of Melancholia: Feminism, Psychoanalysis, and the Symbolics of Loss in Renaissance Literature* (Ithaca, NY, 1992).

Schwartz, Jerome, 'Aspects of Androgyny in the Renaissance', in *Human Sexuality in the Middle Ages and the Renaissance*, ed. Douglas Radcliffe-Umstead (Pittsburgh, 1978), 121–31.

Sedley, Stephen (ed.), *The Seeds of Love* (London, 1967).

Sensabaugh, George F., 'John Ford and Platonic Love in the Court', *Studies in Philology* 36/2 (1939), 206–26.

—— 'John Ford Revisited', *Studies in English Literature, 1500–1900*, 4/2 (1964), 195–216.

—— *The Tragic Muse of John Ford* (Stanford, CA, 1944).

Sharon-Zisser, Shirley, *Critical Essays on Shakespeare's* A Lover's Complaint: *Suffering Ecstasy* (Aldershot, 2006).

Sharpe, Kevin, *Criticism and Compliment: The Politics of Literature in the England of Charles I* (Cambridge, 1987).

Sherman, Stuart P., 'Stella and The Broken Heart', *Proceedings of the Modern Languages Association*, 24 (1909), 274–85.

Showalter, Elaine, *The Female Malady: Women, Madness and English Culture, 1830–1980* (London, 1987).

—— 'Hysteria, Feminism, and Gender', in Sander L. Gilman *et al.* (eds.), *Hysteria Beyond Freud* (Berkeley, 1993), 286–344.

—— *Hystories: Hysterical Epidemics and, Modern Media* (New York, 1998).

—— 'Representing Ophelia: Women, Madness, and the Responsibilities of Feminist Criticism', in Patricia Parker and Geoffery Hartman (eds.), *Shakespeare and the Question of Theory* (New York, 1985), 77–94.

Simkin, Stevie (ed.), *Revenge Tragedy. New Casebooks* (Basingstoke, 2001).

Simmons, J. L., 'Diabolical Realism in Middleton and Rowley's *The Changeling*', *Renaissance Drama*, NS 11 (1980), 135–70.

Simon, Bennett, *Mind and Madness in Ancient Greece: The Classical Roots of Modern Psychiatry* (Ithaca, NY, 1978).

Skultans, Vieda, *English Madness: Ideas on Insanity, 1580–1890* (London, 1979).

Small, Helen, *Love's Madness: Medicine, the Novel, and Female Insanity 1800–1865* (Oxford, 1996).

Smith, Bruce R., *Homosexual Desire in Shakespeare's England: A Cultural Poetics* (Chicago, 1991).

Solomon, Michael, *The Literature of Misogyny in Medieval Spain: The Arcipreste de Talavera and the Spill*, Cambridge Studies in Latin American and Iberian Literature, 10 (Cambridge, 1997).

Somerset, Anne, *Unnatural Murder: Poison at the Court of James I* (London, 1988).

Soufas, T. S., *Melancholy and the Secular Mind in Spanish Golden Age Literature* (Columbia, MO, 1990).

Stallybrass, Peter, 'Patriarchal Territories: The Body Enclosed', in Margaret Ferguson, Maureen Quilligan, and Nancy Vickers (eds.), *Rewriting the*

Renaissance: The Discourses of Sexual Difference in Early Modern Europe (Chicago, 1986), 123–42.

Stavig, Mark, *John Ford and the Traditional Moral Order* (Madison, 1968).

Steggle, Matthew, *Richard Brome: Place and Politics on the Caroline Stage* (Manchester, 2004).

Stephens, Dorothy, *The Limits of Eroticism in Post-Petrarchan Narrative: Conditional Pleasure from Spenser to Marvell* (Cambridge, 1998).

Stone, Lawrence, *The Family, Sex and Marriage in England, 1500–1800* (New York, 1977).

Strong, Roy, *The Tudor and Stuart Monarchy: Pageantry, Painting, Iconography. II Elizabethan* (Woodbridge, 1995).

Summers, Claude J., and Ted-Larry Pebworth (eds.), *Renaissance Discourses of Desire* (Columbia, MO, and London, 1993).

Sutherland, Sarah P., *Masques in Jacobean Tragedy* (New York, 1983).

Sutton, Juliet, 'Platonic Love in Ford's *The Fancies, Chaste and Noble*', *Studies in English Literature, 1500–1900*, 7/2 (1967), 299–309.

Tallis, Frank, *Love Sick* (London, 2004).

Thomas, Keith, *Religion and the Decline of Magic* (Harmondworth, 1971).

Tuana, Nancy, 'The Weaker Seed: The Sexist Bias of Reproductive Theory', in Tuana (ed.), *Feminism and Science* (Bloomington, IN, 1989), 147–71.

Ure, Peter, 'Cult and Initiates in Ford's *Love's Sacrifice*,' *Modern Language Quarterly*, 11 (1950) 298–306.

Veith, Ilza, *Hysteria: The History of a Disease* (Chicago, 1965).

Vice, Sue, 'Addicted to Love', in Lynne Pearce and Jackie Stacey (eds.), *Romance Revisited* (London, 1995), 117–27.

Vickers, Brian, *Occult and Scientific Mentalities in the Renaissance* (Cambridge, 1984).

Voaden, Rosalynn, 'The Language of Love: Medieval Erotic Vision and Modern Romance Fiction', in Lynne Pearce and Jackie Stacey (eds.), *Romance Revisited* (London, 1995), 117–27.

Wack, Mary Frances, 'From Mental Faculties to Magical Philters: The Entry of Magic into Academic Medical Writings on Lovesickness, 13th–17th Centuries', in Donald Beecher and Massimo Ciavolella (eds.), *Eros and Anteros: The Medical Traditions of Love in the Renaissance*, University of Toronto Italian Studies, 9 (Toronto, 1992), 9–32.

—— *Lovesickness in the Middle Ages: The Viaticum and its Commentaries* (Philadelphia, 1990).

—— 'Lovesickness in Troilus', *Pacific Coast Philology*, 19 (1984), 55–61.

Walker, Julia M., 'Spenser's Elizabeth Portrait and the Fiction of Dynastic Epic', *Modern Philology*, 90 (1992), 172–99.

Wall, Wendy, *The Imprint of Gender: Authorship and Publication in the English Renaissance* (Ithaca, NY, 1993).

—— 'Struggling into Discourse: The Emergence of Renaissance Women's Writing', in Margaret Patterson Hannay (ed.), *Silent But for the Word: Tudor Women as Patrons, Translators, and Writers of Religious Works* (Kent, OH, 1985), 238–56.

Wear, Andrew, *Knowledge and Practice in English Medicine* (Cambridge, 2000).

Weller, Barrry, '*The Two Noble Kinsmen*, the Friendship Tradition, and the Flight from Eros', in Charles H. Frey (ed.), *Shakespeare, Fletcher and The Two Noble Kinsmen* (Columbia, MO, 1989), 93–108.

Wells, Marion A., *The Secret Wound: Love-Melancholy and Early Modern Romance* (Stanford, CA, 2007).

Wickham, Glynne, '*The Two Noble Kinsmen* or *A Midsummer Night's Dream*, Part II?', in G. R. Hibbard (ed.), *The Elizabethan Theatre*, 7 (1977), 167–96.

Williams, Katherine E., 'Hysteria in Seventeenth-Century Case Records and Unpublished Manuscripts', *History of Psychiatry*, 1 (1990), 383–401.

Wind, Edgar, *Pagan Mysteries in the Renaissance* (Oxford, 1967, repr. 1980).

Wiseman, Susan J., 'Representing the Incestuous Body' in Stevie Simkin (ed.), *Revenge Tragedy* (Basingstoke, 2001), 208–28.

Wood, Charles T., 'The Doctors' Dilemma: Sin, Salvation and the Menstrual Cycle', *Speculum*, 56 (1981), 710–27.

Wymer, Rowland, *Suicide and Despair in the Jacobean Drama* (Brighton, 1986).

Yates, Frances A., *Astraea: The Imperial Theme in the Sixteenth Century* (London, 1975).

—— *The Art of Memory* (London, 1966).

Index

Abu Jafar Ahmed Ibn Ibrahim ibn Ali
    Khalid, *Provisions* 14–15, 21–2
Adams, Joseph, *Diseases of the Soule* 38
Adelman, Janet 67, 73
Alciati, Andrea, *Emblemata* 101
Alday, John 16, 26
Alexander VI, Pope 203
Anderson, Donald K., Jr 148
Arabic medicine 14, 61, 196–7
Aretaeus of Cappadocia 61
Ariadne 115–16
Ariosto, Ludovico, *Orlando Furioso* 205
Aristophanes, *Symposium* 132
Aristotle 14, 21, 47–8, 135
Arnald of Villanova, *De amore heroico* 22
Ashelford, Jane 41
Aubrey, John, *Brief Lives* 28
Avicenna 21, 26, 197

Babb, Lawrence 43
Bacon, Francis
    'Narcissus' 130
    'Of Revenge' 9, 114
Bakhtin, Mikhail 202
Bancroft, Richard, bishop of London 65
Barnes, Barnabe, *The Devil's
    Charter* 202, 203
Bates, Catherine 6
Beaumont, Francis
    The Coxcomb (with John Fletcher) 206
    The Maid's Tragedy (with John
        Fletcher) 44, 112–18, 169–70
        Aspatia 9, 94, 111, 112–18, 126
        Evadne 44, 112–14, 117, 169–70
        King 44, 112, 117, 169–70
Beecher, Donald 14, 15, 19–20, 21, 42
Bembo, Pietro 131, 156
Bergeron, David 144
Berry, Philippa 7
Bersani, Leo 196
Bessarion, Basilios, *In calumniatorem
    Platonis* 135
Bible, The 109, 199–200, 202–3, 205

Boaistuau, Pierre, *Theatrum Mundi* 16,
    17–18, 26
Brabant, women of 51
Brackley, Elizabeth, *The Concealed
    Fancies* 108–11
Bradwell, Stephen 64
brain 21–2, 25
Brathwait, Richard, *The Golden
    Fleece* 202–3
Breton, Nicholas
    Grimellos Fortunes 67–8
    Madde Letters 205
Brewer, Anthony, *Love-Sick King* 175
Bright, Timothie, *Treatise* 14, 15
Brome, Richard
    The Antipodes 70–2, 180
    The Court Beggar 174–5
    The Sparagus Garden 102
Broom, Wendell 154
Brown, Robert 193
Bruno, Giordano 131, 133
    The Heroic Frenzies 136–7
Bueler, Lois 140, 141
Burbridge, Roger 126
Burks, Debora 169
Burton, Robert, *The Anatomy of
    Melancholy* 5, 6, 14, 16, 28,
    39–40, 70, 79, 98–9, 147, 197–8,
    211
    and fixation 18, 23, 177, 178, 179,
        180, 185
    and green sickness 51, 79
    and *Inamorato* 34, 37
    and Neoplatonism 129, 141
    and phlebotomy 19
    and seed 25
    and sexual cures 172

Campion, Thomas, 'Faine would I
    wed' 55
Carew, Thomas 59
carpe diem tradition 47, 53; *see also* cures
    for lovesickness

Carter, Angela, 'John Ford's *'Tis Pity She's a Whore*' 145
Castiglione, Baldassare, *The Courtier* 133, 137, 156
causes of lovesickness
  beauty 26–7; *see also* fixation (below)
  blood 2, 20, 21, 26–7, 34, 122, 159, 172–3, 179
  diet 18–19
  the humours 2, 14, 18–19, 20–1, 92, 160, 165
  fixation 17–18, 20–5, 163–4, 175, 176, 177–90, 192
    'dramatic' cures of 180–5; *see also* phantasms
  movement of the planets 18–19
  the occult 15
  seed 2, 19, 25–6, 73, 74, 77, 87, 95, 103, 165, 172–3, 176, 179
Cavendish, Jane, *The Concealed Fancies* 108–11
Cavendish, Margaret, duchess of Newcastle, *True Relation* 98, 108
Cavendish, William, duke of Newcastle 108
Chamberlain, Robert, *The Swaggering Damsell* 105
Chapman, George
  Blind Beggar 21
  Monsieur D'Olive 102
  The Widowes Teares 104–5
Charles I, king of England 150, 154
Charney, Maurice 72
Chaucer, Geoffrey, *The Knight's Tale* 80
Cherchi, Paulo 205
Chloris 75, 86
chlorosis 49, 75; *see also* green sickness
Clark, Sandra 117, 206
class distinctions 5, 8, 39–42, 44, 58, 81–3, 96–100, 105, 108, 208–10
  and blood 209
Clifford, Lady Anne 97
Coëffeteau, F. N., *Table* 15, 16, 29
coitus, *see* cures for lovesickness
Cokain, Aston, 'A Satyre' 56
Colet, John 133
Constantine the African, *Viaticum* 14, 21
Coulianu, Ioan P. 22–3

Cowley, Abraham
  The Guardian 203–4
  'Platonick Love' 141–2
Crawford, Patricia, 'Attitudes to Menstruation' 200
Culler, Jonathan 1
Culpeper, Nicholas, *A Directory for Midwives* 77
cures for lovesickness
  the 'bed trick' 24, 81, 173–4, 175
  clysters 19
  coitus 19, 23–6, 31–3, 81, 87–90, 121, 159–61, 163, 172–6, 208
  diet 18–19, 20
  disgust 192–211; *see also* misogyny
  exercise 20
  humiliation 185–90
  music 19
  the occult 18–19, 189
  phlebotomy 19, 50, 163–72, 175, 181, 201
  showing of menstrual blood 190, 194–9, 201, 205–11
  sleeping habits 20
  'theatrical' cures 177–85
  travel 20
  vomits 19

Dante Alighieri, *Puragtory* 205
Davenant, William
  The Cruel Brother 167–8
  The Platonick Lovers 131, 150, 154–61
    Buonateste 27, 154, 157–9, 160
    Theander 154–7, 158–60
  The Temple of Love 150–4, 158, 159–60
Dekker, Thomas
  Honest Whore 21, 67, 166
  Northward Hoe 68
Democritus 98
Diana (goddess) 85–7, 158
diarrhoea 30
Dido 115
Dixon, Laurinda S. 32, 46, 92
Donne, John 38
  'The Ecstasy' 27
  'The Canonization' 142
Douglas, Mary 201

Dowland, John, *Second Booke of Songes or Ayres* 100
Drayton, Michael
  Poly-Olbion 66
  'Shores Wide to King Edward the Fourth' 43
dress 98–101, 106–7, 109–11; *see also* performance of grief
Duncan-Jones, Katherine 204–5
Durer, Albert, *Melancholia I* 38, 98

Eagleton, Terry 33–4
Ibn Eddjezzar, *see* Abu Jafar Ahmed Ibn Ibrahim ibn Ali Khalid
Elizabeth I, queen of England 16–17, 97–8
Elizabeth of Bohemia 97
Ellman, Maud 124
emasculation 3, 5–6, 44, 103, 164, 185–90, 194–5, 196, 210–11
  and Platonic love 139–40, 150–2, 156, 161
Enterline, Lynn 95
Erasmus, Desiderius 133
Eunapius of Sardes, *De Vitis Philosophorum et Sophistarum* 196
Eyles, Elizabeth 61
Ezell, Margaret 111

Falkland, Viscount 28
Farr, Dorothy 140
female lovesickness 1–5, 7–10, 13, 36, 91–6, 102–11, 187–90
  and female complaint 8–10, 31–2, 94
  historical examples 16–17, 30–1, 96–101
  and intellectual melancholy 8, 10, 93–4, 96–100
  relation to other maladies 4, 46–90 (esp. 52–3), 93, 95
  see also Beaumont and Fletcher's Aspatia; Ford's Penthea; Shakespeare and Fletcher's Jailer's Daughter; Shakespeare's Ophelia; Spenser's Britomart
Ferrand, Jacques, *Erotomania* 18, 36, 51, 68–9, 70, 197, 206

Ficino, Marsilio 96, 131
  Commentary on Plato's Symposium on Love 26, 130, 132–3, 134–6, 144, 159
Finke, Laurie A. 147
Findlay, Alison 170
Fleetwood Habergham, Mrs, 'The Seeds of Love' 36
Flesher, Miles, *Cupids Messenger* 42
Fletcher, John 80
  The Elder Brother (with Philip Massinger) 49, 54, 56–8
  The Faithful Shepherdess 206
  The Humorous Lieutenant 206
  The Loyal Subject 206
  The Mad Lover 174, 175
    Memnon 23, 175, 207–10
  The Maid in the Mill (with William Rowley) 206
  Monsieur Thomas 206
  The Nice Valour (with Thomas Middleton) 24, 170–2, 174, 176
  A Very Woman (with Philip Massinger) 170, 171–2, 181–2
  see also Francis Beaumont; William Shakespeare
Flora 75, 86
flowers 36, 72–5, 76–7, 84–8, 90, 110–11, 113, 192
Francis, duke of Anjou 97
Fregosos, Giovan Battista, *L'anteros* 25
Freud, Sigmund 9, 96, 114, 123, 195–6
Ford, John
  The Broken Heart 1, 10, 17, 106, 118–26, 165
    Orgilus 1, 118–19, 165
    Penthea 1, 94, 118–26
  A Line of Life 126
  Love's Sacrifice 42–3, 187–8
  The Lover's Melancholy 54, 104 182–5, 190
  The Queen 186–7, 188
  'Tis Pity She's a Whore 17, 131, 140–9, 150
    Annabella 141, 144
    Giovanni 140–9
Ford, John (film-maker) 145

Forker, Charles 140–1
Fracastoro, Girolamo 173–4
furor uterinus, *see* uterine fury

Galen of Pergamum 14, 20, 25, 61, 69, 200
Gaudy, Philip 16–17
George of Trebizond 135
Gerard of Berry 21–2
Gifford, William 123–4
Gilbert, Sandra, and Susan Gubar 199
Gilman, Sander 11
Girard, Rene 124
Glapthorne, Henry, *The Ladies Priviledge* 56
Glover, Mary 64–5
Goffe, Thomas, *The Tragedy of Orestes* 103
Gordon, Bernard de 205
  De conservatione vitae humanae 197
Graham, Elspeth 98
green sickness 4–5, 46–60, 73, 74, 75, 79, 82, 85, 86–7, 90, 95
  coitus (as cure) 48, 50–2, 55–60, 201
  against hysteria 61–3, 66
  and lovesickness 4, 46–8, 50–3
  and menstruation 49–50, 55, 60, 74, 201–2
  and pregnancy 50
  and seed 49–53, 201
  symptoms 49–50
Greene, Robert, *Mamillia* 56
Gregerson, Linda 130

Hackett, Helen 97
Hall, John, 'Platonick Love' 139
hallucinations, *see* phantasms
Haly Abbas, *see* Ibn al-Jazzar
Hannay, Margaret 97, 107
Harding, Samuel, *Sicily and Naples* 103–4, 105–6, 175, 180–1
Harrington, Lucy, countess of Bedford 98–100
Hart, James, *Klinike* 16
Harvey, Gideon, *Morbus Anglicus* 197, 198–9
heart 16–17, 127, 207

Heath, Robert, 'On the Report of Clarastella's Death' 138
Heilbrun, Carolyn 143
Henrietta Maria, queen of England 134, 138, 150–1, 154
Henry, prince, son of James I 32
Herbert, Edward, Lord Cherbury 38
  'The Green-Sickness Beauty' 59–60
  'Platonick Love' 138
Herbert, Mary (née Sidney) 97
  Triumph of Death 107–8
Hercules 14
heroic melancholy 3, 4, 39–40, 92
Herrick, Robert, 'To the Virgins to Make Much of Time' 53
Heywood, Thomas
  Amphrisa 106–7
  Gunaikeion 166
  A Woman Killed with Kindness 120–1
Hill, R. F. 184
Hilliard, Nicholas
  Man Among the Flowers 104
  Unknown Man 38
Hippocrates of Kos 20, 61, 200
Hogan, A. P. 143–4
Homer 14
Honthorst, Gerard van, *Lucy Harrington* 98–9
Hopkins, Lisa 108
Howell, James 151
  Epistolae 138
Huebert, Ronald 116
humanism 44–5, 94
humiliation 18, 163–4; *see also* cures for lovesickness
humours 152; *see also* causes of lovesickness
Hutchinson, Colonel John 28–30, 41–2
Hutchinson, Lucy, *Memoirs* 28–30, 41–2, 97
Hutton, Sarah 133
Hypatia of Alexandria 196–7
hysteria 4–5, 46–8, 60–8, 90, 92, 95
  causes 60–1
  coitus (as cure) 48, 62–3
  and lovesickness 4, 46–8, 63–4
  and menstruation 61
  performance of 67–8
  and seed 61–3
  and witchcraft 64–5

incest 143–9
insomnia 17, 30–1

Jackson, Elizabeth 64–5
Jayne, Sears 133
Ibn Al-Jazzar 14
St. John Chrysostum 197
Jones, Ann Rosalind 8, 137, 147, 162
Jonson, Ben
  The Alchemist 203
  The Case is Altered 106
Jordan, Constance 137
Jorden, Edward, *A Briefe Discourse* 61,
  62–3, 64–5

Katz, David S. 201
Kaufmann, R. J. 140
Kerrigan, John 112
Kick, Simon, *Elegantly Dressed Young
  Woman* 100–1
King, Helen 50, 51, 61
Klindienst, Patricia 116
Knevet, Ralph, *Rhodon and Iris* 104
Kramer, Heinrich and Jacob Sprenger,
  Malleus Maleficarum 65
Kraye, Jill 134, 135
Kristeva, Julia 149
Kyd, Thomas, *The Spanish Tragedy*
  103

Lacan, Jacques 7
Laqueur, Thomas 11
Laertius, Diogenes, *Lives of the
  Philosophers* 135
Lamb, Mary Ellen 96
Lange, Johannes, *Medicinalium
  epistolarum miscellanea* 52
Laurentius, Andreas, *Preservation of the
  Sight* 5–6, 19, 23, 34, 97, 163,
  178, 179–81
Leech, Clifford 123–4
Lemnius, Levinus, *Touchstone* 14
Lenton, Francis, *Characters* 200
Lévi-Strauss, Claude 143
Lewis, C. S. 130
liver 2, 16, 26, 51, 87, 91, 92, 95,
  156
lovesickness
  and display 13, 27–8, 94, 96, 104–5;
    see also dress; performance of grief

see also causes of lovesickness; cures for
  lovesickness; female lovesickness;
  male lovesickness
Lucretius Carus, Titus 196
  De rerum natura 192–5
Lust's Dominion 21
Lyly, John
  Endimion 21
  Midas 41
  Sappho and Phao 36, 37, 42, 108

McCabe, Richard 149
MacDonald, Michael 65, 90
McFarland, Ronald 46, 60
McMullan, Gordon 86–7
madness 3, 12, 48, 51, 63–4, 69, 70–1,
  72–8, 79, 81, 83, 88, 90, 106,
  122–5, 173–4, 199
magic 15, 29, 151–3, 160, 201
male lovesickness 4, 5–7, 91–3, 95–6,
  103–4
  historical examples 28–30, 32–3,
    37–8
  see also Davenant's Theander;
    emasculation; Fletcher's Memnon;
    Ford's Giovanni; Ford's Orgilus;
    heroic melancholy
Manuche, Cosmo, *The Loyal Lovers* 105
Mares, F. H. 203
Marlowe, Christopher 38, 147
Marmion, Shakerly, *Hollands
  Leaguer* 102
marriage 28, 30–3, 63, 79, 81–2, 85, 87,
  109–11, 119–20, 173, 188
  and green sickness 50–1, 56–9
  and platonic love 130, 137, 139, 143,
    150–1, 154, 156, 160–2
Marston, John, *The Dutch
  Courtesan* 102, 176
Mary Magdalen 94–5
masochism 3, 6–7, 8–10, 12, 112–26,
  188, 208
Massé, Michelle 9
Massinger, Philip, *The Emperour of the
  East* 104; *see also* John Fletcher
Medea 14, 94
menstruation 47, 49–53, 55, 60, 61, 73,
  74, 77, 79, 87, 88, 137, 190,
  191–211
Micale, Mark 65

Middleton, Thomas
  The Changeling (with William
    Rowley) 168–9
  Women Beware Women 143
  see also John Fletcher
Milton, John, *Comus* 186
misogyny 3, 51, 108, 118, 166, 190,
    191–211
Moffett, Thomas, *Silkwormes* 203
Montaigne, Michel de, *Essays* 144
Morris, Brian 126

Nabbes, Thomas, *Microcosmus* 103
Napier, Richard 30–3, 40, 49–50, 96–7
  and Jane Travell 30–1
  and Mr Fettyplace 32–3
  and Robert Malins 28
  and Thomas May 30
narcissism 7, 127–8, 131, 140–9
Narcissus 127–8, 130, 145; *see also*
    narcissism
Nashe, Thomas, *The Unfortunate
    Traveller* 66
Neely, Carol 5, 46, 79, 88, 89–90
Neill, Michael 121–2
Neoplatonism 2, 4, 10, 33, 83, 107,
    127–162 (esp. 131–40), 184–5,
    195, 196
  Cambridge School of 134
  and Christianity 134–5
  and gender 92, 130
  and green sickness 50–1
  and misogyny 136–7
  and narcissism 131, 141–9
  and sublimation of sexual desire 7,
    138–9
Norland, Howard 117
Numidian lion 208, 210
Nussbaum, Martha 194

O'Hara, Diane 28
Oliver, Isaac, *Man with a Background of
    Flames* 38
Orbison, Tucker 140
Ortner, Sherry 199
Osborne, Dorothy 98
Ovid 75, 196
  Ars amatoria 42
Oxenbridge, Daniel, *General
    Observations* 70

Paré, Ambroise, *Workes of the Famous
    Chirugion* 69
Paster, Gail Kern 202
Peaps, William, *Love, In its Extasie* 104
Peterson, Kaara L. 46–7, 73, 74, 77, 90
Pierce, Robert, *Bath Memoirs* 61
Percy, Henry, earl of Northumberland 38
Percy, Lucy 97
performance of grief 1, 27–8, 28–30,
    32–3, 33–45, 93–101, 106,
    109–11, 112–18, 122–6
Petrarch
  Canzoniere 107
  Trionfo della Morte 107–8
Petrarchan tradition 4, 7, 21, 26–7, 98,
    107, 109, 134, 148, 191–2, 195,
    207
  and green sickness 50–1, 59
  and platonic love 134, 136
Phaedra 14, 94
phantasms 22–5, 89, 137, 177, 179–80,
    183
phlebotomy, *see* cures for lovesickness
Pico della Mirandella, Giovanni 131, 135
Plater, Felix 63
  A Golden Practice of Physick 62
  Platerus Histories 69–70, 172–3
Plato 14, 130, 131, 133, 135, 157–8
  Phaedrus 128, 132
  see also Neoplatonism; Platonic love
Platonic love 128, 129 31, 145, 150–62
  cult of 134, 138–9, 151
  deriders of 138–40, 156
  and homosexuality 134–6, 150
  and madness 148
  see also Neoplatonism
Pliny the Younger 201
Porter, Roy 11, 65

Rambouillet, Marquise de 138
rape 166–8, 170, 174–5
*A Rational Account of the Natural
    Weaknesses of Women* 49
Rasi, Muhammad ibn Zakariya, *see*
    Rhazes
revenge 8–9, 112–18, 122–6, 148–9,
    170
Rhazes 14
Roberts, Joan Warthling 106
Rose, Mary Beth 195

Rowlands, Samuel, *The Melancholie Knight* 34–5
Rowley, William, *see* John Fletcher; Thomas Middleton
Rousseau, G. S. 64, 93, 103

Salerno, school of 14
Sandys, George, 'Lamentations of Jeremiah' 203
Sappho 14, 94; *see also* John Lyly
Schiesari, Juliana 92–3, 96
Scot, Reginald, *The Discoverie of Witchcraft* 64
seed
  and blood 25–6, 85–6, 165–6, 209
  and gender 95
  see also menstruation; causes of lovesickness
Ibn Seena, *see* Avicenna
Sensabaugh, George 140
Showalter, Elaine 3, 58, 77, 92, 95–6
Shakespeare, William 80
  Antony and Cleopatra 187
    Cleopatra 7–8, 76
    Enobarbus 17
  As You Like It 34
  Hamlet 36–7, 56, 59, 72–9, 90
    Hamlet 23, 36–7, 72, 75, 76, 92, 93, 112
    Ophelia 10, 36–7, 46–7, 72–9, 80, 81, 83, 87–8, 90, 92, 94, 106, 111, 112, 118, 122, 123
  Henry IV, Part 2 54
  King Lear 17
    King Lear 17, 66–7, 93, 195, 199, 211
  Love's Labours Lost 33
  Macbeth 80, 149
  Merchant of Venice 37
  Merry Wives of Windsor 21
  A Midsummer Night's Dream 84
  Much Ado About Nothing 103
  Othello 36, 113–14
    Desdemona 36, 77, 113–14
  Pericles 56, 143
  The Rape of Lucrece 44, 115, 117, 166–7, 168
  Romeo and Juliet 56
  'Sonnet 1' 127–8

'Sonnet 18' 204
'Sonnet 129' 211
Twelfth Night 91–2, 93, 176
The Two Noble Kinsmen (with John Fletcher) 24–5, 73, 78–90, 112, 174, 175
  Arcite 80–1, 84–5, 89
  Emilia 78, 80–1, 83–7, 89
  Jailer's Daughter 24–5, 73, 78–83, 87–90, 112
  Palamon 78, 80–2, 84–5, 89
Titus Andronicus 43–4
and the 'dark lady' sonnets 204–5
Shirley, James
  Changes: or Love in a Maze 56
  A Lady of Pleasure 188–9
  St Patrick for Ireland 102–3
Sidney, Sir Philip 136, 205
  Astrophil and Stella 21, 107
  New Arcadia 7
    Pyrocles 7, 36
  Old Arcadia 185
    Basilius 24
Sidney, Sir Robert 37–8
Simon, Bennett 63, 68
Skultans, Vieda 95, 102
Small, Helen 3
Socrates 135
Soranus 61
Spenser, Edmund
  The Faerie Queene 186, 205
    Britomart 127–30, 141
  Fowre Hymns 107
  The Shepheardes Calender 135–6
sperm, *see* seed
Stampa, Gaspara 8
starvation 118–26
Stavig, Mark 140
Steggle, Matthew 71
Stephens, Dorothy 108–9
Stevenson, Matthew
  'To My Lillie White Leda' 203
  'A Visit' 54
stoicism 121–6
Strong, Roy 37, 38
Suckling, John
  'Letter 52' 176, 205–6
  'Letter 53' 206
  'Upon A. M.' 175
Suda, The 196

suicide 18, 52, 82–3, 117–18, 149,
172
and self-mastery 118–26
Swift, Jonathan, 'The Lady's Dressing
Room' 191–4

Temple, Sir William 98
Theseus 115–16
Tofte, Robert, 'Laura' 97
Tomkis, Thomas, *Albumazar* 68
Traversari, Ambrogio 134–5
Turner, Paul 209

uterine disorders 3, 5, 46–90, 73–4, 77;
see also green sickness, hysteria,
and uterine fury
uterine fury 46–8, 68–72, 74, 79,
90
coitus (as cure) 70–2
and seed 69

Vaughan, William, *Directions for
Health* 25, 52, 173–4, 175,
178–9, 182, 197
Veith, Ilza 64–5

Wack, Mary 3, 95
Walkington, Thomas, *Optick Glasse* 14
Waller, Gary 8
Webster, John
Appius and Virginia 21
The Duchess of Malfi 1
The White Devil 103
Whitney, Geoffrey, *A Choice of
Emblems* 186
Whythorne, Thomas, *Autobiography* 41
Wickham, Glynne 89
Williams, Katherine 61, 63
Wiseman, Susan 142–3
womb, *see* green sickness; hysteria; uterine
disorders; and uterine fury
Wright, Thomas, *Minde* 14
Wroth, Mary 8
Urania 97
Wyatt, Sir Thomas
'Sonnet 26' 21
'Sonnet 47' 27

Zephyrus 75
Zwinger, Theodor, *Theatrum humanae
vitae* 197